Davis's Manual of Critical Care Therapeutics

D0218165

Davis's Manual of Critical Care Therapeutics

Kathleen Miller Baldwin, RN, PhD, CEN, CCRN
Post-Doctoral Trainee in Nursing Intervention
University of Utah College of Nursing
Salt Lake City, Utah

Christine Seftchick Garza, RN, PhD
Assistant Professor of Nursing
Texas Woman's University
Dallas, Texas

Rita N. Martin, MSN, RN
Clinical Instructor of Nursing
Texas Woman's University
Dallas, Texas

Susan Sheriff, RN, PhD
Assistant Professor of Nursing
Texas Woman's University
Dallas, Texas

Grace A. Hanssen, MS, RN
Clinical Instructor of Nursing
Texas Woman's University
Dallas, Texas

 F. A. Davis Company, Philadelphia

F. A. Davis Company
1915 Arch Street
Philadelphia, PA 19103

Copyright © 1995 by F. A. Davis Company

All rights reserved. This book is protected by copyright. No part of it may be reproduced, stored in a retrieval system, or transmitted in any form or by any means, electronic, mechanical, photocopying, recording, or otherwise, without written permission from the publisher.

Printed in Canada

Last digit indicates print number: 10 9 8 7 6 5 4 3 2

Publisher, Nursing: Robert G. Martone
Nursing Acquisitions Editor: Joanne Patzek DaCunha
Production Editor: Glenn L. Fechner
Cover Designer: Steven R. Morrone

As new scientific information becomes available through basic and clinical research, recommended treatments and drug therapies undergo changes. The authors and publisher have done everything possible to make this book accurate, up to date, and in accord with accepted standards at the time of publication. The authors, editors, and publisher are not responsible for errors or omissions or for consequences from application of the book, and make no warranty, expressed or implied, in regard to the contents of the book. Any practice described in this book should be applied by the reader in accordance with professional standards of care used in regard to the unique circumstances that may apply in each situation. The reader is advised always to check product information (package inserts) for changes and new information regarding dose and contraindications before administering any drug. Caution is especially urged when using new or infrequently ordered drugs.

Library of Congress Cataloging in Publication Data

Davis's manual of critical care therapeutics / Kathleen M. Baldwin . . . [et al.].

    p.   cm.

    Includes bibliographical references and index.

    ISBN 0-8036-0574-9

    1. Intensive care nursing — Handbooks, manuals, etc. 2. Critical care medicine — Handbooks, manuals, etc. I. Baldwin, Kathleen M. II. F. A. Davis Company. III. Title: Manual of critical care therapeutics.

    [DNLM: 1. Critical Care — handbooks. 2. Nursing Care — handbooks. 3. Critical Care — nurses' instruction. WY 39 1995]

RT120.I4D38   1995

610.73′61 — dc20

DNLM/DLC

for Library of Congress   94-37605

                                                CIP

Authorization to photocopy items for internal or personal use, or the internal or personal use of specific clients, is granted by F.A. Davis Company for users registered with the Copyright Clearance Center (CCC) Transactional Reporting Service, provided that the fee of $.10 per copy is paid directly to CCC, 222 Rosewood Dr., Danvers, MA 01923. For those organizations that have been granted a photocopy license by CCC, a separate system of payment has been arranged. The fee code for users of the Transactional Reporting Service is: 8036-0574/95 0 + $.10.

Preface

The *Davis's Guide to Critical Care Therapeutics* is a concise, easy to use reference for the critical care nurse or nursing student. Its pocket size and outline format make information readily available at the bedside for quick look-ups. The selection of the forty-six health problems in this book was the result of much analysis of the major reasons for admission to the intensive care unit.

Each health problem monograph is designed to assist the reader in understanding the pathophysiology of the disorder so he or she can fully comprehend why the client exhibits the specific signs and symptoms, what treatments work and why they work, and which nursing interventions are most appropriate. Several useful appendices were selected to enhance the book's usefulness as a reference.

Kathleen Miller Baldwin

Acknowledgments

For my husband, Steve. Thank you for understanding me and loving me even though I wouldn't get off your computer.

For the nursing staff of the Medical/Respiratory Intensive Care Unit at Parkland Memorial Hospital. Thank you for allowing this old ER nurse to be part of your team for the past three years.

KB

For Gumaro and Jenna. Thank you for enduring the mega stress generated by this "creative venture." I appreciate the loan of your Medical Grand Rounds and textbooks and the precious time spent critiquing my work. Most importantly, I thank both of you for still speaking to me. My work is dedicated to you.

CG

For Jay. Thank you for buying me the new computer, showing me how to use it, cooking great meals, and continuing to have faith in me.

For Lindsay and Bailey. Thank you for being patient with Mom. You are wonderful helpers and the joy of my life.

For my family . . . This book will always be here because of your help. In memory of my mother, whose own nursing career inspired mine greatly.

RM

For Rick, Rachel, and Taylor. Many thanks for your support and encouragement.

SS

Consultants

Linda S. Baas, RN, PhD, CCRN
Assistant Professor
University of Cincinnati College of Nursing
and Health
Cincinnati, OH

Charold L. Baer, RN, PhD, FCCM, CCRN
Professor and Chair
Oregon Health Sciences University
Portland, OR

Jéanne M. Bouvette-Risey, RN, MSN, CNS
Neuroscience Clinical Nurse Specialist
Ochsner Foundation Hospital
New Orleans, LA

Barbara A. Brown, RN, MN
Professor
Community College of Allegheny County
Pittsburgh, PA

Nancy G. Evans, RN, BSN, CGRN
Nurse Manager — Gastroenterology
Daniel Freeman Memorial and Marina Hospitals
Inglewood, CA

Teresa Heise Halloran, RN, MSN, CCRN
Clinical Care Services Director
Memorial Hospital
Bellville, IL

Rosemary L. Hoffman, RN, MSN
Instructor
West Penn Hospital School of Nursing
Pittsburgh, PA

Sande Jones, RN,C, MSN, MSEd
Clinical Nurse Specialist, Medical/Special
    Immunology
Mount Sinai Medical Center
Miami Beach, FL

Mary Ann Nasuta, RN, MS in Ed, MSN
Associate Professor
Mohawk Valley Community College
Utica, NY

Marilyn N. Pase, RN, MSN
Assistant Professor
New Mexico State University
Las Cruces, NM

Brenda K. Shelton, RN, MS
Critical Care Clinical Nurse Specialist
Johns Hopkins Oncology Center
Baltimore, MD
Towson State University Division of Health
    Sciences
Baltimore, MD

Linda Tamburri, RN, MS, CCRN
Clinical Nurse Specialist
Critical Care Medicine
Robert Wood Johnson University Hospital
New Brunswick, NJ

Contents

8. Psychosocial Aspects **589**

Appendices **629**

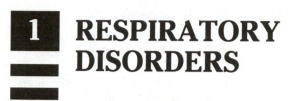

RESPIRATORY DISORDERS

1

Acute Respiratory Failure Type I: Adult Respiratory Distress Syndrome

Acute respiratory failure type I, which occurs in adult respiratory distress syndrome (ARDS), is characterized by intrapulmonary right-to-left shunt (unoxygenated venous blood moves into the arterial circulation across the pulmonary capillary bed) and results in severe, refractory arterial hypoxemia without hypercapnia. ARDS is a rapidly progressive, well-recognized syndrome that can follow any medical or surgical condition and can potentially affect pulmonary function, whether or not there is underlying pulmonary disease.

Mortality rates from ARDS are greater than 50%. Associated organ failure increases mortality significantly. ARDS is the most common cause of non – injury associated death from trauma. It is also known as shock lung, traumatic wet lung, stiff lung, posttraumatic massive pulmonary collapse, blast lung, congestive atelectasis, Da Nang lung, pulmonary contusion, high-permeability pulmonary edema, postperfusion lung, and noncardiogenic pulmonary edema.

Etiology/Pathophysiology

1. ARDS occurs after direct lung injury or indirect systemic insult. However, the exact mechanism of pathologic change is unclear. No single element or common mechanism has been identified.
2. Patients with direct lung injury or sepsis are at greatest risk for developing ARDS.
3. The progression of ARDS varies in each patient but results in grave illness.
4. Initial insult is followed by increased pulmonary shunting, increased dead space, decreased compliance, and worsening hypoxemia despite inspiration of high percentages of oxygen.
5. Symptoms develop 1 – 7 days after the initial injury or insult. Most patients develop symptoms within the first 3 days.
6. Capillary leak syndrome from disruption of the capillary endothelium results in leaking and accumulation of fluid, protein, and cellular material in the interstitium causing noncardiogenic pulmonary edema.
7. Decreased surfactant activity allows fluid to enter the alveoli resulting in alveolar collapse (atelectasis). This increases shunting and worsens hypoxemia.
8. Hyaline membrane is formed and causes stiffening of the lungs, which decreases compliance, increases shunting, and increases hypoxemia.

Four Stages of Adult Respiratory Distress Syndrome

Stage I	*Stage II*	*Stage III*	*Stage IV*
Acute injury (12–24 h after injury)	Latent period (lasts 6–48 h)	Acute respiratory failure	Severe respiratory failure
Lungs sound clear	Increased work of breathing	Tachypnea and dyspnea	Severe hypoxemia unresponsive to therapy
Normal chest X-ray	Minor chest X-ray changes	Diffuse infiltrates	
Tachycardia Hyperventilation	Hemodynamic instability	Progressive pulmonary insufficiency	Acidosis with severe hypoxemia
Hypocarbia	Deteriorating arterial blood gases (widening A-aO$_2$)	100% inspired oxygen needed	Acute respiratory distress
Respiratory alkalosis	Hyperventilation	Mechanical ventilation needed	Acute pulmonary edema
	Respiratory alkalosis with hypoxemia	Crackles on auscultation	Decreased sensorium

Assessment/Analysis

ASSESSMENT FINDINGS

Subjective

1. History of a preceding event that could cause lung damage
2. Dyspnea
3. Anxiety

Objective

1. Initial hyperventilation occurs (a normal compensatory mechanism to hypoxemia)
2. Severe dyspnea
3. Nasal flaring
4. Use of accessory muscles of respiration
5. Diaphoresis
6. Tachypnea
7. Vocal fremitus (palpable vibration)
8. Dullness to percussion over all lung fields
9. Reduced lung expansion on auscultation
10. Crackles upon auscultation
11. Bronchovesicular breath sounds over most lung fields
12. Hypotension

SUPPORTING TEST FINDINGS

Laboratory Tests

1. Arterial blood gases (ABGs)
   Abnormality: Persistently decreased PaO_2 despite increasing high concentrations of inspired oxygen
   Initially decreased $PaCO_2$ that eventually increases
   Initial alkalosis followed by acidosis
2. White blood cell (WBC) count
   Abnormality: Increased if infection present

Diagnostic Tests

1. Chest X-ray
   Abnormality: Initially, patchy infiltrates with irregular borders that often progress to total "white out" of the lung as a result of diffuse infiltrates

2. Hemodynamic monitoring
   Abnormality: Increased cardiac output (CO) but may decrease with positive end-expiratory pressure (PEEP)
   Decreased or normal pulmonary capillary wedge pressure (PCWP)
   Increased pulmonary artery pressure (PAP)
3. Pulmonary function tests
   Abnormality: Significantly decreased functional residual capacity (FRC)
   Decreased tidal volume
   Increased respiratory rate and effort
   Increased peak inspiratory pressures
   Decreased compliance
   Increased dead space
   Right-to-left (intrapulmonary) shunt
4. SvO_2
   Abnormality: Decreased
5. Capnography
   Abnormality: Ventilation/perfusion mismatch
6. Pulse oximetry
   Abnormality: Decreased oxygen saturation

Planning/Intervention

COLLABORATIVE MANAGEMENT

Procedures

1. Monitor patients at risk for the onset of ARDS so that early intervention can occur.
2. Assist with treatment of the primary disorder that preceded the onset of ARDS because this leads to improvement in pulmonary status.
3. Prevent further damage to the alveoli and support oxygenation by:
   a. Obtaining serial ABGs and monitoring the values
   b. Assisting with intubation and beginning mechanical ventilation for:
      1) Respiratory rate >30 bpm
      2) PaO_2 <55 mm Hg on room air
      3) Retention of CO_2
   c. Initiating one of the types of mechanical ventilation used in ARDS as ordered:

1) Assist control with PEEP. Indications for PEEP are as follows:
   a) PaO_2 <60 mm Hg on an FiO_2 >50%
   b) pH <7.25
   c) $PaCO_2$ >45 mm Hg
2) Intermittent mandatory ventilation with or without synchronization (IMV/SIMV)
3) Pressure-controlled with inverse ratio ventilation
d. Extracorporeal membrane oxygenation (ECHO) is currently under evaluation as a treatment for ARDS. Its use is very controversial in adults.

Drug Therapy

1. Steroids
   Examples: cortisone (Cortone)
   hydrocortisone (Solu-Cortef)
   Action: Improve outcome of patients who develop ARDS following fat embolism when given early in the course of the syndrome
   Caution: Do not discontinue abruptly
   Decreases wound healing
   Increases susceptibility to infection
2. Prostaglandins
   Examples: PGE_1
   Action: May interrupt the development of ARDS
   Experimental at present
3. Fluid replacement
   Examples: crystalloids (Ringer's lactate, normal saline)
   colloids (hetastarch, blood, blood products)
   Action: Maintains adequate intravascular volume
   Provides sufficient cardiac output
   Maintains tissue perfusion
   Caution: Observe closely for pulmonary edema
4. Antibiotics
   Examples: cephalosporins
   aminoglycosides
   Action: Most frequently used drugs in the treatment of ARDS; bacteriocidal
   Broad-spectrum drugs that kill gram-positive and gram-negative aerobic and anaerobic bacteria; used to prevent or to treat existing infections
   Caution: Should not be used indiscriminately

Can cause superinfection, ototoxicity, and nephro-toxicity

5. Bronchodilators
   Examples: aminophylline (theophylline)
   Action: Dilates bronchioles; reduces bronchospasm
   Caution: Aminophylline accumulates in the body and may reach toxic levels
6. Nonsteroidal anti-inflammatory drugs (NSAIDs)
   Example: ibuprofen (Advil)
   Action: Alters cellular metabolism to reduce pulmonary hypertension and hypoxemia
   Caution: Precise effects of this drug in patients with ARDS are unknown
7. Diuretics
   Examples: furosemide (Lasix)
      bumetanide (Bumex)
      mannitol
   Action: Increases urine excretion used to treat oliguria
   Caution: Can cause hypokalemia and dehydration
8. Sedatives
   Examples: lorazepam (Ativan)
      diazepam (Valium)
      midazolam (Versed)
   Action: Depresses the central nervous system (CNS), pro-ducing sedation and relief of anxiety
   Caution: Can cause respiratory depression
9. Paralytics
   Examples: pancuronium (Pavulon)
      vecuronium (Norcuron)
   Action: Paralyzes skeletal muscle
   Caution: Results in apnea; airway must be effectively managed
      Can cause difficulty with weaning
      Additional medications need to be given for pain or anxiety

NURSING MANAGEMENT

Monitoring and Managing Clinical Problems

1. Gas Exchange: impaired
   a. Monitor for and treat increasing respiratory distress leading to increasing hypoxemia.

1) Monitor serial ABG results and report abnormalities.
2) Monitor serial chest X-ray reports for increasing infiltrates.
3) Auscultate lungs every 4 hours for decreased breath sounds, crackles, and/or rhonchi.
4) Continuously measure oxygen saturation by pulse oximetry and report values less than 90%.
5) Administer bronchodilators as ordered.
6) Monitor for air hunger, tachypnea, restlessness, and confusion, which indicate increasing respiratory distress.

b. Monitor for and promote effective ventilation while on mechanical ventilator.
1) Reassess lung sounds every 4 hours and as needed.
2) Suction every 2 hours and as needed to remove sputum and promote a clear airway.
3) Measure compliance frequently and report decreases.
4) Measure peak pressures and report increases.
5) Sedate the patient as needed to control ventilator fighting. Paralytics also may be necessary.
6) Monitor serial ABGs for effectiveness of mechanical ventilation and report abnormalities.
7) Decrease FiO_2 to <50% as quickly as possible to prevent oxygen toxicity.
8) If the patient is on PEEP, remember PEEP holds alveoli open thereby increasing functional residual capacity, decreasing shunting, and decreasing hypoxemia. But, PEEP can:
   a) Decrease cardiac output
   b) Increase the chance of oxygen toxicity
   c) Cause fluid overload
   d) Cause barotrauma
   e) Cause gastric distention

2. Fluid Volume Excess or Deficit—Monitor for and promote effective fluid volume status.
a. Assist with insertion of a hemodynamic monitoring catheter and measure cardiac output, PCWP, PAP, systemic vascular resistance, stroke volume, and central venous pressure (CVP), as ordered.

    b. Measure hourly urine output and report output <30 mL/h.

    c. Observe for signs of fluid overload (onset of S_3 gallop rhythm, increasing pulmonary crackles and rhonchi, edema, weight gain, intake greater than output) and report positive findings.

    d. Observe for signs of dehydration (weight loss, low cardiac output, tachycardia, intake less than output, tenting of skin) and report positive findings.

    e. Cautiously give intravenous (IV) fluids to prevent fluid overload but maintain adequate fluid volume.

3. Airway Clearance: ineffective — Promote effective ventilation and airway clearance when the patient is not on mechanical ventilation.

    a. Encourage coughing and deep breathing every 2 hours.

    b. Encourage use of incentive spirometry.

    c. Assist the patient with turning every 2 hours.

    d. Suction the patient, as needed.

    e. Reassess breath sounds every 4 hours to identify areas of decrease or onset of crackles and/or rhonchi.

    f. Perform chest percussion and postural drainage, as needed, for areas of decreased breath sounds.

4. Gas Exchange: impaired, high risk for — Identify patients at risk for ARDS and:

    a. Prevent fluid overload or deficit.

    b. Filter all blood and blood products.

    c. Prevent nosocomial infections.

        1) Maintain strict aseptic technique when performing procedures such as suctioning and dressing changes.

        2) Wash hands frequently.

        3) Minimize the number of invasive procedures and lines.

    d. Prevent aspiration by inserting a nasogastric or orogastric tube, elevating the head of the bed, if possible, and preventing vomiting.

    e. Maintain a patent airway by assisting the patient with turning, coughing, deep breathing, incentive spirometry, chest percussion, and postural drainage.

5. Injury: high risk for — Monitor for and manage complications seen in patients with ARDS.
   a. Pulmonary fibrosis
      1) This condition is diagnosed when the patient recovers from ARDS, but has residual, impaired lung function.
      2) Monitor for fibrotic changes noted on chest X-ray.
      3) Monitor serial ABGs and continuous pulse oximetry for abnormalities.
   b. Oxygen toxicity
      1) Occurs when high concentrations of oxygen are given for a prolonged period of time. Reduce FiO_2 to <50% as soon as possible. Changes can occur within 24 hours when oxygen concentrations >50% are used. Monitor all patients on FiO_2 >50% closely for signs and symptoms.
      2) Prevention is the key. Maintain meticulous respiratory hygiene so that patients may be weaned from high percentages of oxygen as quickly as possible.
      3) Recognize and report the onset of signs and symptoms that are variable, difficult to recognize, and include substernal soreness, cough, sore throat, dyspnea, painful inspiration, and nasal congestion.
      4) Observe patients closely for increasing respiratory distress and hemoptysis from alveolar endothelial edema and destruction and hemorrhage into the alveoli.
      5) Promote effective secretion mobilization by using deep-breathing and coughing exercises, incentive spirometry, chest percussion, and postural drainage, as needed, to decrease the length of time and percentage of oxygen needed.
      6) Administer bronchodilators, as ordered, to promote an effective airway and decrease the length of time and percentage of oxygen necessary.
   c. Pulmonary barotrauma (spontaneous pneumothorax, pneumomediastinum)
      1) This may occur with PEEP.
      2) Be alert for increases in peak pressures and decreases in lung compliance.
      3) Assess for subcutaneous emphysema on the chest frequently.

       4) Keep equipment for immediate chest-tube insertion at bedside.

       5) Obtain a stat, portable chest X-ray if a pneumothorax is suspected (may see a rise in peak pressure, decrease in compliance, unequal chest wall movement, decreased or absent breath sounds over the pneumothorax).

       6) Auscultate breath sounds every 4 hours.

   d. Malnutrition

       1) Obtain a nutritional consult on all ventilator-dependent patients.

       2) Institute enteral feeding (the preferred method) as soon as possible to prevent malnutrition.

       3) Begin total parenteral nutrition if the patient is unable to tolerate enteral feeding.

       4) Monitor serum albumin to assess nutritional state.

       5) Weigh daily and report decreases.

Monitoring, Managing, and Preventing Life-Threatening Emergencies

1. ARDS is a life-threatening emergency that is often rapidly fatal.
2. Multisystem organ failure
   a. Monitor patients at risk and recognize signs of onset during the early phases.
       1) Assess for risk factors.
       2) Be alert for early warning signals such as:
         a) Increased or decreased temperature
         b) Increasing heart rate
         c) Tachypnea (increased respiratory rate)
         d) Increased or decreased WBC count
         e) Subtle changes in sensorium
       3) Report findings suggestive of multisystem organ failure.
   b. Prevent organ injury
       1) Provide ventilatory support by intubation and mechanical ventilation.
       2) Control body temperature to adjust for hyperthermia or hypothermia.
       3) Institute ordered treatment to reverse acidosis.
       4) Monitor for progression of disease.

    a) Assess for subtle changes that may indicate deterioration from the hyperdynamic phase to the hypodynamic phase.

    b) Measure hemodynamic parameters frequently and report changes.

    c) Compare all assessment findings with patient's baseline findings to identify alterations in previously uninvolved organ systems.

    d) Analyze changes in laboratory values to determine alteration in organ function.

    e) Monitor the patient's responses to medications and treatments, and report significant findings.

c. Provide supportive care.

  1) Control the infection.

    a) Obtain a specimen of all secretions for analysis.

    b) Prepare the patient for surgical intervention to remove sources of infection.

    c) Promote an aseptic environment to prevent concomitant (nosocomial) infections.

      1] Use aseptic technique when providing care.

      2] Monitor invasive tube sites for signs and symptoms of infection.

      3] Wash hands frequently.

      4] Monitor serial WBCs for signs of infection.

      5] Culture suspicious secretions from the patient.

      6] Immediately report signs and symptoms of infection.

      7] Monitor the patient's temperature every 4 hours and more frequently if fever develops.

      8] Administer medications ordered to prevent or fight infection, and monitor response to them.

  2) Arrest and reverse the progress of the syndrome.

    a) Prevent translocation of bacteria from the gut with enteral feeding of glutamine, an immunonutrient that maintains gut integrity and stimulates the immune system.

    b) Prepare for continuous arteriovenous hemodiafiltration (CAVHD), which has been used successfully in trauma patients.

    c) Recognize complications.

    1] Skin breakdown
      a] Use pressure-relieving devices (e.g., pads, mattresses, specialty beds) to prevent breakdown.
      b] Turn the patient every 2 hours, if possible.
      c] Assess the skin every 4 hours to identify and intervene in the early stages of breakdown.
      d] Consult the enterostomal therapy nurse for definitive treatment of skin breakdown.
    2] Third spacing of fluid (movement into the extravascular spaces)
      a] Assess the patient every 4 hours for edema, ascites, or anasarca.
      b] Weigh the patient daily and report significant increases.
      c] Accurately measure intake and output, and report significant disparities.
      d] Monitor lung sounds every 4 hours and report changes.
      e] Administer ordered diuretics to increase urine output.
  3) Provide metabolic support.
    a) Measure oxygen consumption with increased flow until lactic acid level returns to normal.
    b) Provide adequate nutrition. Enteral route is preferred over parenteral, using a formula that is high in protein and has medium-chain triglycerides for lipids.
3. Cardiogenic shock
  a. Monitor for hemodynamic instability.
    1) Continuously monitor hemodynamic parameters to evaluate the cardiovascular response to treatment.
    2) Titrate fluids and inotropic agents to maintain a systolic blood pressure of at least 80 mm Hg.
    3) Place the patient in modified Trendelenburg position.
    4) Continuously monitor blood pressure to determine the cardiovascular response to treatment.

      5) Monitor cardiac rhythm for tachycardia and life-threatening ventricular arrhythmias (ventricular tachycardia and/or fibrillation).

  b. Promote adequate oxygenation.

      1) Administer supplemental oxygen, as ordered.

      2) Obtain specimens for and monitor results of serial ABGs and hemoglobin and report abnormalities.

      3) Monitor capillary refill and monitor skin color to assess peripheral perfusion.

      4) Maintain a patent airway and adequate ventilation. Administer supplemental oxygen to ensure that sufficient oxygen is delivered to the lungs.

  c. Monitor for altered organ and tissue perfusion.

      1) Monitor for signs of acute renal failure as evidenced by decreased urine output and elevated renal function tests. Continuously monitor urinary output via catheter to evaluate renal function.

      2) Monitor for ARDS as evidenced by a falling arterial oxygen concentration and shunting of blood in the lungs.

      3) Auscultate bowel sounds to monitor for gastroparesis, and observe for the presence of bright-red or coffee-ground nasogastric tube drainage that could indicate stress ulceration.

      4) Check temperature every 4 hours to monitor for hypothermia or hyperthermia.

      5) Monitor for decreased alertness and attention span, drowsiness, or increased sleeping, indicating downward changes in the level of consciousness.

  d. Provide enteral nutrition.

Acute Respiratory Failure Type II: Acute Exacerbation of Chronic Obstructive Pulmonary Disease

Acute respiratory failure type II is defined as a sudden progressive deterioration of ABGs to an arterial oxygen tension (PaO_2) of 50 mm Hg or less (hypoxemia) and an arterial carbon dioxide tension ($PaCO_2$) of 50 mm Hg or more (hypercapnia) in patients with underlying chronic pulmonary disease. In this disorder, adequate amounts of oxygen cannot be supplied to the body, and sufficient amounts of carbon dioxide cannot be removed from the body to prevent acidosis. Acute respiratory failure type II is a relatively common complication and a major cause of death in patients with acute exacerbations of chronic pulmonary disease.

Etiology/Pathophysiology

1. Acute respiratory failure type II may be caused by infection (the most common cause), heart failure, chest trauma, pulmonary embolism, or pneumothorax. It usually develops over 2–3 days and may be rapidly fatal.
2. The following four major mechanisms cause hypoxemia in acute respiratory failure type II:
   a. Hypoventilation
   b. Impaired diffusion
   c. Ventilation-perfusion mismatch
   d. Intrapulmonary shunting
3. Two major mechanisms cause hypercapnia in acute respiratory failure type II. They are:
   a. Impaired carbon dioxide elimination due to alveolar hypoventilation
   b. Ventilation-perfusion mismatch

Assessment/Analysis

ASSESSMENT FINDINGS

Subjective

1. History of chronic obstructive pulmonary disease (COPD)
2. History of a sudden increase or decrease in sputum production
3. Shortness of breath
4. Headache
5. Fatigue

Objective

1. Restlessness, confusion, somnolence, or coma
2. Dyspnea (may or may not be present)
3. Increased respiratory rate to >25 bpm
4. Altered breathing patterns
   a. Paradoxic breathing—abdomen falls rather than rises during inspiration
   b. Respiratory alternans—intercostal muscles and dia-

   phragm   work   asynchronously   rather   than
   synchronously
c. Active contraction of abdominal muscles with
   respiration
d. Pursed-lip breathing — prolonged expiratory phase
5. Cough with sputum production
6. Cyanosis
7. Nasal flaring
8. Papilledema
9. Sitting upright in a leaning-forward position
10. Diaphoresis; cool, clammy skin
11. Tachycardia with bounding pulses
12. Cold extremities
13. Hyperresonance on chest percussion
14. Decreased lung expansion
15. Presence of vocal fremitus
16. Irregular cardiac rhythm
17. Decreased breath sounds
18. Crackles or wheezes
19. Rhonchi or gurgles

SUPPORTING TEST FINDINGS

Laboratory Tests

1. ABGs
   Abnormality: Increased $PaCO_2$ >50 mm Hg
      Decreased PaO_2 <50 mm Hg
      Increased bicarbonate level
      Decreased pH (acidosis) in the previously compen-
   sated patient
2. Red blood cells (RBCs)
   Abnormality: Increased due to polycythemia
3. Sputum culture
   Abnormality: Bacterial growth in 24–48 hours
4. White blood cells (WBCs)
   Abnormality: Increased, indicating infection

Diagnostic Tests

1. Chest X-ray
   Abnormality: Pneumonia, bronchitis, or atelectasis with
   evidence of underlying chronic pulmonary disease

2. Pulmonary function tests (PFTs)
   Abnormality: Increased functional residual capacity (FRC)

   Increased residual volume (RV) (When increased alone, reflects bronchitits; if increased with total lung capacity [TLC], reflects emphysema)

   Increased TLC

   Decreased vital capacity (VC) and forced expiratory volume (FEV)

Planning/Intervention

COLLABORATIVE MANAGEMENT

Procedures

1. Improve ventilatory dynamics.
   a. Evaluate respiratory muscles for fatigue and response to treatment.
   b. Stimulate the respiratory drive and treat CO_2 narcosis with medication.
   c. Assist with intubation and instituting mechanical ventilation, which is used as a last resort when conservative treatment has failed to correct the acute respiratory acidosis.
   d. Draw serial arterial blood gases (ABGs) to evaluate the effectiveness of treatment, as ordered.
2. Correct hypoxemia.
   a. Administer ordered oxygen using low FiO_2 for patients dependent on the hypoxic respiratory drive.
   b. Draw serial ABGs to evaluate the effectiveness of treatment, as ordered.
   c. Carefully titrate the FiO_2 to ABG results.
   d. Administer ordered bronchodilators to improve air flow and lessen hypoxemia.
3. Treat the underlying cause of the acute exacerbation.
   a. Administer ordered antibiotics to treat infection, if present.
   b. Assist with adjustment of drug regimen to facilitate improved ventilation with emphysema.
   c. Monitor closely for improvement or deterioration, and report findings as needed.

Drug Therapy

1. Respiratory stimulants (controversial)
   Examples: doxapram (Dopram)
   almitrine hydrochloride
   Action: Stimulates aortic and carotid bodies to increase ventilation
   Caution: Can cause seizures, dyspnea, and hypertension
2. Antibiotics
   Examples: penicillin (Duracillin)
   gentamycin (Garamycin)
   ceftriaxone (Rocephin)
   Action: Bacteriocidal
   Broad-spectrum drugs kill aerobic and anaerobic gram-positive and gram-negative bacteria
   Caution: Can cause allergic reaction, possibly even anaphylaxis
   Monitor serum gentamycin levels to prevent nephrotoxicity and ototoxicity
3. Bronchodilators
   Example: aminophylline (theophylline)
   Action: Improves air flow and ventilation by decreasing bronchospasms
   Caution: Hepatic dysfunction and congestive heart failure (CHF) may require dosage adjustments; can cause toxicity; monitor serum aminophylline levels
4. Inhalational bronchodilators
   Examples: iprantropium bromide (Atrovent)
   salbutamol
   Action: Bronchodilation without systemic anticholinergic effects
   Caution: Can cause nervousness, cough, and nausea
5. Steroids
   Examples: cortisone (Cortone)
   hydrocortisone (Solu-Cortef)
   methylprednisolone (Solu-Medrol)
   Action: Suppresses the normal immune response and inflammation
   Caution: Use is controversial
   Reduces the ability of the lungs to clear bacteria
   Can cause gastrointestinal bleeding
6. Mucolytic agents
   Example: acetylcysteine (Mucomyst)

Action: Degrades mucous, allowing for easier mobilization and expectoration

Caution: Can cause nausea and vomiting, bronchospasm

7. Antipyretics

Examples: acetaminophen (Tylenol)
aspirin (Bayer)

Action: Lowers fever by inhibiting production of prostaglandins

Caution: Overdose of acetaminophen can cause hepatic necrosis

Can cause gastrointestinal bleeding

NURSING MANAGEMENT

Monitoring and Managing of Clinical Problems

1. Gas Exchange: impaired — Monitor for and manage impaired gas exchange.
   a. Evaluate serial ABG results.
   b. Auscultate breath sounds every 4 hours and as needed.
   c. Assess respiratory rate and rhythm every 4 hours and as needed.
   d. Assess nailbeds and mucous membranes for cyanosis.
   e. Observe for respiratory distress and report positive findings.
   f. Monitor continuous pulse oximetry and/or Svo_2, and report abnormalities.
   g. Administer oxygen therapy, as ordered.
2. Breathing Pattern: ineffective — Monitor for and manage ineffective breathing pattern.
   a. Observe for hypoventilation.
   b. Assess respiratory rate and rhythm frequently.
   c. Observe for signs of respiratory distress and respiratory muscle weakness, and report positive findings.
   d. Elevate head of bed to assist breathing.
   e. Have emergency equipment available for intubation and mechanical ventilation, if needed.
   f. Sedate and/or paralyze (used in extreme cases) as needed to prevent ventilator fighting.
3. Airway Clearance: ineffective — Monitor for and manage ineffective airway clearance.
   a. Deliver humidified oxygen to decrease mucosal drying.

b. Perform endotracheal suctioning with preprocedure and postprocedure FiO$_2$ of 100% oxygen.

d. Encourage coughing and deep breathing.

e. Perform chest percussion and postural drainage to assist mobilization of secretions, as needed.

f. Change patient's position frequently to help mobilize secretions.

g. Administer incentive spirometry to increase lung expansion and prevent atelectasis.

4. Aspiration: high risk for — Monitor for and manage aspiration.

a. Monitor temperature every 4 hours and report elevations.

b. Auscultate lung sounds every 4 hours and report changes.

c. Keep head of bed elevated if patient is on enteral feeding to decrease the potential for aspiration.

d. Test for aspiration of tube feeding by adding food coloring to enteral feedings (this procedure is controversial; may cause allergic reactions to the dye) or testing suctioned secretions for glucose.

e. Monitor color and consistency of suctioned sputum and report changes.

f. Monitor serial WBCs for increases indicating infection.

g. Monitor daily chest X-rays for evidence of aspiration pneumonia.

5. Infection: high risk for — Monitor for and manage infection.

a. Monitor temperature every 4 hours and report elevations.

b. Auscultate breath sounds routinely and report alterations.

c. Monitor serial WBCs and report increased values.

d. Report change in color, consistency, and/or amount of sputum.

e. Obtain sputum specimen and send to laboratory for culture, as ordered.

f. Administer ordered antibiotics and monitor patient's response to them.

g. Medicate for fever, as needed.

6. Self-Care Deficit: feeding, bathing/hygiene, dressing/

grooming, toileting — Monitor for and manage self-care deficits.

   a. Observe for dyspnea with exertion when patient is performing daily care.

   b. Assist with daily care, if needed, to prevent dyspnea.

   c. Perform care activities throughout day, rather than clustered together, to prevent dyspnea.

   d. Consult social services to plan for home care assistance, if needed.

7. Nutrition: altered, less than body requirements — Promote adequate nutrition.

   a. Consult nutritional services to evaluate nutritional status.

   b. Perform calorie counts to ensure adequate nutrition.

   c. Allow for rest periods if dyspnea occurs during eating.

   d. Monitor the patient for anorexia, an adverse effect of many of the medications used to treat this disease. Administer medicine around mealtime.

   e. Give high-calorie, high-protein snacks if needed.

   f. Request an order for enteral or parenteral feedings if patient is unable to consume adequate nutrition.

8. Breathing Pattern: ineffective — Promote adequate ventilation/oxygenation.

   a. Administer the correct amount of oxygen by using either a Venturi mask or nasal cannula. A nasal cannula can increase patient compliance.

   b. Place patient in position of comfort (patients are usually most comfortable with the head of bed elevated).

   c. Perform incentive spirometry, as ordered.

   d. Encourage coughing and deep breathing to clear secretions.

   e. Monitor serial ABGs and chest X-rays to assess ventilation/oxygenation parameters.

9. Injury: high risk for — Recognize and treat complications of mechanical ventilation.

   a. Barotrauma — Chronic lung disease and mechanical ventilation may combine to increase the risk of pneumothorax or tension pneumothorax.

     1) Assess breath sounds every 4 hours.

     2) Note changes in ventilator parameters, particu-

larly increases in peak pressures and decreases in exhaled volumes.
3) Check bilateral chest expansion hourly.
4) Obtain a stat chest X-ray if there is a question of pneumothorax or tension pneumothorax.
5) Keep supplies needed for chest-tube insertion readily available for immediate use, if necessary.
b. Cardiac arrhythmias
1) Continuously monitor for ventricular arrhythmias and report their occurrence.
2) Administer medication, as ordered, to treat arrhythmias.
c. Difficulty in weaning
1) Assess for prerequisites for successful weaning.

Prerequisites for Successful Weaning

Sufficient respiratory muscle strength to maintain ventilation
Sufficient respiratory drive to support ventilation
Ability to maintain arterial oxygenation
Successful treatment of the acute condition that precipitated the event
Adequate level of consciousness to understand what is happening
Correction of nutritional deficits
Psychological readiness to wean

---

2) Assist with testing for the ability for weaning.
3) Monitor respiratory pattern closely following extubation and report abnormalities.
4) Monitor ABGs closely following extubation and report abnormalities.
5) Be prepared for reintubation should weaning become unsuccessful.
6) Because of the difficulty of weaning patients with chronic pulmonary disease from mechanical ventilation, some patients are discharged home on ventilators. Prepare patient and family to manage care at home, if necessary.

Monitoring, Managing, and Preventing Life-Threatening Emergencies

1. Respiratory arrest
   a. Monitor patient closely for inability to sustain adequate ventilation.
      1) Auscultate breath sounds hourly.
      2) Obtain frequent ABGs to monitor oxygenation status.
      3) Watch close for cyanosis, pallor, diaphoresis, or air-hunger.
   b. Assist with emergency intubation and manage airway through intubation and mechanical ventilation.
   c. Begin cardiopulmonary resuscitation immediately to treat any arrhythmias that occur with the respiratory arrest.
2. Difficulty with intubation
   a. Maintain adequate oxygenation between attempts to intubate.
   b. Be prepared for immediate tracheostomy if intubation attempts fail.
3. Tension pneumothorax and mediastinal shift
   a. Observe for and immediately report tension pneumothorax.
   b. Set up for immediate needle decompression using a 14- to 16-gauge needle at the second intercostal space, midclavicular line on affected side.
   c. Prepare for chest tube insertion.
   d. Monitor chest drainage color, consistency, and amount. Report signs of hemorrhage.
   e. Monitor chest drainage for air leaks. These will either close within the first few days after injury or require surgical repair.
   f. Assess breath sounds frequently for reexpansion.
   g. Monitor serial ABGs and chest X-ray reports to determine successful reexpansion.

Status Asthmaticus

Status asthmaticus, a medical emergency that may be life-threatening, refers to a severe, unrelenting asthma attack that is refractory to hydration and the usual bronchodilator therapy, including beta-adrenergic agents and aminophylline. Onset of symptoms of asthma is usually during childhood (3–8 years) with boys more affected than girls in the early years; after adolescence both sexes are affected equally.

Patients with asthma vary widely in their clinical presentation, from mild wheezing to status asthmaticus, and symptoms may worsen as time passes.

Etiology/Pathophysiology

1. Etiology
   a. There may be a genetic predisposition to produce increased amounts of immunoglobulin E (IgE) which, when released from mast cells, causes sensitivity to environmental antigens.
2. Pathophysiology
   a. A lack of or defect in adenylate cyclase on the cell membrane, which reduces formation of 3′, 5′-cyclic AMP (adenosine monophosphate) from adenosine triphosphate (ATP), results in partial beta-receptor blockade, producing hyperresponsiveness of the bronchial tree to immunologic, physical, chemical, and psychic stimuli.
   b. When IgE combines with an antigen, histamine and slow-reacting substance are released and possibly induce bronchospasm and bronchial edema.
   c. Epithelial structural changes may allow increased permeability to irritants and allergens. Cilial injury inhibits ciliary function and makes clearing secretions more difficult. An abnormally increased parasympathetic tone to the airway smooth muscle may cause bronchospasm.
   d. Decreased responsiveness or blockade of beta$_2$-receptor activity inhibits bronchodilation, and increases responsiveness to alpha-receptor and cholinergic-receptor activity, promoting bronchoconstriction.
   e. Widespread bronchoconstriction results in:
      1) Hypoxemia
      2) Airway narrowing
      3) Air trapping
      4) Increased functional residual capacity (FRC)
      5) Decreased vital capacity (VC)
      6) Increased dead space
      7) Increased airway resistance
      8) Increased work of breathing
      9) Hypoventilation
      10) Hypercapnia, normocapnia, or hypocapnia
      11) Local areas of atelectasis resulting in increased shunting

f. Wheezing increases as airway flow is restricted by bronchospasm, edema, and hypersecretion of mucus, however, wheezing does not always indicate a diagnosis of asthma, nor do all asthmatics wheeze.

g. The work of breathing increases because intrapulmonary airways are narrower during expiration than inspiration. FRC increases and more negative pressure is needed to produce the same tidal volume.

h. Long-standing asthma produces lung changes similar to emphysema including:
   1) Hypertrophy of the smooth muscle layer
   2) Thickening of the basement membrane of the respiratory epithelium
   3) Hypertrophy and hyperplasia of mucous glands
   4) Increase in the number of goblet cells
   5) Eosinophilic infiltrates within the bronchial wall

3. Risk of complications
   a. Those with hypercapnia who:
      1) are elderly
      2) are young adults (late teens through early twenties)
      3) are black
      4) have a history of a previous episode of respiratory failure that required mechanical ventilation
      5) have a history of recent (within 1 year) hospitalization for asthma
      6) experience symptomatic bronchospasm for more than 24 hours, but underestimate or deny the severity of disease
      7) have bronchospasm requiring high-dose steroids

Assessment/Analysis

ASSESSMENT FINDINGS

Subjective

1. History of asthma
2. History of increased use of beta$_2$-agonists with little or no responsiveness
3. History of gradual or sudden onset of symptoms
4. Increasing dyspnea, coughing, and wheezing
5. Difficulty expectorating thick, tenacious sputum

6. Exhaustion
7. Fear
8. Dizziness

Objective

1. Severe dyspnea
2. Dyspnea on exertion — difficulty walking and talking (able to speak only 2–3 words at a time)
3. Intercostal retractions and accessory muscle use
4. Decreased chest-wall movement
5. Barrel chest (if asthma is a chronic problem)
6. Prolonged expiratory phase of respiration
7. Shallow breathing
8. Nasal flaring
9. Nasal inflammation
10. Restlessness and agitation
11. Sits upright and leans forward to help breathing
12. Progressive fatigue leading to exhaustion
13. Cyanosis or flushing of the upper body
14. Flushed, moist, diaphoretic skin
15. Signs of dehydration (e.g., dry mucous membranes, poor skin turgor)
16. Nausea and vomiting
17. Abdominal pain from severe coughing
18. Harsh cough that eventually becomes productive for large amounts of clear, white, green, or grey sputum
19. Hyperresonance on percussion
20. May have pulsus paradoxus (decrease in systolic blood pressure of 10 mm Hg or more during inspiration)
21. Vocal and/or rhonchial fremitus (palpable vibration)
22. Low position of diaphragm with reduced excursion
23. Wheezing on inspiration and/or expiration (absence of wheezing implies minimal air movement and may precede respiratory arrest)
24. Diminished breath sounds (AN OMINOUS SIGN)
25. Expiratory stridor

SUPPORTING TEST FINDINGS

Laboratory Tests

1. White blood cell (WBC) count
   Abnormality: Increased eosinophils

Increased total WBC count with infection present
2. Arterial Blood Gases (ABGs)
   Abnormality: May see normal or increased $PaCO_2$, PaO_2, and pH
3. Theophylline levels
   Abnormality: Outside of the therapeutic range
4. Sputum cultures
   Abnormality: Presence of eosinophils
   Infective organisms present in bacterial infections

Diagnostic Tests

1. Chest X-ray
   Abnormality: Nonspecific findings; may show increased anterior-posterior diameter
2. Pulmonary function tests (PFTs)
   Abnormality: Decreased VC (Forced VC of <1 L)
   Increased functional residual capacity
   Increased residual volume (RV)
   Decreased forced expiratory volume (FEV) (<600 mL)
3. Electrocardiogram (ECG)
   Abnormality: May show right-axis deviation, right bundle branch block, or supraventricular tachycardia

Planning/Intervention

COLLABORATIVE MANAGEMENT

Procedures

1. Maintain adequate ventilation/oxygenation.
   a. Administer humidified oxygen.
   b. Give medications to induce bronchodilation to correct severely reduced peak inspiratory flow, forced VC, and FEV.
   c. Be prepared for emergency intubation and mechanical ventilation.
2. Correct abnormal gas exchange.
   a. Monitor serial ABGs closely.
   b. Correct acidosis with hyperventilation or medications.
   c. Relieve bronchospasm.

1) Administer corticosteroids and bronchodilators, as ordered.
2) Relieve mucosal edema with medications, as ordered.
3) Administer nebulizer treatments with beta$_2$-selective agonists, as ordered.
3. Clear airway secretions.
   a. Rehydrate with intravenous (IV) fluid, as ordered.
   b. Administer mucolytics to liquefy and promote expectoration of mucus, as ordered.

Drug Therapy

1. Bronchodilators
   Examples: albuterol or salbutamol (Proventil)
       metaproterenol (Alupent)
       terbutaline (Brethaire)
       epinephrine (Adrenalin)
       aminophylline (theophylline)
   Action: Relaxes bronchial smooth muscle
   Cautions: Can cause tachycardia, hypertension, and tremors
2. Anticholinergics
   Examples: ipratropium bromide (Atrovent)
   Action: Bronchodilation
   Caution: Can cause worsening of glaucoma, urinary retention, dry mouth, and tachycardia
3. Corticosteroids
   Examples: beclomethasone dipropionate (Beclovent)
       flunisolide (AeroBid)
       triamcinolone (Azmacort)
       methylprednisolone (Depo-Medrol)
   Action: May potentiate the action of bronchodilators
   Caution: Can cause mouth and throat irritation
       Increased risk of infection
4. Mucolytics
   Examples: acetylcysteine (Mucomyst)
   Action: Degrades mucus allowing easier mobilization and expectoration
   Caution: Can cause nausea and bronchospasm
5. Oxygen therapy
   Action: Relieves hypoxemia
   Caution: Use low-flow devices with patients who are chronic CO_2 retainers

6. Fluid replacement
   Examples: normal saline solution
   Action: Corrects dehydration
   May help thin bronchial secretions and facilitate mucous
   expectoration
   Caution: Can cause fluid overload and congestive heart
   failure (CHF)
7. Antibiotics
   Examples: cefuroxime (Zinacef)
   gentamycin (Garamycin)
   penicillin V (Pen Vee K)
   Action: Bacteriocidal broad-spectrum drugs that kill aerobic and anaerobic gram-positive and gram-negative
   organisms
   Caution: Can cause renal toxicity, ototoxicity, and allergic
   reaction
   Use those antibiotics with sensitivity to the bacteria
   causing the infection

NURSING MANAGEMENT

Monitoring and Managing Clinical Problems

1. Breathing Pattern: ineffective—Monitor for ineffective
   breathing and promote effective breathing.
   a. Encourage patient to relax neck and shoulder
      muscles.
   b. Teach the patient pursed-lip breathing.
   c. Place the patient in high Fowler's position.
   d. Turn the patient every 2 hours.
   e. Suction the airway, as needed.
   f. Provide frequent mouth care.
   g. Administer ordered oxygen therapy.
   h. Administer ordered bronchodilators.
   i. Administer aspirin and nonsteroidal anti-inflamma-
      tory drugs with caution, as they may precipitate an
      asthma attack in some patients.
2. Gas Exchange: impaired—Monitor for and prevent impaired gas exchange.
   a. Monitor serial ABGs for acidosis.
   b. Monitor effectiveness of oxygen therapy with pulse
      oximetry and maintain SaO_2 of >85%.
   c. Be prepared for emergency intubation and mechani-
      cal ventilation, if necessary.
   d. Monitor respiratory rate and tidal volume frequently.

   e. Place the patient in a comfortable position (usually sitting up, leaning forward with arms supported and shoulders elevated). Provide an over-bed table and pillows for support.

   f. Monitor for complications of mechanical ventilation, such as barotrauma and pneumothorax.

3. Activity Intolerance — Monitor for and prevent activity intolerance.

   a. Assess vital signs to determine how the patient is tolerating activity.

   b. Observe for dyspnea when giving care and allow patient to rest if dyspnea occurs.

   c. Space activities of daily living throughout the day to decrease activity-related dyspnea.

   d. Assist the patient with activities if dyspnea occurs.

4. Infection: high risk for — Monitor for infection.

   a. Monitor temperature every 4 hours.

   b. Monitor WBCs for elevation.

   c. Use strict aseptic technique to decrease the risk for nosocomial infections.

   d. Observe body secretions for signs of infection and culture suspicious material.

   e. Administer ordered antibiotics.

   f. Maintain adequate nutrition to ensure optimal healing.

5. Fluid Volume Deficit: high risk for — Monitor for dehydration.

   a. Monitor hourly intake and output, and report discrepancies.

   b. Weigh patient daily.

   c. Monitor serial serum electrolytes, hematocrit, and hemoglobin for signs of dehydration.

   d. Promote fluid and electrolyte balance.

      1) Monitor IV fluid administration.

      2) Accurately monitor intake and output.

      3) Encourage oral fluid intake and report inability to take fluids orally.

      4) Assess frequently for edema.

6. Airway Clearance: ineffective — Promote removal of airway secretions.

   a. Perform chest physiotherapy (postural drainage, percussion, and vibration) to mobilize secretions.

    b. Encourage deep breathing and coughing every 4 hours.

    c. Assess for skin turgor and inspect mucous membranes for signs of adequate hydration.

    d. Administer inhalation treatments of bronchodilators.

7. Fatigue — Promote rest and sleep.
    a. Provide a calm, quiet environment.
    b. Cluster patient-care activities to allow for periods of rest.
    c. Avoid sedation during acute attacks.

8. Nutrition: altered, less than body requirements — Promote adequate nutrition.
    a. Assist with feeding, if necessary.
    b. Monitor caloric intake.
    c. Monitor serum albumin levels to determine malnutrition.
    d. Monitor weight daily.
    e. Suggest family bring food from home if the patient does not like hospital food.
    f. Suggest parenteral or enteral nutrition, if needed.
    g. Auscultate for the presence of bowel sounds and medicate to prevent constipation.

9. Cardiac Output: decreased, high risk for — Recognize signs and symptoms of decreased cardiac output.
    a. Assist with insertion of hemodynamic monitoring catheter and measure cardiac output and cardiac index, as ordered.
    b. Assess vital signs hourly for tachycardia and hypotension.
    c. Check peripheral perfusion every 4 hours and report decreased pulse amplitude or lengthened capillary refill time.
    d. Monitor continuously for ECG changes and arrhythmias, and report significant findings.

Monitoring, Managing, and Preventing of Life-Threatening Emergencies

1. Status asthmaticus is, in and of itself, a life-threatening emergency.
2. Bronchospasm
    a. Measure respiratory rate frequently. Report increases in rate and in the work of breathing.

  b. Auscultate breath sounds and report increasing wheezing or coughing.
  c. Observe for signs of respiratory distress (e.g., tachypnea, intercostal retraction, anxiety, air hunger, and diaphoresis).
  d. Monitor serial ABGs for hypocapnia, which may precede bronchospasm.
  e. Administer ordered bronchodilators.
  f. Administer ordered oxygen therapy.
  g. Administer ordered respiratory treatments.
  h. Be prepared for emergency intubation and mechanical ventilation.
3. Respiratory failure
  a. Monitor for increasing respiratory distress leading to increasing hypoxemia.
    1) Monitor serial ABG results and report abnormalities.
    2) Monitor serial chest X-ray reports.
    3) Auscultate lungs frequently for decreased breath sounds, crackles, and/or rhonchi.
    4) Apply pulse oximeter and continuously measure oxygen saturation.
    5) Administer ordered bronchodilators.
    6) Observe for signs of respiratory distress (e.g., tachypnea, intercostal retraction, anxiety, air hunger, and diaphoresis).
  b. Prepare for immediate intubation if necessary.
  c. Monitor for effective ventilation while on mechanical ventilator.
    1) Assess lung sounds frequently.
    2) Suction as needed to remove sputum and promote a clear airway.
    3) Measure pulmonary compliance frequently and report decreases.
    4) Measure peak pressures and report increases.
    5) Sedate the patient as needed to control ventilator fighting. Paralytics also may be necessary.
    6) Monitor serial ABGs for effectiveness of mechanical ventilation. Indications for positive end-expiratory pressure (PEEP) include:
      a) PaO_2 <60 mm Hg on an FiO_2 >50%
      b) pH <7.25

       c) $Paco_2$ >45 mm Hg

   7) Decrease Fio_2 to <50% as quickly as possible to prevent oxygen toxicity.

   8) If the patient is on PEEP, remember that PEEP holds alveoli open, thus increasing FRC, decreasing shunting, and decreasing hypoxemia. But, PEEP can:

       a) Decrease cardiac output (CO)

       b) Increase the chance of oxygen toxicity

       c) Cause fluid overload

d. Monitor fluid volume status.

   1) Hemodynamically measure CO frequently.

   2) Measure hourly urine output and report output <30 mL/hr.

   3) Observe for signs of fluid overload (e.g., new S_3, increasing pulmonary crackles and rhonchi, edema, weight gain, intake greater than output) and report positive findings.

   4) Observe for signs of dehydration (e.g., weight loss, low CO, intake greater than output, tenting of skin) and report positive findings.

Pulmonary Embolism

A pulmonary embolism (PE) is a blood clot (thromboembolus), fat globule (fat embolus), air bubble (air embolus), or any other material (such as a sheared catheter tip, amniotic fluid, calcium, infected tissue, or tumor fragment) that has migrated to the lung from elsewhere in the body, lodged in the circulation within the lung, and interrupted blood flow to an area of lung tissue. The size of embolus and the extent of obstruction determines the severity of lung tissue injury and amount of lung function affected. Large emboli often result in immediate cardiopulmonary collapse and death. Massive pulmonary embolus is a major cause of sudden, unexpected death.

Etiology/Pathophysiology

1. Risk factors for PE
   a. Phlebitis—deep vein thrombosis (DVT) in the legs and pelvis. An estimated 95% arise from DVT.
   b. Smoking
   c. Oral contraceptive use
   d. Immobilization
   e. Trauma
   f. Carcinoma—frequently of the breast, lungs, and viscera
   g. Pregnancy and childbirth
   h. Cardiac disease, especially congestive heart disease and atrial fibrillation
   i. Polycythemia vera
   j. Diabetes mellitus
   k. Varicose veins
   l. Previous pulmonary embolus
   m. Obesity
   n. Major abdominal or orthopedic surgery
2. Types of emboli
   a. Thromboembolus
      1) Virchow's triad for development of venous thrombosis
         a) Venous stasis of blood
         b) Coagulation abnormalities (hypercoagulable state)
         c) Vessel-wall damage or abnormalities
      2) Frequent complication of prolonged bed rest
      3) Preventable
      4) Once a thrombus forms, it may dislodge spontaneously or be jarred lose by sudden movement.
      5) Resolves by absorption and fibrinolysis within hours or days.
   b. Fat embolus
      1) Causes
         a) Long-bone fractures (especially tibia and femur)
         b) Sternal splitting procedures
         c) Use of extracorporeal membrane oxygenation (ECMO) during cardiac bypass surgery
         d) Trauma to subcutaneous fat

    2) Believed to occur more often than diagnosed clinically

    3) Occurs 12–24 hours after traumatic injury

    4) Pressure gradients between the intravascular and interstitial spaces cause fat globules to enter the circulation.

    5) Capillary obstruction from fat globules is thought to be the cause of the petechiae that occur following fat embolism.

    6) Lipases in the plasma break the fat globule down until it is small enough to be removed by phagocytosis. Low-dose heparin may stimulate lipase activity.

  c. Air embolus

    1) Causes

      a) Surgery in the peritoneal cavity resulting in intraperitoneal air

      b) Air in IV lines

      c) Pulmonary artery balloon rupture

      d) Tubal insufflation

      e) Uterine douching

      f) Hemodialysis

      g) Neck surgery

      h) Nasal sinuses irrigation

      i) Chest trauma

      j) Rapid decompression

      k) When deep inspiration is taken while central venous catheter is left open to air

    2) A 100-cc dose of air is lethal.

    3) Air usually enters the circulation through the venous system.

3. The three main effects of pulmonary embolism are:

  a. Increased amount of pulmonary dead space. It occurs in the early stages as a result of ventilation-perfusion mismatch.

  b. Loss of surfactant. Surfactant is reduced because of decreased blood flow to surfactant-producing cells. Altered surfactant production results in alveolar collapse, atelectasis, shunting of blood, and hypoxemia.

  c. Decreased lung volume resulting from atelectasis

4. Emboli may travel through the venous or arterial system.

5. Right lung involved more than left; lower lobes more than upper

6. The most rapidly fatal emboli are 7–8 mm in diameter. Those <4 mm rarely cause clinical problems.
7. Pulmonary artery hypertension (a result of the release of chemical mediators after PE that cause vasoconstriction and thereby increase pulmonary vascular resistance) occurs with a mechanical occlusion of 50% or more of the pulmonary vascular bed and may lead to right ventricular failure.
8. Bronchoconstriction and bronchospasm can occur from the release of serotonin from platelets that surround the embolus and from other chemical mediators.
9. Since the lungs have a dual blood supply—the pulmonary arterial system and the bronchial arterial system— good collateral circulation decreases tissue hypoperfusion and tissue death after pulmonary embolism.

Assessment/Analysis

ASSESSMENT FINDINGS

Subjective

1. May have vague and nonspecific complaints which often result in misdiagnosis.
2. Calf or leg tenderness
3. Sudden onset of dyspnea (most common complaint)
4. Pleuritic chest pain (with large emboli)
5. History of one or more risk factors for development of PE

Objective

1. Range from none (with small emboli) to cardiovascular collapse (with large emboli)
2. May see any or all of the following:
   a. Tachypnea
   b. Profuse perspiration
   c. Cyanosis
   d. Cough possibly with hemoptysis
   e. Syncope
   f. Slight temperature elevation
   g. Signs of phlebitis—positive Homan's sign (pain in the calf with dorsiflexion of the foot)
   h. Splinting of the affected side and dullness on percussion over the involved lung area

    i. Anxiety, apprehension, and restlessness caused by hypoxemia

    j. Weakness

    k. Nausea and vomiting

    l. Nonspecific crackles in the lungs

    m. Wheezing (asthma-like symptoms)

    n. Pleural friction rub and/or pleural effusion

    o. Signs of right ventricular overload: fixed splitting of the second heart sound, right-sided S_4, murmur over the lung field, hepatomegaly, and jugular vein distension

    p. Atrial arrhythmias

    q. Hypotension

    r. Tachycardia

    s. Ventricular gallop rhythm

    t. Cardiopulmonary arrest

3. In addition, a patient with fat embolism may also exhibit the following:

    a. Onset of symptoms within hours or up to 4 days, most commonly before the third day

    b. Petechial rash usually on chest, shoulders, and axilla, which appears within 24 hours

4. In addition, a churning sound may be heard on auscultation in a patient with air embolism in the right ventricle.

SUPPORTING TEST FINDINGS

Laboratory Tests

1. ABGs
   Abnormality: In massive PE:
       Decreased PaO_2
       Increased $PaCO_2$
       Respiratory acidosis

2. Serum lipase
   Abnormality: Elevated in patients with fat embolus the third day after injury

3. White Blood Cell (WBC) count
   Abnormality: Generally normal, but may be slightly elevated

4. Serum lactic dehydrogenase (LDH)
   Abnormality: May be elevated

5. Serum bilirubin
   Abnormality: May be elevated
6. Fibrin split products
   Abnormality: May have increased levels
7. Prothrombin time (PT)
   Abnormality: Prolonged when patient on warfarin (Coumadin) therapy
8. Partial thromboplastin time (PTT)
   Abnormality: Prolonged when patient on heparin therapy

Diagnostic Tests

1. Pulmonary angiogram (most definitive test)
   Abnormality: Isolated areas of malperfusion
2. Lung scan (most frequently done test)
   Abnormality: Abnormal distribution of gas within the lung
3. Chest X-ray
   Abnormality: None, even with massive PE
       Used to rule out other causes of chest pain
4. Hemodynamic monitoring
   Abnormality: Sudden increase in PAP, right arterial pressure (RAP), right ventricular end-diastolic pressure
       Sudden decrease in CO
5. Electrocardiogram (ECG)
   Abnormality: New right-axis deviation
       New right bundle branch block
       Prominent P waves
       ST elevation in the precordial leads
       In massive PE: Deep S waves in lead I
       Q waves in lead I
       Inverted T waves in lead III
6. Pulmonary function tests (PFTs)
   Abnormality: Decreased vital capacity (VC)
       Decreased ratio of 1-second forced expiratory volume (FEV) to forced VC
       Decreased diffusing capacity
7. Capnography
   Abnormality: Sudden rise in arterial to alveolar pressure of CO_2 ($P(A\text{-}a)CO_2$) without a sudden fall in cardiac output (CO)

Planning/Intervention

COLLABORATIVE MANAGEMENT

Procedures

1. For all types of emboli
   a. Provide cardiopulmonary support, as indicated.
      1) Institute mechanical ventilation if respiratory failure occurs.
      2) Provide oxygen therapy.
      3) Administer ordered volume expanders to improve CO.
      4) Assist with insertion of central line to monitor hemodynamic parameters.
   b. Prevent occurrence or recurrence.
      1) Prepare patient for insertion of intracaval filter or umbrella used to trap emboli in the vena cava, as ordered.
      2) Administer ordered prophylactic anticoagulant therapy for patients at risk for PE.
         a) Low-dose heparin therapy
         b) Daily aspirin
         c) Promote early ambulation for patients on bed rest.
         d) Apply antiembolic stockings to patients requiring prolonged bed rest.
         e) Elevate legs.
         f) Prepare patient for early surgical repair of fractures.
2. For thromboemboli
   a. Initiate and monitor anticoagulation intravenously with heparin followed by oral administration of warfarin (Coumadin).
      1) Administer loading dose of 5,000–15,000 U of heparin IV bolus. Follow with IV heparin drip and adjust to keep PTT between 1.5–2.5 times the normal baseline. Continue therapy for 8–10 days. Give a loading dose of warfarin 2–3 days prior to discontinuing heparin followed by a daily dose based on the PT results.
   b. Prepare patient for clot removal.

1) Administer ordered thrombolytics to directly lyse the clot.
2) Prepare patient for pulmonary embolectomy, as indicated.

Drug Therapy

1. Anticoagulants
   Examples: sodium heparin (heparin)
       warfarin (Coumadin)
   Action: Decreases clotting ability of blood thereby preventing thromboembolus
   Caution: May cause occult and overt bleeding
       Heparin — monitor PTT closely to assess anticoagulation; antidote is protamine sulfate
       Coumadin — monitor PT closely to assess anticoagulation; antidote is vitamin K
2. Volume expanders
   Examples: Low-molecular-weight dextran, albumin, and hetastarch
   Action: Replaces fluids to treat hypovolemia: colloids recommended; low-molecular-weight dextran thought to prevent continuing thrombosis
   Caution: Can cause fluid overload
3. Inotropic agents
   Examples: dopamine (Intropin)
       dobutamine (Dobutrex)
       norepinephrine (Levophed)
   Action: Improves myocardial contractility; increases cardiac output, improves hypotension
   Caution: Increases myocardial oxygen consumption; may worsen hypokalemia and arrhythmias (**Note:** Isoproterenol contraindicated in pulmonary emboli because it increases myocardial oxygen consumption and decreases coronary blood flow)
4. Diuretics
   Examples: furosemide (Lasix)
       bumetanide (Bumex)
       mannitol (Osmitrol)
   Action: Increases urine excretion
   Caution: Can cause hypokalemia and dehydration
5. Opioid analgesics

Examples: morphine (Duramorph)
    meperidine (Demerol)
    hydromorphone (Dilaudid)
Action: Depresses pain-impulse transmission to relieve associated chest pain
Caution: May cause sedation and respiratory depression

6. Thrombolytics
Examples: streptokinase (Streptase)
    tissue plasminogen activator (Activase)
Action: Dissolves clot thereby restoring blood flow to the ischemic portion of the lung; most effective when clot less than 3 days old
Caution: May cause uncontrolled bleeding and arrhythmias; experts feel more research needed before widespread clinical application

7. Corticosteroids
Example: hydrocortisone (Solu-Cortef)
Action: Stabilizes capillary walls thereby decreasing fluid shifts out of the vasculature, reducing interstitial pulmonary edema following fat embolus
Caution: May cause hypokalemia, hypernatremia, nausea, and petechiae
    Increases risk of gastrointestinal bleeding

8. Bronchodilators
Example: aminophylline (theophylline)
Action: Relieves bronchoconstriction
Caution: May cause tachycardia and anxiety; toxicity may occur; monitor blood levels closely

NURSING MANAGEMENT

Monitoring and Managing Clinical Problems

1. All types of emboli
   a. Breathing Pattern: ineffective, high risk for — Monitor for signs of respiratory distress.
      1) Observe for dyspnea and tachypnea, anxiety, apprehension, and restlessness.
      2) Check nailbeds for pallor or cyanosis.
      3) Be prepared to institute mechanical ventilation, if necessary.
      4) Apply pulse oximeter and continuously monitor oxygen saturation.

       5) Obtain specimens and monitor serial arterial blood gases (ABGs).

  b. Gas Exchange: impaired — Promote activities to improve ventilation.

      1) Encourage coughing and deep breathing.

      2) Administer ordered oxygen.

      3) Observe for respiratory distress with patient-care activities, interrupt care if it occurs, and space activities to prevent recurrence of respiratory distress.

      4) Elevate the head of the bed.

      5) Auscultate the lungs every 4 hours for abnormalities and report significant findings.

      6) Assist with incentive spirometry, as indicated.

2. Thromboembolism

  a. Fluid Volume Deficit: high risk for — Monitor patient for side effects of anticoagulant therapy.

      1) Assess for and prevent overt bleeding.

        a) Check injection sites for bleeding.

        b) Apply pressure to venipuncture sites until bleeding stops.

        c) Observe for bleeding from the gums following mouth care.

        d) Check for nosebleeds.

        e) Avoid using a razor blade for shaving. If needed, use an electric razor.

      2) Assess for and prevent occult bleeding.

        a) Check for blood in the urine and stool.

        b) Administer antacids to prevent stress ulceration.

        c) Observe for bruising and hematomas, especially at injection sites.

        d) Monitor for decreasing hemoglobin and hematocrit.

      3) Keep protamine sulfate or vitamin K available as an antidote for excessive bleeding.

      4) Monitor PTT or PT to assess anticoagulation.

  b. Tissue Perfusion, altered: peripheral, high risk for — Promote nursing actions to prevent venous stasis.

      1) Apply antiembolic stockings or sequential compression device.

        a) Sequential compression devices provide cyclic

compression and relaxation periods which closely approximate muscle contraction. The most effective type of antiembolic device.

b) Elastic hose and ace bandage wraps compress superficial veins in the legs and prevent venous stasis. These are the most useful for ambulatory patients.

2) Assist with active and passive exercises.
3) Avoid venipuncture in the legs.
4) Do not forcibly irrigate clotted IV lines.
5) Administer anticoagulants, as ordered.
6) Prevent dehydration.
7) Elevate legs to promote venous return.
8) Instruct patient not to cross legs.
9) Instruct patient not to keep knees bent while in bed.

3. Fat embolus
   a. Injury, high risk for — Promote patient-care activities that prevent fat embolism.
      1) Splint fractures as soon as possible.
      2) Avoid overmanipulation of the fracture.
      3) Administer ordered corticosteroids.
   b. Injury, high risk for — Monitor for signs and symptoms of fat embolus.
      1) Observe for subtle changes in the level of consciousness.
      2) Observe for signs and symptoms of respiratory distress.
      3) Monitor urine and sputum for fat globules.
      4) Observe skin for petechiae.
   c. Pain — Promote patient comfort.
      1) Relieve pain with ordered analgesics. Prevent emotional distress by placing the patient in a quiet, calm environment.
      2) Place patient on bed rest with the head of bed elevated.
      3) Assist with activities of daily living.

4. Air embolus
   a. High risk for injury — Institute interventions to optimize chances for aspiration of the air embolus
      1) Place patient on left side in head down position so air will float into the right atrium

    2) Prepare for aspiration of the air from the right atrium via central line inserted into the right atrium

5. High risk for injury—Pulmonary infarction
   a. Uncommon
   b. Usually seen in patients with underlying pulmonary disease
   c. Results in significant lung consolidation from hemorrhage
   d. Causes pleuritic pain
   e. May necrose, become infected, and form a lung abscess. Healing results in fibrosis and scar tissue

Monitoring, Managing, and Preventing Life-Threatening Emergencies

1. Pulmonary embolism is, in and of itself, a life-threatening emergency
2. Cardiopulmonary arrest
   a. Call for help
   b. Begin cardiopulmonary resuscitation
   c. Follow with advanced cardiac life support
3. Hemorrhage following anticoagulation therapy or thrombolytic therapy
   a. Monitor for physical finding of blood loss
      1) tachycardia with a faint, thready pulse
      2) tachypnea
      3) hypotension in recumbent position or postural hypotension
      4) cool, pale or cyanotic, clammy skin
      5) poor skin turgor with dry mucous membranes
      6) lethargy, confusion, or obtundation
      7) decreased urine output
      8) increasing abdominal girth
      9) rigid abdomen
      10) guaiac positive stools or nasogastric drainage, and blood per rectum, vagina, urinary meatus, emesis or peritoneal lavage
   b. Monitor serial hemoglobin and hematocrit for decreasing values
   c. Monitor serial hemodynamic parameters for decreased central venous pressure, pulmonary artery

pressure, pulmonary capillary wedge pressure, and cardiac output; report significant findings
d. Prevent hemorrhage by
   1) Applying direct pressure over bleeding sites
   2) Administering blood products such as fresh frozen plasma

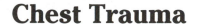

Chest Trauma

Chest trauma includes injury to the heart and great vessels, lungs, lower airways, bony thorax, and diaphragm (see Cardiovascular Trauma in Chapter 2, "Cardiovascular Disorders").

Injuries to the lungs include pneumothorax (closed, open, and tension), hemothorax (see Cardiovascular Trauma), and pulmonary contusion. Injuries to the lower airways include obstruction (partial and complete), tracheobronchial tears, and tracheoarterial and tracheoesophageal fistulas.

Bony thorax injuries include fractures of the ribs or sternum. Multiple rib fractures can result in a flail chest. Rupture of the diaphragm also can be caused by chest trauma.

Chest trauma includes most of the life-threatening injuries seen in patients and is the second leading cause of death caused by trauma.

Etiology/Pathophysiology

1. Blunt trauma is most often caused by impact with the steering wheel in motor vehicle accidents.
2. Survivors experience many postevent complications.

Types of Chest Trauma

Type of Injury	Cause	Pathophysiology	Comments
Simple, closed pneumothorax	Most commonly fractured rib Blunt or penetrating trauma Spontaneous rupture of blebs High intrathoracic pressures with mechanical ventilation	Air, fluid, or blood collects in the pleural space causing loss of normal negative intrathoracic pressure and resulting in lung collapse	May or may not require chest tube depending on size
Open pneumothorax (sucking chest wound)	Penetrating chest injury (common combat injury) Central venous catheter insertion	Atmospheric air flows into the pleural space causing loss of normal intratho-	Degree of seriousness depends on the site of the wound

Type of Injury	Cause	Pathophysiology	Comments
	Chest surgery	racic pressure and resulting in lung collapse	
Tension pneumothorax	Penetrating chest injury with air-sealed chest opening Lung laceration from fractured rib, especially when associated with mechanical ventilation Chest-tube occlusion or malfunction	Air accumulates in closed intrathoracic cavity, creating increased pressure, which results in shifting of mediastinum and displacement of major vessels; this decreases venous return to the heart and causes cardiovascular collapse	Can rapidly progress to death without treatment
Pulmonary contusion	Usually follows blunt chest injury	Impact can rupture lung tissue and vessels,	Young people are at higher risk because

Continued

Types of Chest Trauma— *Continued*

Type of Injury	*Cause*	*Pathophysiology*	*Comments*
		bronchioles, and alveoli	chest wall is more flexible
			Severity varies from mild to life threatening
			May progress to atelectasis and ARDS
Obstruction (complete or partial)	Tongue or foreign body	Unconsciousness following trauma leads to relaxation of the tongue muscle, inability to clear foreign bodies, and obstruction	Can be life threatening if not recognized
Tracheobronchial tears	Blunt or penetrating chest trauma	Force of blow to chest can cause complete or incomplete circumferential tears, most	

Type of Injury	Cause	Pathophysiology	Comments
		commonly of the mainstem bronchi near the carina Results in subcutaneous emphysema around the area that may extend into the chest and arms	
Tracheal fistula	Chest trauma Endotracheal or tracheal cuff erosion from an overinflated cuff or incorrect positioning of the airway	An opening between the trachea and the esophagus or an artery is created by erosion or trauma	Tracheoarterial fistula is often fatal and most commonly involves the right carotid, lower thyroid, or innominate artery Tracheoesophegeal fistula results in air and fluid or food

Continued

Types of Chest Trauma — *Continued*

Type of Injury	*Cause*	*Pathophysiology*	*Comments*
			moving between the lungs and stomach
Flail chest	Blunt chest injury	Free-floating sections of ribs broken away from the rib cage cause the chest to move paradoxically (depresses on inspiration and expands on expiration) Airflow in the lungs decreases and dead space increases	May be posterior, anterior, or lateral
First or second rib fracture	High-impact chest trauma	Application of significant outside force	Considered the hallmark of severe trauma

Type of Injury	Cause	Pathophysiology	Comments
		causes fracture	
Middle rib fracture (single or multiple)	Blunt trauma	Impact with an outside force causes fracture	4–10 are the most common fractures as they are the most exposed
Lower rib fracture	Blunt trauma	Impact with an outside force causes fracture	Free-floating ribs are located here
Sternal fracture	Significant blunt chest injury	Impact with a tremendous amount of outside force causes fracture	Can result in complete separation of the sternum from the rib cage
Diaphragmatic rupture	Blunt chest injury	Diaphragm tears allowing abdominal organs to herniate into the chest cavity	May be life threatening

Assessment/Analysis

ASSESSMENT FINDINGS

Subjective

1. History of a mechanism of injury consistent with thoracic trauma
2. Patient may report chest pain, agitation, and fear.
3. The chief complaints vary with type of injury.

Objective

CLOSED PNEUMOTHORAX

1. Dyspnea, tachypnea, and respiratory distress are present.
2. Cyanosis and crepitus may be present.
3. Diminished or absent breath sounds over the site
4. Hyperresonance (high-pitched sound) over affected site
5. A sudden drop in PaO_2 on arterial blood gases (ABGs)

OPEN PNEUMOTHORAX — Signs and symptoms of a closed pneumothorax plus:

1. Obvious injury at affected site
2. Sucking sound on inspiration at affected site
3. Subcutaneous emphysema in upper chest and neck
4. Signs of reduced venous return — neck vein distension, tachycardia

TENSION PNEUMOTHORAX — Signs and symptoms of a closed pneumothorax plus:

1. Asymmetric chest movement
2. Tracheal deviation to the unaffected side
3. Signs of reduced venous return — neck vein distension, tachycardia
4. Signs of shock — decreased blood pressure, tachycardia
5. Muffled heart sounds

PULMONARY CONTUSION

1. Initially, few symptoms unless injury is large. Usually patients complain of chest pain.

2. Contusions or abrasions to the skin over the site
3. Tachypnea and hemoptysis
4. Dyspnea resulting from falling pulmonary compliance and increasing airway pressure
5. Ineffective cough with copious secretions
6. Fever may develop.
7. Moist crackles and local areas of wheezing
8. Decreased PaO_2 and pH on ABGs
9. Evidence of injury on X-ray after 24 hours

PARTIAL OBSTRUCTION

1. Audible air movement
2. Accessory muscle use — sternal retractions
3. Cough
4. Tachycardia
5. Cyanosis
6. Decreased PaO_2 and pH on ABGs

COMPLETE OBSTRUCTION

1. Inability to talk followed rapidly by unconsciousness
2. Cyanosis
3. Absence of air movement progressing to apnea without treatment
4. Tachycardia, deteriorating to pulselessness without treatment

TRACHEOBRONCHIAL TEARS

1. Tachypnea, dyspnea, and cyanosis
2. Cough with hemoptysis
3. Cervical and mediastinal subcutaneous emphysema
4. Positive Hamman's sign — crepitus (crunching sound) heard synchronously with the heartbeat
5. When chest tube is in place, a continuous air leak is heard. Dyspnea increases when suction is applied to the chest drainage system.

TRACHEOARTERIAL FISTULA

1. Sudden onset of hemoptysis, dyspnea, tachypnea caused by hemorrhage into the airway
2. Blood pressure drops, pulse increases, shock develops, and cardiopulmonary arrest occurs without treatment.

TRACHEOESOPHAGEAL FISTULA

1. Increased pulmonary secretions containing gastric contents
2. Coughing with swallowing
3. Constant gastric distension

FLAIL CHEST

1. Dyspnea and tachypnea
2. Splinting with respirations
3. Paradoxic chest-wall movement with respirations
4. Cyanosis
5. Point tenderness
6. Diminished or absent breath sounds over the affected area

RIB FRACTURES

1. Dyspnea and tachypnea
2. Splinting with respirations
3. Rapid, shallow respirations
4. Crepitus over affected area
5. Unwillingness to cough deeply
6. Fracture evident on X-ray

STERNAL FRACTURES

1. Progressively increasing pain during inspiration
2. Contusions and abrasions over affected area
3. Palpable step-off deformity (area of depressed bone) over affected area
4. Tenderness and crepitus on palpation

DIAPHRAGMATIC RUPTURE

1. Severe pain radiating to the shoulder
2. Dyspnea
3. Decreased breath sounds
4. Signs of shock may be present — hypotension, tachycardia, pale clammy skin.

SUPPORTING TEST FINDINGS

Laboratory Tests

1. Hematocrit and hemoglobin (H&H)
   Abnormality: Decreased — hemorrhage-induced hypovolemia
2. White blood cell (WBC) and differential
   Abnormality: Increased WBC count, neutrophils, bands, monocytes, and lymphocytes; infection present
3. ABGs
   Abnormality: Hypoxemia — ineffective ventilation (PaO_2 <80 mm Hg)
   Hypercapnia — ineffective ventilation ($PaCO_2$ >45 mm Hg)
   Respiratory acidosis — ineffective ventilation (pH <7.35) (HCO_3 22 – 26 mEq/L)
4. Blood type and cross or type, screen, and hold
   Abnormality: In extreme emergencies, untyped and uncrossmatched blood (0 negative) or type specific, but uncrossmatched, blood may be given

Diagnostic Tests

1. Hemodynamic monitoring
   Abnormality: Cardiac output (CO) <4 L/min
   Pulmonary artery pressure (PAP) <20/8 mm Hg
   Pulmonary mean pressure <10 mm Hg
   Wedge pressure <8 mm Hg
   Central venous pressure <2 mm Hg
2. Continuous blood pressure monitoring via arterial line or automatic cuff
   Abnormality: Mean arterial blood pressure <90 mm Hg
3. Chest X-ray
   Abnormality: Evidence of pulmonary contusion 24 hours after injury
4. Ventilation — perfusion scan
   Abnormality: Ventilation-perfusion mismatch
5. Computed tomography scan of the chest
   Abnormality: Evidence of injury
6. Pulmonary function tests (PFTs)
   Abnormality: Evidence of decreased lung function
   Tidal volume <500 mL

Inspiratory reserve volume <3000 mL
Residual volume (RV) <1200 mL
Vital capacity (VC) <4500 mL

Planning/Intervention

COLLABORATIVE MANAGEMENT

Procedures

1. Provide pain relief.
   a. Assist with intercostal nerve blocks—for fractures of up to three ribs.
   b. Monitor thoracic epidural anesthesia—for greater than three rib fractures and for flail chest.
   c. Administer ordered IV narcotics.
   d. Apply transcutaneous electrical nerve stimulation (TENS) unit, if ordered.
2. Maintain adequate oxygenation.
   a. Assist with insertion of endotracheal tube and institute mechanical ventilation, as ordered.
   b. Monitor controlled ventilation with controlled positive airway pressure (CPAP) or positive end-expiratory pressure (PEEP) for pulmonary contusion, multiple fractured ribs, and flail chest.
   c. Assist with needle decompression followed by chest-tube insertion to reexpand pneumothorax.
   d. Prepare patient for surgical repair of any traumatic injury.
   e. Prepare patient for diagnostic bronchoscopy to determine the extent of injury.
3. Prevent infection.
   a. Collect needed specimens and send to laboratory for analysis.
   b. Administer ordered antibiotics. Before the source is identified at least a two-drug combination should be given. When the source is identified, therapy may be tailored to the cause.
4. Open-chest cardiac massage in massive chest trauma may be used as a "last ditch" effort to save life. It is rarely successful.

Drug Therapy

1. Volume expanders — Controversy exists regarding fluid replacement. Generally, if blood loss is the cause of hypovolemia, blood should be replaced.

   Examples: Crystalloids — Should be used judiciously in the presence of major lung injury; Ringer's, Ringer's lactate (plain Ringer's is used if the patient has a chance of returning to aerobic metabolism), and normal saline are the common ones used

   Blood or blood products — Packed red blood cells (RBCs), whole blood, autotransfusion, and synthetic blood products may be used as the primary means of volume reexpansion in acute lung injury to minimize the chance of fluid overload and pulmonary edema

   Action: Increases intravascular volume

   Used to replace lost intravascular volume, with caution exercised to prevent fluid overload

   Caution: Can cause hypervolemia and pulmonary edema

2. Antibiotics

   Examples: cephalosporins: ticarcillin (Timentin), ceftazidime (Fortaz)

   aminoglycosides: gentamycin (Garamycin), tobramycin (Nebcin)

   Action: Bacteriocidal; broad-spectrum antibiotics which kill aerobic and anaerobic gram-negative and gram-positive bacteria

   Caution: Can cause renal failure, allergic reaction, and ototoxicity

3. Analgesics

   Examples: morphine (Duramorph)

   meperidine (Demerol)

   hydromorphone (Dilaudid)

   Action: Depresses pain impulse transmission

   Caution: Can cause sedation, respiratory depression, and drug dependency

4. Sedatives

   Examples: lorazepam (Ativan)

   diazepam (Valium)

   midazolam (Versed)

   Action: Depresses the central nervous system producing sedation and relief of anxiety

Caution: Can cause respiratory depression and psychological dependence
   Tolerance can develop
5. Anesthetics
   Examples: lidocaine (Xylocaine)
          bupivacaine (Marcaine)
          procaine
   Action: Provides local anesthesia to relieve pain associated with chest trauma
      May be given by block or via epidural catheter
   Caution: Can cause hypersensitivity, toxicity, and prolonged anesthesia

NURSING MANAGEMENT

Monitoring and Managing of Clinical Problems

GENERAL PROBLEMS

1. Airway Clearance: ineffective, high risk for — Monitor for inadequate expectoration of excretions.
   a. Encourage coughing, deep breathing, and incentive spirometry to ensure the expectoration of secretions to decrease chances for infection.
   b. Assess the adequacy of pain control frequently so patient can deep breath and cough with minimal discomfort.
   c. Auscultate lungs frequently for areas of atelectasis and for abnormal sounds, and report findings.
   d. Monitor WBC to determine onset of infection.
   e. Monitor temperature every 4 hours to identify early onset of infection.
2. Breathing Pattern: ineffective — Monitor for ineffective ventilation.
   a. Observe for any signs of respiratory distress (tachypnea, dyspnea, pallor, cyanosis, and anxiety) and report any positive findings.
   b. Monitor serial ABGs and chest X-ray results to monitor response to treatment.

    c. Perform frequent lung assessment. Identify and report new abnormalities.

    d. Administer supplemental oxygen, as ordered.

3. Gas Exchange: impaired — Monitor for inadequate oxygenation.

    a. Auscultate breath sounds frequently.

    b. Observe for peripheral cyanosis.

    c. Assess for change in mental status frequently.

    d. Monitor serial ABGs for signs of hypoxemia and hypercapnia.

    e. Monitor ventilator parameters for decreased compliance and increased peak pressures.

4. Pain — Promote pain relief.

    a. Medicate liberally with pain medicine, especially before patient movement or breathing exercises.

    b. Assess adequacy of pain medication and report undermedication and poor pain control.

DIAGNOSIS OF SPECIFIC PROBLEMS

1. Simple, closed pneumothorax:

    Tissue Perfusion, altered: pulmonary — Promote reexpansion of the lung. No treatment is required if the pneumothorax is less than 20%.

    a. Assist with chest-tube insertion.

    b. Monitor chest drainage color, consistency, and amount. Report signs of hemorrhage.

    c. Monitor chest drainage for air leaks. These will either close within the first few days after injury or require surgical repair.

    d. Assess breath sounds frequently for reexpansion.

    e. Monitor serial ABGs reports and serial chest X-ray reports to determine successful reexpansion.

2. Open pneumothorax:

    Tissue Perfusion, altered: pulmonary — In addition to nursing actions for simple, closed pneumothorax, recognize complications from occlusion of the wound.

    a. Immediately apply a sterile occlusive dressing over the wound using the three-sided tape method.

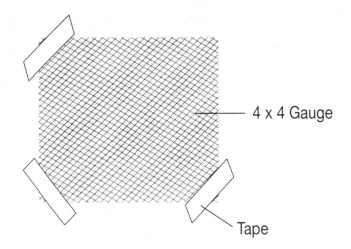

4 x 4 Gauge

Tape

b. Observe closely for signs and symptoms of the development of a tension pneumothorax (tracheal deviation, jugular vein distension, acute distress) once wound is occluded. If these occur, uncover the wound and summon the physician.
c. Prepare patient for surgery to clean, debride, and close the wound.
3. Tension pneumothorax:
Tissue Perfusion; altered: pulmonary — In addition to nursing actions for simple, closed pneumothorax, ensure early recognition of the complication of mediastinal shift.
a. Observe for and immediately report tension pneumothorax.
b. Assist with immediate needle decompression using a 14- to 16-gauge needle at the second intercostal space, midclavicular line on affected side.
c. Assist with chest-tube insertion.
4. Pulmonary contusion:
Gas Exchange: impaired — Monitor for pulmonary deterioration and prevent ARDS.
a. Prepare for possible intubation and controlled ventilation using CPAP and PEEP.

b. Avoid excess fluid administration. Monitor intake and output closely.

c. If not intubated, monitor closely for signs and symptoms of obstruction.

5. Partial obstruction:
Breathing Pattern: ineffective — Promote removal of the obstruction (often the tongue) and obtain a patent airway.

a. Open the airway with chin lift or jaw thrust method.

b. Insert an oral or nasal airway.

c. Encourage the patient to cough.

d. Suction the patient.

e. Deliver back blows, if necessary.

6. Complete obstruction:
Breathing Pattern: ineffective — Promote adequate ventilation by providing an effective method of ventilation.

a. Attempt to ventilate by repositioning airway.

b. Insert an oral or nasal airway.

c. If this does not help, set up and assist with intubation.

d. If this is ineffective, set up and assist with cricothyroidotomy or tracheostomy.

7. Tracheobronchial tears:
Breathing Pattern: ineffective — Recognize and report evidence of tracheobronchial tears.

a. Examine pleural drainage for evidence of new or increasing air leaks, which may occur for up to 3 or 4 days.

b. Examine the patient for new or expanding subcutaneous air.

c. Assess for development of new pneumothorax or pneumomediastinum.

d. Assist with chest-tube insertion if pneumothorax is present.

e. Assist with emergency bronchoscopy and anticipate possible emergency surgical repair of the tear.

f. Monitor for signs of air embolism:
   1) Sudden deterioration after intubation in the absence of bleeding
   2) Neurologic signs in the absence of head injury

g. Intervene quickly if signs occur:
   1) Place patient in Trendelenburg position.

2) Assist with cardiocentesis (insertion of a needle into the heart) to remove the air.

h. Post repair — Protect the airway with gentle suctioning and appropriate neck positioning.

8. Tracheal fistulas:

Injury: high risk for — Monitor cuff pressure to prevent their occurrence, but recognize them if they do occur.

a. Prevent overinflation of the endotracheal or tracheal tube cuff. Auscultate over the trachea for a slight air leak every 4 hours.

b. Maintain correct position of the head and neck to protect the airway.

c. Tracheoarterial fistula — often a fatal event. Observe for a pulsing tracheostomy tube as a sign of possible occurrence. If bleeding occurs, overinflate the cuff to tamponade the vessel. Summon the physician. Prepare for immediate surgical repair.

d. Tracheoesophageal fistula — Check pulmonary secretions for gastric contents. Observe for coughing after swallowing. Test sputum with glucose test strips. A positive test indicates aspiration. Prepare for a methylene blue test. Have the patient swallow the dye. Presence of the dye in sputum indicates a positive test.

9. Flail chest:

Breathing Pattern: ineffective — Recognize and report evidence of flail chest.

a. Observe for paradoxic chest movement.

b. Stabilize flail first by applying external splinting with sandbags or internal splinting with controlled mechanical ventilation and CPAP or PEEP.

c. Observe for the onset of pulmonary edema (dyspnea, moist crackles, rhonchi, frothy secretions).

10. Rib fractures:

Breathing Pattern: ineffective — Recognize the potential complications of hemorrhage and respiratory distress and intervene quickly.

a. First and second rib fractures — Assess for concomitant injury to the organs of the chest and the spinal cord (fracture and/or paralysis).

b. Fracture of the middle ribs — Assess for concomitant injury to the lungs or tracheobronchial tree or the heart and great vessels.

   c. Fracture of the lower ribs — Assess for concomitant injury to the kidneys (hematuria, bruising to the flanks), injury to the spleen if the injury is on the left side (hemorrhage resulting in shock), and injury to the liver if the injury is on the right (increased liver enzymes, jaundice, shock from hemorrhage).

11. Sternal fracture:
    Breathing Pattern: ineffective — Recognize signs of respiratory distress and intervene quickly.
   a. Monitor for respiratory distress, hemorrhage followed by shock, and cardiac arrhythmias.
   b. Institute cardiopulmonary resuscitation measures, as needed.

12. Ruptured diaphragm:
    Breathing Pattern: ineffective — Recognize signs of respiratory distress and intervene, as needed.
   a. Assess for and report bowel sounds heard in the chest cavity.
   b. If present, decompress stomach with nasogastric tube.
   c. Prepare the patient for surgical repair.

Monitoring, Managing, and Preventing of Life-Threatening Emergencies

1. Respiratory failure
   a. Monitor for increasing respiratory distress leading to increasing hypoxemia.
    1) Monitor serial ABG results and report abnormalities.
    2) Monitor serial chest X-ray results.
    3) Auscultate lungs frequently for decreased breath sounds, crackles, and/or rhonchi.
    4) Apply pulse oximeter and continuously measure oxygen saturation.
    5) Administer bronchodilators, as ordered.
    6) Monitor for air hunger, tachypnea, restlessness, and confusion indicating increasing respiratory distress.
   b. Have emergency resuscitation equipment nearby and assist immediate intubation, if necessary.
   c. Monitor for effective ventilation while on mechanical ventilator.

1) Reassess lung sounds frequently.
2) Suction, as needed, to remove sputum and promote a clear airway.
3) Measure compliance frequently and report decreases.
4) Measure peak pressures and report increases.
5) Sedate the patient, as needed, to control ventilator fighting. Paralytics also may be necessary.
6) Monitor serial ABGs for effectiveness of mechanical ventilation. Indications for PEEP are:
   a) PaO_2 <60 mm Hg on an FiO_2 >50%
   b) pH <7.25
   c) $PaCO_2$ >45 mm Hg
7) Decrease FiO_2 to <50% as quickly as possible to prevent oxygen toxicity.
8) If the patient is on PEEP, remember PEEP holds alveoli open thus increasing functional residual capacity, decreasing shunting, and decreasing hypoxemia. But, PEEP can:
   a) Decrease CO
   b) Increase the chance of oxygen toxicity
   c) Cause fluid overload
d. Monitor fluid volume status.
   1) Measure CO frequently.
   2) Measure hourly urine output and report output <30 mL/hr.
   3) Observe for signs of fluid overload (new S_3, increasing pulmonary crackles and rhonchi, edema, weight gain, intake greater than output) and report positive findings.
   4) Observe for signs of dehydration (weight loss, low CO, intake less than output, tenting of skin) and report positive findings.
   5) Administer IV fluids to prevent fluid overload but maintain adequate fluid volume.
2. Hemorrhage
   a. Monitor for physical findings of blood loss such as:
      1) Tachycardia with a faint, thready pulse
      2) Tachypnea
      3) Hypotension in recumbent position or postural hypotension
      4) Cool, pale, or cyanotic clammy skin

     5) Capillary refill greater than 3 seconds
     6) Poor skin turgor with dry mucous membranes
     7) Lethargy, confusion, or obtundation
     8) Decreased urine output
     9) Increasing abdominal girth
    10) Rigid abdomen
    11) Guaiac positive stools or nasogastric drainage, blood per rectum or vagina, urinary meatus, emesis, or peritoneal lavage

  b. Monitor serial hematocrit and hemoglobin levels for decreasing values.

  c. Monitor serial hemodynamic parameters for decreased central venous pressure, PAP, pulmonary capillary wedge pressure, and CO. Report significant findings.

  d. Prevent hemorrhage by:
     1) Applying direct pressure over bleeding sites
     2) Preparing patient for selective angiography with embolization or laparotomy
     3) Not removing impaled objects before surgery
     4) Applying medical anti-shock trousers (MAST) for pelvic fractures
     5) Administering fresh frozen plasma

3. Tension pneumothorax and mediastinal shift
  a. Monitor for signs of increasing respiratory distress and intervene quickly.
     1) Observe for and immediately report tension pneumothorax.
     2) Assist with immediate needle decompression using a 14- to 16-gauge needle at the second intercostal space, midclavicular line on affected side.
     3) Assist with chest-tube insertion.
     4) Monitor chest drainage color, consistency, and amount. Report signs of hemorrhage.
     5) Monitor chest drainage for air leaks. These will either close within the first few days after injury or require surgical repair.
     6) Assess breath sounds frequently for re-expansion.
     7) Monitor serial blood gas reports and serial chest X-ray reports to determine successful reexpansion.

4. Pulmonary emboli

a. Monitor for signs of respiratory distress.
   1) Observe for dyspnea and tachypnea.
   2) Assess nailbeds for pallor or cyanosis.
   3) Observe for anxiety, apprehension, and restlessness.
   4) Have emergency resuscitation equipment nearby and be prepared to institute mechanical ventilation, if necessary.
   5) Apply pulse oximeter and continuously measure oxygen saturation with continuous pulse oximetry.
   6) Obtain specimens for ABGs and monitor results for significant changes.
b. Promote activities to improve ventilation.
   1) Encourage coughing and deep breathing.
   2) Observe color and consistency of expectorated secretions, particularly hemoptysis.
   3) Administer oxygen as ordered.
   4) Observe for respiratory distress with patient care activities, interrupt care if it occurs, and space activities to prevent recurrence of respiratory distress.
   5) Elevate the head of the bed.
   6) Auscultate the lungs frequently for abnormalities and report findings.
   7) Assist with incentive spirometry.
c. Monitor patient for side effects of anticoagulant therapy.
   1) Assess for and prevent overt bleeding.
      a) Check injection sites for bleeding.
      b) Apply pressure to venipuncture sites until bleeding stops.
      c) Observe for bleeding from the gums following mouth care.
      d) Observe for nose bleeds.
   2) Assess for and prevent occult bleeding.
      a) Check for blood in the urine and stool.
      b) Administer antacids to prevent stress ulceration.
      c) Observe for bruising and hematomas especially at injection sites.
      d) Monitor hemoglobin and hematocrit for decreasing values.

       3) Keep protamine sulfate (heparin antidote) or vita-
min K (coumadin antidote) available for bleeding.

       4) Monitor lab studies to assess anticoagulation.

  d. Promote nursing actions that prevent venous stasis.

       1) Apply antiembolic stockings.

          a) Sequential compression devices provide cyclic compression and relaxation periods which closely approximate muscle contractions. They are the most effective type of antiembolic stocking for the intensive care unit (ICU) patient.

          b) Elastic hose and ace bandage wraps compress superficial veins in the legs and prevent venous stasis there. They are difficult to apply and remove in the ICU setting. They are most useful in the ambulatory patient.

       2) Assist with active and passive range-of-motion exercises.

       3) Avoid venipuncture in the legs.

       4) Do not forcibly irrigate clotted IV lines.

       5) Administer anticoagulants as ordered.

       6) Promote adequate fluid intake to prevent dehydration.

       7) Elevate legs to promote venous return.

       8) Instruct patient not to cross legs.

       9) Instruct patient not to keep knees bent while in bed.

2 CARDIOVASCULAR DISORDERS

Acute Myocardial Infarction

Acute myocardial infarction (AMI) is damage to myocardial tissue due to lack of blood flow to the tissue, resulting in permanent loss of contractility to this portion of myocardial muscle.

Risk Factors for Myocardial Infarction

Uncontrollable

Sex and age	Men have a greater chance for myocardial infarction (MI) before 50 years of age. Women increase their risk after menopause; and actually have more severe problems post MI.
Race	Blacks have a higher incidence of hypertension, which is a risk factor for infarction.
Genetics	Familial history could be a genetic connection or a social connection concerning eating habits.
Geographics	A higher incidence of heart disease is found in Western industrialized nations, colder climates, and lower altitudes.
Hyperglycemia	Compliant, controlled diabetics have a higher risk for cardiovascular disease and MI than the general population.

Controllable

Hypertension	Blood pressure >140/90 mm Hg. A high risk factor in women.
Smoking	Cigarettes.
Hyperlipidemia	Low-density lipoprotein is the most dangerous of lipoproteins for predicting coronary artery disease. Value >130 mg/dL: high risk for coronary heart disease. High-density-lipoprotein value <35 mg/dL: high risk for coronary heart disease.
Diet	High in salt, fat, sugar, alcohol, and caffeine.
Type A behavior	Aggressiveness, competitiveness, constant attempt to accomplish more in less time.
Lifestyle	Sedentary.

Etiology/Pathophysiology

1. Causes
   a. Coronary atherosclerosis: A buildup of plaque in the coronary circulation, occurring over a long period
   b. Coronary thrombosis: Acute onset of a blood clot in the coronary artery, occluding blood flow
   c. Coronary artery vasospasm: Actual vasoconstriction of the coronary artery, caused by drugs, or of unknown etiology
   d. Profound hypotension: Extremely low blood pressure leading to oxygen starvation of coronary muscle
   e. Cardiac trauma: Any trauma to the cardiac muscle that deprives the cardiac muscle of blood, and subsequently oxygen
2. More commonly a combination of coronary atherosclerosis and either thrombus or spasm
3. Chest pain occurs when myocardial cells are ischemic, or are not receiving enough oxygen, and local metabolic changes are occurring.
   a. Types of chest pain
      1) Ischemic pain
         a) Stable angina: Occurs at a predictable workload of the heart and is easily controlled with rest or nitroglycerin
         b) Unstable angina: Also known as preinfarction angina or acute coronary insufficiency; indicates a change in the architecture of the coronary atherosclerotic lesion; a medical emergency
      2) Injury pain
         a) Variant angina
            1] Also known as Prinzmetal's angina
            2] Coronary artery spasms occurring at rest, causing severe pain
            3] Controlled with nitroglycerin and/or calcium channel blockers
            4] Variant angina in women is caused not by an obstruction, but by coronary spasm.
            5] Variant angina in men is caused by an obstruction.

    b) Myocardial infarction (MI) pain
        1] Description: Dull, aching, deep, strangling, tightness, squeezing, crushing, pressure, heaviness
        2] Location: Substernal, down the arms (primarily left) radiating into the neck, jaw, teeth, and back
        3] Duration: Lasts longer than 15–30 minutes
        4] Relieved by morphine (rest and nitroglycerin ineffective)
        5] Pain variances
            a] Women describe pain more vaguely than men.
            b] The elderly, diabetic, or hypertensive patient may have a peripheral neuropathy or altered sensorium, thus masking the pain sensation.

4. AMI may be seen concurrently with a cerebrovascular accident.
5. Pathophysiology
   a. When myocardial tissue is deprived of oxygen, cells quickly revert to anaerobic metabolism, which produces less energy and more lactic acid.
   b. This process adversely affects regional wall motion, impairing myocardial contraction. Forward flow of blood is reduced, and left ventricle and atrium pressures increase, leading to pulmonary congestion.
   c. In response to the buildup of lactic acid and decrease in oxygen, the heart muscle becomes irritable. Areas of the conduction system may alter impulse transmission, resulting in arrhythmias.
   d. If oxygen is not restored to the myocardial cells within approximately 20 minutes, cellular necrosis or death begins, and continues for 4–6 hours. These dying cells become edematous and rupture, allowing enzymes to escape into the bloodstream. This causes elevation in cardiac enzymes and isoenzymes the first few days after infarction.
   e. In the first 24 hours, the myocardium appears essentially normal, with some bruising; however, white blood cells are drawn to the area of damage.
      1) If the damage does not affect the entire wall depth, it is called a subendocardial infarction.

    2) A transmural infarction causes damage through the full thickness of the heart wall.

  f. By the third to fifth day after infarction, macrophages begin removing the necrotic tissue. At this point, the myocardial wall is fairly thin, and very susceptible to myocardial rupture; this is especially important to the transmural, anteroseptal, or apical infarction patient.

  g. During the second week, necrotic muscle is replaced by fibrous connective tissue and blood vessels. This process of remodeling continues for several weeks, during which time there may be lengthening and stretching of the muscle fibers. There also may be an expansion of the injured area and a thickening of the uninfarcted wall, causing an uncoordinated contraction and relaxation (or systole and diastole). This dyskinesis, or abnormal wall motion, subsequently produces a decreased cardiac output (CO) and congestion of blood within the heart and cardiopulmonary tree.

  h. The remodeling process is influenced by the size of the infarction, the healing process, and the amount of stress placed on the ventricles.

    1) This pathologic process is slowed by limiting the infarction size through reperfusion, immediately after obstruction, with thrombolytic therapy.

    2) The healing process has been shown to be delayed with the use of steroidal therapy.

    3) The reduced CO from the weakened postinfarct heart stimulates the sympathetic compensatory mechanisms of the body. Rather than improve CO, vasoconstriction increases systemic vascular resistance, and afterload, ultimately increasing the workload of the heart.

Assessment/Analysis

ASSESSMENT FINDINGS

Subjective

1. Chest pain that may or may not radiate to the arms, shoulders, or neck.

2. Weakness, fatigue

Objective

1. Dyspnea

Nursing Alert

Be mindful of possible acute myocardial infarction with any elderly patient presenting with a chief complaint of dyspnea, regardless of a history of lung or heart congestion. Some patients may have a decreased pain sensation due to peripheral neuropathy (as in diabetes). Chest pain is not always the hallmark of cardiac problems.

2. Nausea, vomiting (commonly seen with inferior infarctions)
3. Decreased level of consciousness
4. Temperature elevation
5. Blood pressure lability (either increased or decreased)
6. Heart sounds
   a. Softer S_1 and S_2 heart sounds
   b. Newly developed S_4 heart sounds or becomes louder with pain
   c. S_3 heart sound indicating ischemia and developing ventricular failure
   d. Transient pericardial friction rub or systolic murmur
7. Crackles heard in lung bases

SUPPORTING TEST FINDINGS

Laboratory Tests

1. Cardiac enzymes — Creatine kinase (CK).
   Abnormality: Increased with myocardial and skeletal muscle damage. Increase begins 4 – 8 hours after injury, peaks in 12 – 24 hours, and returns to normal within 2 – 4 days.
2. CK isoenzymes MM or CK_3
   Abnormality: Increased after AMI
3. CK isoenzymes MB or CK_2
   Abnormality: Increases 3 – 36 hours after AMI; peaks within 24 hours after injury

4. Aspartate aminotransferase (Serum glutamic oxaloacetic transaminase)
   Abnormality: Increases 8–12 hours after injury; peaks within 36–48 hours; and returns to normal within 3–4 days
5. Lactic dehydrogenase (LDH)
   Abnormality: Increases within 2–4 days after injury; returns to normal within 8–14 days
6. LDH isoenzymes LDH_1 and LDH_2
   Abnormality: LDH_1 increases to a higher level than LDH_2 (LDH flip pattern) within 12–72 hours after injury
7. White blood cell (WBC) count
   Abnormality: Increases within 48 hours after injury
8. Erythrocyte sedimentation rate
   Abnormality: Increases 2–4 days after injury

Diagnostic Tests

1. 12-lead electrocardiogram (ECG)
   Abnormality: ST depression and/or T-wave inversion during chest pain indicates ischemia
   ST-segment elevation indicates AMI or coronary spasm
   Development of Q waves indicates infarction
   Infarction can also be present without a Q-wave, and is common in diabetics, women, and the elderly
2. Cardiac monitoring
   Abnormality: Sinus node dysfunction—Sinus bradycardia
   Atrioventricular blocks
   Atrial fibrillation or flutter
   Premature ventricular contractions, supraventricular tachycardia, ventricular tachycardia or fibrillation
3. Hemodynamic monitoring
   Abnormality: Increased pulmonary artery pressure (PAP) and pulmonary capillary wedge pressure (PCWP)
   Decreased CO
4. Cardiac catheterization
   Abnormality: Coronary artery occlusion
   Decreased contractility or ejection fraction
   Myocardial wall dysfunction

Valvular dysfunction
Increased chamber pressures

5. Technetium pyrophosphate heart scan
   Abnormality: "Hot spots" indicate areas of myocardial damage; most sensitive within 1–3 days

6. Thallium 201 scan
   Abnormality: "Cold spots" indicate areas of myocardial damage. Most sensitive in the first 24 hours after injury

7. Multiple gated acquisition scan
   Abnormality: Decreased wall motion and ejection fraction

8. Echocardiography
   Abnormality: Left or right ventricular wall motion abnormality, suggesting compromised blood flow

9. Doppler flow study: Two-dimensional echocardiography
   Abnormality: Mitral valve regurgitation, as a result of papillary muscle failure
   Ventricular septal perforation

10. Electrophysiologic studies
    Abnormality: Prolonged or shortened conduction intervals
    Prolonged refractory or recovery periods

11. Digital subtraction angiography
    Abnormality: Dyskinetic wall motion
    Coronary artery bypass graft occlusion
    Decreased ejection fraction
    Presence of aneurysms, tumors, plaque, or emboli

12. Magnetic resonance imaging
    Abnormality: Infarcted myocardium
    Calcified valves

Planning/Intervention

COLLABORATIVE MANAGEMENT

Procedures

1. Reduce myocardial oxygen consumption.
   a. Maintain bed rest.

    b. Administer ordered medications.
      1) Nitrates
      2) Opioids
      3) Beta-blockers
      4) Calcium channel blockers (with coronary vasospasm)
      5) Sedatives
    c. Assist with insertion of intra-aortic balloon pump, as needed.
    d. Assist with insertion of ventricular assist device, as needed.
2. Increase myocardial oxygen supply.
    a. Administer ordered supplemental oxygen.
    b. Administer ordered medications.
      1) Thrombolytics
      2) Aspirin
      3) Anticoagulants
    c. Prepare patient for percutaneous transluminal coronary angioplasty (PTCA), as needed.
    d. Assist with insertions of intra-aortic balloon pump or ventricular assist device, as needed.
    e. Prepare patient for open heart surgery, as indicated.
3. Assess for and prevent further cardiovascular damage.
    a. Monitor vital signs every 2 hours, and as indicated.
    b. Obtain 12-lead ECG, as ordered.
    c. Place patient on continuous cardiac monitoring.
    d. Insert an intravenous (IV) line and infuse fluids to keep vein open.
    e. Administer ordered medications.
      1) Antiarrhythmias
      2) Nitrates
      3) Diuretics
      4) Inotropic agents
    f. Assist with insertion of central lines, as indicated.
    g. Prepare patient for cardiac catheterization or PTCA.
    h. Assist with insertion of external or transvenous pacemaker, as indicated for second- or third-degree heart block.
    i. Prepare patient for coronary artery bypass graft (CABG) surgery, as indicated.

Drug Therapy

1. Thrombolytics

   Examples: tissue plasminogen activator (Activase)
   streptokinase (Streptase)
   anistreplase (Eminase)

   Action: Dissolves blood clots obstructing coronary arteries

   Caution: (See Nursing Alert)

Nursing Alert

Use extreme caution or not at all in patients experiencing:
- Internal bleeding
- Recent trauma, surgery, or cardiopulmonary resuscitation
- Recent head trauma or history of neurovascular disorder
- Uncontrolled hypertension
- Pregnancy
- Liver or kidney disease
- Prior allergic reaction to thrombolytic therapy

2. Nitrates

   Example: nitroglycerin (Nitro-bid, Nitrostat)

   Action: Reduces cardiac workload by peripheral vasodilation, thus decreasing preload and afterload

   Vasodilates coronary arteries, thereby reducing the angina caused by spasm; if the injured area is small, vasodilation of collateral arteries will compensate blood flow to the injured area.

   Caution: Can cause headache, hypotension, poor tissue perfusion, and stimulate a reflex tachycardia, which can cause an increased myocardial oxygen demand.

3. Opioid analgesics

   Example: Morphine sulfate (Duramorph)

   Action: Relieves severe pain and anxiety

   Reduces workload of the heart by decreasing afterload and venous return to the heart

   Caution: Can cause hypotension and bradycardia, particularly in infarction of the inferior wall of the left ventricle and right coronary artery

4. Antiarrhythmics
   Examples: lidocaine
   Action: Increases the electrical stimulation threshold in the ventricular conduction system, thereby reducing ventricular arrhythmias
   Caution: Can cause seizures and postural hypotension

5. Anticoagulants/Platelet inhibitors
   Example: heparin sodium (Heparin)
      aspirin (Bayer)
      dipyridamole (Persantine)
   Action: Slows clumping of platelets and inhibits blood clot formation
   Caution: Can cause excessive bleeding

6. Beta-blockers
   Example: metoprolol tartrate (Lopressor)
      atenolol (Tenormin)
   Action: Decreases myocardial oxygen consumption by decreasing heart rate, blood pressure, and CO
   Caution: Can exacerbate bradycardia, heart failure, or shock

7. Angiotensin-converting enzyme (ACE) inhibitors.
   Example: captopril (Capoten)
   Action: Reduces afterload and progressive dilation of the ventricle post-MI in patients with a 40% or less ejection fraction
   Caution: Captopril is the only ACE inhibitor that has been recommended at present. The others have not yet been tested.

8. Inotropic agents
   Example: dobutamine (Dobutrex)
   Action: Augments coronary circulation by increasing CO and decreasing PAP and systemic vascular resistance
   Caution: Increases myocardial oxygen consumption
      May worsen hypokalemia and arrhythmias

9. Magnesium
   Example: magnesium sulfate
   Action: Reduces serious arrythmias post-MI
   Caution: Monitor serum magnesium levels closely

Research Update

The following exogenous free radical scavenger drugs are being researched for their potential benefit for patients with AMI:

- Allopurinol (Zyloprim)
- Mannitol (Osmitrol)
- Superoxide dismutase
- Nonsteroidal anti-inflammatory drugs (Motrin)

NURSING MANAGEMENT

Monitoring and Managing Clinical Problems

1. Tissue Perfusion, altered peripheral
   a. Monitor tissue perfusion.
      1) Assess for chest pain using a scale of 0 to 10, with 10 being the most severe.
         a) Have the patient describe the pain.
         b) Note the location of the pain and where it radiates.
         c) Note any activity that occurred before the onset of the pain.
      2) Place patient on a cardiac monitor and note the presence, increases in, and type of arrhythmias.
      3) Monitor blood pressure, CO, cardiac index, PAP, PCWP, as indicated.
      4) Assess the skin for cyanosis, pallor, coolness, and moisture.
      5) Obtain specimens for arterial blood gas (ABG) analysis and monitor results for significant changes.
      6) Apply pulse oximeter and continuously monitor arterial oxygen saturation.
      7) Assess for dyspnea.
      8) Auscultate lungs for presence of adventitious sounds (crackles).
      9) Monitor urine output, noting trends over several hours and days.
      10) Assess level of consciousness, noting any change in mentation and behavior.

11) Assess all extremity pulses, color, and temperature; assess for presence of Homan's sign.
12) Obtain specimens for cardiac enzymes and isoenzymes, and monitor results.

b. Promote tissue perfusion.
1) Limit activity, as ordered.
2) Slowly progress activity as directed by the cardiac rehabilitation criteria.
3) Administer ordered inotropic agents, vasodilators, and calcium channel blockers, and monitor patient response to treatment.
4) Schedule nursing activities to allow for ample rest periods.
5) Administer ordered supplemental oxygen.
6) Administer ordered pain medication and antianxiety agents to alleviate pain and anxiety, and monitor for patient response to treatment.
7) Administer ordered antiarrthymics, as indicated.
8) Administer ordered anticoagulants.
9) Provide comfort measures, such as massage, to increase relaxation.

2. Cardiac Output: decreased
a. Assess CO.
1) Monitor blood pressure for hypotension or hypertension.
2) Palpate point of maximal impulse for presence of a thrill or heave.
3) Auscultate the heart for presence of any murmurs, extra heart sounds, or rubs.
4) Assess hemodynamic parameters for increased PAP, PCWP, and central venous pressure and decreased CO and cardiac index.
5) Monitor for cardiac arrhythmias, indicating myocardial irritability.
6) Assess for further decrease in CO evidenced by:
   a) Shortness of breath
   b) Moist lung sounds
   c) Decreased blood pressure
   d) Extra heart sounds
   e) Jugular vein distention
   f) Pulsus alternans (amplitude of pulse changes with each beat)

g) Elevated PCWP
h) Decreased CO and cardiac index
b. Decrease myocardial workload.
1) Maintain bed rest with bedside commode, as patient's condition permits.
2) Administer medications to maintain blood pressure, as indicated.
3) Administer ordered supplemental oxygen.
4) Prepare for insertion of intra-aortic balloon pump.
5) Administer ordered beta-blockers in hyperdynamic patient.
c. Recognize complications.
1) Hyperdynamic state—Compensatory mechanism causing tachycardia and hypertension
2) Hypotension—Decreased blood pressure due to either hypovolemia or decreased CO
3) Reocclusion post-PTCA, thrombolytic therapy, or CABG
4) Bleeding after cardiac procedure
5) Reperfusion injury and arrhythmias

Monitoring, Managing, and Preventing Life-Threatening Emergencies

1. Cardiogenic shock
   a. Monitor for hemodynamic instability.
   1) Monitor ABGs and hemoglobin, and report significant changes.
   2) Monitor capillary refill and skin color changes to assess peripheral perfusion.
   3) Continuously monitor hemodynamics to determine patient response to drug therapeutics.
   4) Monitor cardiac rhythm for tachycardiac and life-threatening ventricular arrhythmias.
   b. Promote adequate oxygenation.
   1) Maintain a patent airway and adequate ventilation, and monitor patient's response to treatment.
   2) Administer ordered supplemental oxygen.
   3) Titrate fluids and inotropic agents to maintain a systolic blood pressure of at least 80 mm Hg.
   4) Position the patient in modified Trendelenburg position (head flat with legs elevated at 45 degrees).

   c. Monitor for altered organ and tissue perfusion.
- 1) Monitor for decreased urine output and elevated renal function tests, possibly indicating acute renal failure.
- 2) Monitor for a falling arterial oxygen concentration, possibly indicating adult respiratory distress syndrome.
- 3) Monitor for decreased alertness and attention span, drowsiness, and excessive sleeping indicating a deterioration in the level of consciousness.

2. Cardiopulmonary arrest
   a. Call for help.
   b. Begin cardiopulmonary resuscitation.
   c. Follow with advanced cardiac life support.

3. Pulmonary embolism
   a. Monitor for signs of respiratory distress.
- 1) Dyspnea and tachypnea
- 2) Pallor or cyanosis of the nailbeds
- 3) Anxiety, apprehension, and restlessness
- 4) Decreasing oxygen saturation
- 5) Changing arterial blood gas values

   b. Promote activities to improve ventilation.
- 1) Encourage coughing and deep breathing.
- 2) Observe color and consistency of expectorated secretions. Hemoptysis may occur.
- 3) Administer ordered supplemental oxygen.
- 4) Observe for respiratory distress with patient care activities, interrupt care if it occurs, and space activities to prevent recurrence.
- 5) Initiate mechanical ventilation, as indicated.
- 6) Elevate head of the bed.
- 7) Auscultate lungs and report adventitious sounds.

   c. Administer ordered anticoagulants and monitor for patient response to treatment and adverse effects.
- 1) Observe injection sites and apply pressure to stop bleeding, as indicated.
- 2) Monitor nose and gums for bleeding during and after care.
- 3) Obtain specimens and monitor results of coagulation studies to assess response to treatment.

Myocardial Infarction

Type	Affected Artery	Affected Area	ECG Findings	Complications	Special Treatment
Anterior infarction	Left coronary artery or branches	Anterior portion, left ventricle Two thirds of ventricular septum Bundle of His, right and left branches	V3/V4: Q waves V2/V6 R wave progression missing	Crackles in lungs Shortness of breath Increased PCWP S_3 heart sound Decreased blood pressure Cardiac monitor: Sinus tachycardia Premature ventricular contractions Blocks: Right and left bundle branch blocks	Monitor hemodynamics Monitor for heart blocks Administer inotropic agents and vasodilators, as ordered Prepare for possible pacemaker insertion

Continued

Myocardial Infarction — Continued

Type	Affected Artery	Affected Area	ECG Findings	Complications	Special Treatment
				Mobitz type II Complete heart block Papillary muscle rupture, as evidenced by (1) decreased blood pressure; (2) crackles; new systolic murmur at 4th to 5th intercostal space, left of the sternum	

Anteroseptal infarction	Left coronary artery Left anterior descending artery	Anterior wall, left ventricle Intraventricular septum	V1/V4: Q waves, poor R wave progression		
Inferior infarction	Right coronary artery Dominant left circumflex artery	Inferior or diaphragmatic left ventricular wall A-V node Sinus node	II, III, aVR: new or deeper Q waves, ST-segment elevation, or T wave inverted	Symptomatic bradycardia with nausea, vomiting, syncope, bronchospasm, tracheal burning Cardiac monitor: Sinus bradycardia Sinus arrest Progressive A-V block: First-degree block	Observe for bradycardia and heart block Treat symptomatic bradycardia and heart block: Administer atropine Prepare for pacemaker insertion Administer ordered oxygen

Continued

Myocardial Infarction— *Continued*

Type	Affected Artery	Affected Area	ECG Findings	Complications	Special Treatment
				Second-degree block Mobitz type I Third-degree block Atrial arrhythmias: Atrial fibrillation Atrial flutter Premature atrial contractions	
Posterior infarction	Right coronary artery Circumflex artery	Posterior left ventricle	V1/V2: Reciprocal changes;	Decreased blood pressure Crackles in lungs	Administer ordered atropine and

Right ventricular infarction	Distal right coronary artery	Right ventricle Left ventricle, inferior wall	ST-segment depression; T waves tall, symmetrical, and reversed poles II, III, aVF, V1$_R$ through V6$_R$: ST-segment elevation, Q waves	Neck vein distention Hepatojugular reflux Decreased blood pressure Decreased urine output Skin, cool and clammy Decreased PCWP Increased right atrial pressure Decreased cardiac output	Administer volume expanders if the left ventricle is healthy Administer ordered dobutamine Monitor PCWP Administer ordered oxygen Prepare for pacemaker insertion, as indicated
				Cardiac monitor: Sinus brady-cardia Progressive heart block	isoproterenol Prepare for pacemaker insertion

Continued

Myocardial Infarction — *Continued*

Type	*Affected Artery*	*Affected Area*	*ECG Findings*	*Complications*	*Special Treatment*
Lateral infarction	Circumflex artery Left anterior descending artery	Lateral wall, left ventricle	I, aVL, V5, V6: New or deeper Q waves	Few complications if pure lateral infarction. More complications if coronary circulation is left dominant, or if anterior wall also infarcted If posterior wall involved, expect sinus bradycardia or conduction defects	

*Key: A-V = atrioventricular; PCWP = pulmonary capillary wedge pressure.

Congestive Heart Failure

Congestive heart failure (CHF) is the inability of the heart to pump an adequate amount of blood to the vital organs of the body.

Etiology/Pathophysiology

1. Structural/functional defects
   a. Abnormal pressure loads
      1) Aortic stenosis
         a) A narrowing of the aortic valve between the left ventricle and the systemic circulation
         b) Caused by rheumatic inflammation, congenital defect, or calcification
         c) Decreases the exit for blood leaving the left ventricle
      2) Pulmonic stenosis
         a) A narrowing of the pulmonic valve between the right ventricle and pulmonary artery
         b) Caused by either congenital defect or rheumatic fever
         c) Slows the exit of blood from the right ventricle
      3) Pulmonary hypertension
         a) A pulmonary artery systolic pressure of greater than 30 mm Hg
         b) Caused by cardiac or pulmonary dysfunction, or of unknown etiology
         c) Results in pulmonary congestion
      4) Systemic hypertension
         a) An elevated systemic blood pressure of 140/90 mm Hg or greater
         b) May be idiopathic in origin (or see hypertension)
         c) Results in increased afterload, and a greater resistance to pump blood out of the heart
   b. Abnormal filling of ventricles
      1) Mitral stenosis
         a) Narrowing of mitral opening between the left atrium and left ventricle
         b) Due to rheumatic fever injury, bacterial vegetation, calcification or thrombus formation on valve
         c) Left atrium increases its pumping pressure and eventually hypertrophies in order to maintain its output to the left ventricle
         d) Increased pressure backs up into pulmonary system, causing elevated pulmonary pressures

    2) Tricuspid stenosis
      a) Narrowing of tricuspid valve between the right atrium and right ventricle
      b) Most commonly caused by rheumatic fever
      c) Usually combined with other valvular disorders
      d) Output from right ventricle is lowered due to restriction, resulting in increased pressure in right atrium and eventually systemic venous circulation

c. Abnormal muscle function
    1) Diminished muscle tone of the heart is caused by either alterations caused by injury to the muscle or preload/afterload problems
      a) Cardiomyopathy: Three types
        1] Dilated cardiomyopathy
          a] A dilatation of all four heart chambers
          b] Caused by a decreased calcium uptake by the myocardial cells, which adversely affects contractility of the muscle
          c] Decreases ventricular cardiac output (CO) and increases resting pressure (preload)
        2] Hypertrophic cardiomyopathy (idiopathic hypertrophic subaortic stenosis)
          a] Thickening of the ventricular wall, mitral valve leaflets, and papillary muscles
          b] Thought to be a genetic disorder
          c] Causes a decreased CO and increased left ventricular end diastolic pressure (preload); pressure causes backflow into left atria
        3] Restrictive cardiomyopathy
          a] A stiff ventricle, incapable of satisfactory ventricular filling
          b] Caused by a variety of fibrotic, invasive processes, which make myocardial muscle rigid
          c] The heart is unable to increase its CO when challenged.
      b) Myocarditis
        1] Inflammation of the myocardial muscle
        2] Caused by idiopathic/rheumatoid source

3] Causes failure or arrhythmias, depending on location of inflammation

c) Myocardial infarction (MI) and ventricular remodeling

1] Cardiac muscle tissue dies due to lack of oxygen; this necrotic muscle is replaced by fibrous connective tissue.

2] This replacement tissue lacks the coordination and strength found in the original myocardial tissue.

3] Blood can no longer be pumped as efficiently; CO is decreased, and blood pools in the cardiopulmonary area.

d) Cardiogenic shock

1] A shock state that exists after a significant amount of myocardial necrosis (40%) and decreased CO

2] With decreased CO, urine output and level of consciousness decreases.

3] Despite advanced pharmacotherapy, high mortality results from multisystem organ failure.

d. Abnormal volume load

1) An increased preload is caused by insufficient closure of a valve. Normally this occurs with regurgitant valves, but may occur with stenotic valves that have become incompetent and therefore leak. Because of the increased amount of blood, dilatation and hypertrophy (ventricular remodeling) develop in the chamber into which blood has regurgitated.

a) Aortic regurgitation

1] Chronic regurgitation is caused by congenital defect, infection, and connective tissue diseases.

2] Acute regurgitation is commonly caused by bacterial endocarditis and aortic dissection.

3] Acute regurgitation is most frequently seen in men.

b) Mitral regurgitation

1] Chronic regurgitation is usually caused by rheumatic fever, ischemic heart disease, mitral valve prolapse, or left ventricular dilation.

2] Acute regurgitation usually occurs after papillary muscle rupture secondary to myocardial infarction or dysfunction related to ischemic heart disease, or as a complication of endocarditis.

c) Pulmonic regurgitation

1] Congenital deformity is the primary cause.

2] Pulmonary hypertension also causes pulmonic valve regurgitation.

d) Tricuspid regurgitation

1] The right ventricles hypertrophy and fail due to pulmonary hypertension, intravenous (IV) drug use with infectious endocarditis, or trauma.

2. Pathophysiologic changes

a. CHF occurs because of myocardial muscle or valve dysfunction. The body recognizes a decreased CO, and attempts to compensate via compensatory mechanisms.

1) One mechanism is the release of catecholamines by the adrenal medulla. These catecholamines increase heart rate and contractility, as well as vasoconstrict arterioles and venules. This increased heart rate, contractility, and vasoconstriction improves CO, stroke volume, and venous return.

2) Unfortunately, the catecholamines' vasoconstrictive activity also has the following two undesirable side effects:

a) It makes an already weakened left ventricle work harder to pump blood into the systemic circulation (thus increasing the afterload on the heart).

b) It decreases the blood flow to the kidneys. Altered renal blood flow activates another compensatory mechanism, known as the renin-angiotensin-aldosterone system. With this system alerted, a cascade of events takes place, leading to the reabsorption of water and sodium. This increased fluid initially helps increase CO. But as the myocardial muscle continues to stretch, it loses its elasticity and can no longer deliver the same output.

3) Cardiovascular decompensation is now further complicated by an increased blood volume in the heart (preload).

3. Terms describing CHF

a. CHF is commonly described as either right-sided or left-sided failure. Because the cardiopulmonary system is a closed one, the effects of one-sided heart failure will ultimately affect the other side.

b. Left-sided heart failure occurs when the left ventricle fails to pump the oxygenated blood from the pulmonary circulation to the systemic circulation. This is due to:

1) Left ventricular muscle weakness
   a) Post-MI
   b) Myocardial hypertrophy

2) Increased blood volume before contraction (increased preload)
   a) Volume overload—IV therapy
   b) Volume overload—Renal failure
   c) Valve incompetence

3) Abnormal pressure load
   a) Systemic hypertension—The lack of elasticity of the systemic vessels increases systemic vascular resistance (afterload). Afterload is greater with peripheral hypertension.
      1] In order to maintain an adequate CO, the left ventricle must increase the force of contraction to eject the blood into the hardened vessels of the peripheral vascular system.
      2] This increased contractile force leads to ventricular hypertrophy and increased oxygen requirements.
   b) Valve incompetence—Aortic stenosis results in higher pressures to maintain an adequate CO. This sustained pressure load eventually leads to ventricular dilation and, ultimately, decompensation. Aortic stenosis also can cause regurgitation, increasing the probability of CHF.

   c. Right-sided heart failure is initiated by the following:
     1) Failure of the left ventricle to pump blood into the systemic circulation, causing a backup into the pulmonary vascular system and into the right ventricle via the pulmonary artery
     2) Cor pulmonale due to chronic pulmonary obstructive disease and pulmonary emboli
   d. Other terms used to describe CHF
     1) Forward failure — The heart's inability to eject the blood out of the heart, resulting in poor arterial perfusion of vital organs
     2) Backward failure — Pulmonary and systemic venous congestion caused by a backing up of blood within the cardiopulmonary system
     3) Acute heart failure — Sudden onset of low CO
     4) Chronic heart failure — Prolonged decline in CO, allowing compensatory mechanisms to evolve slowly
     5) High output failure — Inadequate supply of nutrients to the tissues despite normal to accelerated CO, as seen in sepsis
     6) Low output failure — Decreased CO caused by a weakened myocardial muscle, as seen in myocardial infarction

Assessment/Analysis

ASSESSMENT FINDINGS

Comparing Assessment Findings of Right- and Left-Sided Heart Failure

Right	Left
Subjective	
Heaviness of legs	Fatigue
Increased abdominal girth	Anxiety
Inability to wear shoes comfortably	Shortness of breath

Continued

Comparing Assessment Findings of Right- and Left-Sided Heart Failure — *Continued*

Right	*Left*

Subjective

Nocturia
  Behavioral changes due to low cardiac output — easy fatigability, weakness, lethargy, shortened attention span
Vague abdominal discomfort

Objective

Right	*Left*
Tachycardia	Tachycardia
Jugular vein distention	Dyspnea
Ascites	Orthopnea
Jaundice	Paroxysmal nocturnal dyspnea
Paroxysmal nocturnal dyspnea	Coughing, usually dry and hacking in nature
Edema (least reliable sign)	S_3 and/or S_4 heart sounds
Increased anteroposterior chest diameter	Crackles, wheezes on lung auscultation
Accessory muscles used with breathing	Point of maximal impulse >2.5 cm in diameter
Weight gain	Pulsus alternans
S_3 and/or S_4 heart sounds	
Crackles on lung	
Diminished breath sounds	
Hyperresonance of lung sounds low, immobile diaphragm	

DIAGNOSTIC TESTS

Laboratory Tests

1. Arterial blood gases (ABGs)

Abnormality: Decreased pH, reflecting acidosis
     Decreased PaO_2
     Increased $PaCO_2$

2. Prothrombin time
   Abnormality: Prolonged if the liver is involved
3. Serum electrolytes
   Abnormality: Decreased serum sodium in dilutional hyponatremia due to increased fluid volume
       Decreased serum potassium if prolonged use of diuretics
4. Serum bilirubin
   Abnormality: Increased due to failure of normal excretion; caused by acute hepatic venous congestion
5. Serum lactate
   Abnormality: Increased
6. Cardiac enzymes and isoenzymes
   Abnormality: Increased if myocardial damage present
7. Liver enzymes
   Abnormality: Increased with impaired liver function
8. Blood urea nitrogen and serum creatinine
   Abnormality: Increased with renal compromise

Diagnostic Tests

1. Chest X-ray
   Abnormality: Dilated pulmonary blood vessels
       Fluid accumulation in lung fields (increased interstitial markings)
       Ventricular hypertrophy
       Cardiomegaly
2. Electrocardiogram
   Abnormality: Infarction, ischemia
       Arrhythmias (usually atrial in origin due to atrial hypertrophy)
       Ventricular enlargement
3. Echocardiogram/transesophageal echocardiogram
   Abnormality: Valve dysfunction
       Dilation of heart chambers
       Ventricular hypertrophy
       Reduced ejection fractions
       Pericardial effusion
4. Radionuclide studies
   Abnormality: MI seen on cardiac perfusion scan

Abnormal ventricular volumes of both systole and diastole seen on gated radionuclide ventriculography

5. Cardiac catheterization
   Abnormality: Increased pressures within the chambers of the heart, as well as the pulmonary vascular system
   Obstruction of coronary arteries
   Ruptured papillary muscle

6. Hemodynamic monitoring
   Abnormality: Right atrial pressure increased with cardiac failure or fluid overload and decreased with hypovolemia
   Pulmonary capillary wedge pressure (PCWP) increased with cardiac failure or fluid overload and decreased with hypovolemia
   CO and cardiac index decreased with low output failure
   Central venous pressure (CVP) increased with cardiac failure

Planning/Intervention

COLLABORATIVE MANAGEMENT

Procedures

1. Monitor and provide adequate oxygenation to the tissues.
   a. Administer supplemental oxygen: nasal cannula to endotracheal intubation with mechanical ventilation, as indicated.
   b. Assist with and monitor serial chest X-rays.
   c. Apply pulse oximeter and continuously monitor oxygen saturation.
   d. Monitor oxygen saturation to determine patient response to nursing care activities.
   e. Obtain blood specimens for serial ABG analysis, hematocrit and hemoglobin, and serum lactate; monitor results; and report significant changes.

2. Determine etiology of failure and decrease workload on the heart.
   a. Maintain bed rest to spare oxygen consumption.

  b. Maintain cardiac monitor, and report arrhythmias and increased heart rate.
  c. Administer ordered supplemental oxygen, as indicated.
  d. Assist with insertion of central lines, monitor for increases in CVP, pulmonary artery pressure (PAP), and PCWP. Report significant changes.
  e. Obtain measurements of CO and cardiac index with thermodilution catheter. Report the following:
    1) CO <4 L/min
    2) Cardiac index <2.8 L/min per meter squared
  f. Administer ordered diuretics and monitor patient's response to treatment.
  g. Administer vasodilators and closely monitor vital signs to determine patient's response to treatment (May be used in combination with inotropic agents).
  h. Assist with insertion of intra-aortic balloon pump and closely monitor patient for signs of augmentation or complications.
  i. Assist with insertion of arterial line and monitor blood pressure continuously.
3. Increase CO.
  a. Administer ordered inotropic agents and monitor patient's response to treatment (May be used in combination with vasodilators).
  b. Maintain intra-aortic balloon pump to augment stroke volume.

Drug Therapy

1. Vasodilators
   Examples: nitroglycerin (Nitrostat)
       sodium nitroprusside (Nipride)
   Action: Decreases afterload, which helps empty the left ventricle and subsequently decrease pulmonary congestion
   Caution: May cause severe hypotension
       Do not administer bolus dose to patient
   Example: captopril (Capoten)
   Action: Interrupts the conversion of angiotensin I to angiotensin II, a potent vasoconstrictor that normally increases afterload and preload

    Vasodilates arteriolar and venous system, producing a decreased preload and afterload

    Decreases the amount of circulating catecholamines

    Decreases myocardial oxygen demands

Caution: Check serum potassium levels — tend to increase

    Check blood pressure, especially in patients on diuretic therapy — tends to cause hypotension

    Do not use on patients with renal disease or diabetes mellitus

2. Diuretics

    Example: furosemide (Lasix)

    Action: Decreases fluid volume

    Caution: Prolonged use may cause electrolyte imbalance

3. Inotropic agents

    Examples: dopamine hydrochloride (Intropin)

        dobutamine hydrochoride (Dobutrex)

        norepinephrine bitartrate (Levophed)

        amrinone lactate (Inocor)

        digoxin (Lanoxin)

    Action: Increases cardiac muscle contractility and subsequently CO

    Caution: Observe for arrhythmias, increased heart rate, and peripheral vasoconstriction with decreased urinary output

4. Anticoagulant

    Example: heparin sodium (Heparin)

    Action: Prevents formation of emboli, usually seen with atrial arrhythmias or left ventricular aneurysm

    Caution: May cause increased bleeding in the patient with venous congestion and liver dysfunction

5. Opioid analgesics

    Example: morphine sulfate (Durmorph)

    Action: Decreases arterial blood pressure and systemic vascular resistance; vasodilates as well as relieves anxiety and pain

    Caution: Decreases respiratory drive; causes hypotension

NURSING MANAGEMENT

Monitoring and Managing Clinical Problems

1. Cardiac Output: decreased

a. Monitor CO.
1) Assess skin for warmth and dryness.
2) Assess all peripheral pulses and skin temperature every 2 hours, or as indicated.
3) Assess urinary output every hour; relate to IV and oral intake.
4) Monitor hemodynamics and report:
   a) Increased PAP
   b) Increased PCWP
   c) Decreased CO
   d) Decreased cardiac index
   e) Increased CVP
   f) Increased systemic vascular resistance
   g) Increased right atrial pressure
5) Assess level of consciousness.
6) Assess for activity intolerance.
7) Monitor blood pressure in sitting and lying positions, and compare values. Report significant findings.

b. Promote CO.
1) Maintain patency of all hemodynamic monitoring lines.
2) Assist with activities of daily living/comfort measures to prevent over exertion.
3) Administer ordered inotropic agents and assess their effect on the patient's hemodynamic status.
4) Maintain patient on intra-aortic balloon pump. Assess patient status during augmentation for complications.
5) Place patient in semi-Fowler's position, if tolerated.

2. Gas Exchange: impaired
a. Monitor respiratory status.
1) Monitor respiratory rate, depth, and rhythm every 2 hours, or as indicated.
2) Assess lung sounds every 2 hours, noting increase/decrease of moist sounds. Observe and note presence of a cough.
3) Monitor oxygen concentration being administered.
4) Obtain specimens for and monitor serial ABG results as well as chest X-ray reports to determine patient's response to treatment.

    5) Assess level of consciousness and significant changes in patient's behavior.

    6) Monitor skin and mucous membrane for moisture (diaphoresis, sweating) and color (cyanosis, mottling, pallor).

    7) Monitor respiratory secretions for amount, viscosity, and color.

b. Provide for proper oxygenation.

    1) Maintain bed rest.

    2) Schedule nursing care to provide for adequate rest periods.

    3) Elevate head of bed 30–45 degrees if patient tolerates. Position head and neck to prevent obstruction of airway.

    4) Auscultate dependent lung areas for moist lung sounds.

    5) Reposition every 2 hours.

    6) Prepare for emergency intubation as indicated. Keep emergency resuscitation equipment in close proximity.

    7) Add supplemental oxygen to ventilator-controlled airway, as indicated.

    8) Titrate oxygen to maintain adequate PaO_2.

3. Fluid Volume Deficit or Excess

a. Monitor fluid and electrolyte status.

    1) Monitor intake and output.

    2) Monitor hemodynamic pressures and report:

       a) Mean PAP >16 mm Hg

       b) PCWP >12 mm Hg

       c) CO <4 L/min and cardiac index <2.8 L/min per meter squared

    3) Note patient response to diuretics by monitoring hourly urine output.

    4) Observe cardiac monitor and report arrhythmias.

    5) Monitor serial serum electrolyte values and report significant changes.

b. Promote fluid and electrolyte balance.

    1) Administer ordered diuretics.

    2) Administer all IV fluids on infusion pumps or with minidrip infusion sets to prevent fluid overload.

    3) Concentrate IV medications to decrease fluid intake.

4) Restrict water and sodium intake.
5) Weigh daily at same time, on same scale.
6) Treat arrhythmias per hospital protocol.

Monitoring, Managing, and Preventing Life-Threatening Emergencies

1. Rupture of papillary muscle
   a. Report hyperacute pulmonary edema due to mitral valve insufficiency.
   b. Administer ordered vasodilators.
   c. Prepare for emergency insertion of intra-aortic balloon pump, if patient is unable to have immediate valve replacement.
   d. Prepare patient for emergency mitral valve replacement surgery.
2. Rupture of the interventricular septum
   a. This usually occurs after acute myocardial infarction.
   b. Prepare patient for emergency cardiac catheterization.
   c. Anticipate insertion of intra-aortic balloon pump.
3. Pulmonary edema
   a. Monitor for increasing respiratory distress and report:
      1) Increased anxiety, restlessness, deteriorating to lethargy
      2) Increased respiratory rate, heart rate
      3) Decreased blood pressure, increased PAPs
      4) Change in skin color to pallor or cyanosis
      5) Frothy, blood-tinged sputum
      6) Crackles and wheezing upon auscultation
      7) S_3 and S_4 on auscultation
   b. Provide for adequate oxygenation.
      1) Secure a patent airway and reassess continuously.
      2) Elevate the head of bed to 45–90 degrees while lowering the feet, if possible.
      3) Administer morphine sulfate as ordered to vasodilate, and reduce.

Acute Pulmonary Edema

Acute pulmonary edema is a restrictive lung disorder that occurs when hydrostatic pressure in the pulmonary capillaries exceeds intravascular osmotic pressure, resulting in excess serous or serosanguinous fluid accumulation in the pulmonary interstitial or alveolar spaces. It is also known as *backward failure* or *circulatory overload*.

There are two types of acute pulmonary edema. Cardiogenic or high-pressure edema occurs from cardiac dysfunction. Noncardiogenic or normal pressure pulmonary edema occurs from leaking capillaries that are more permeable than normal. (See Chapter 1, "Respiratory Disorders," for information on noncardiogenic pulmonary edema.)

Patients at risk for pulmonary edema include those who have:
1. Increased pulmonary capillary wedge pressure as seen in
   a. Fluid overload

    b. Acute myocardial infarction (AMI)
    c. Decompensating chronic heart failure
    d. Mitral valve disease and severe mitral stenosis
    e. Severe aortic regurgitation and aortic stenosis
    f. Severe hypertension
    g. Massive pulmonary embolism
    h. Central nervous system injuries
    i. Rupture of the chordae tendineae
2. Decreased lymphatic drainage as seen in
    a. Pneumonia
    b. Pulmonary contusion
    c. Microemboli
    d. Increased central venous pressure (CVP)

Etiology/Pathophysiology

1. Acute pulmonary edema reduces the amount of lung tissue available for gas exchange and inhibits gas exchange by impairing the diffusion pathway between the alveolus and capillary. Three factors affect movement of fluid out of capillaries and into the pulmonary interstitial tissue:
   a. Increased capillary permeability, seen in shock and sepsis
   b. Increased hydrostatic pressure in the capillaries, seen in congestive heart failure and fluid overload
   c. Decreased plasma oncotic pressure, seen in cirrhosis and hypoalbuminemia
2. Acute pulmonary edema is caused by increased left atrial and left ventricular pressure and thus is a symptom of some underlying disorder, not a diagnosis. The onset is usually sudden even though the underlying process may have existed for a long time. There are four stages as outlined in the table below.

The Stages of Acute Pulmonary Edema

Stage 1: Interstitial Stage	Stage 2: Alveolar Stage	Stage 3: Bronchial Stage	Stage 4: Final Stage
Lung interstitium swells with fluid as lymphatics cannot absorb excess fluid	Alveolar flooding Decreasing PaO_2 Decreasing $PaCO_2$ Increasing pH Tachypnea Increased venous	Altered surfactant activity Atelectasis Frothy, tenacious, often blood-tinged sputum Crackles on	Tissue hypoxia Hypoventilation Respiratory and metabolic acidosis Increasing $PaCO_2$

Continued

The Stages of Acute Pulmonary Edema — *Continued*

Stage 1: Interstitial Stage	Stage 2: Alveolar Stage	Stage 3: Bronchial Stage	Stage 4: Final Stage
Patient becomes restless and anxious	return to the heart Increased blood volume within the pulmonary capillary bed	auscultation	

Assessment/Analysis

ASSESSMENT FINDINGS

Subjective

1. History of recent AMI
2. Extreme anxiety
3. Extreme shortness of breath

Objective

1. Extreme restlessness and anxiety
2. Orthopnea (breathes better with head elevated)
3. Tachypnea
4. Extreme dyspnea with air hunger
5. Coughing
6. Blood-tinged, frothy sputum
7. Use of accessory muscles for breathing
8. Central and peripheral cyanosis
9. Nasal flaring
10. Diaphoresis with cold, ashen skin
11. Peripheral vasoconstriction resulting in cold extremities and pale to cyanotic nailbeds and mucous membranes
12. Peripheral edema

13. Bubbling crackles on auscultation
14. Wheezing, especially on expiration
15. Hypertension
16. Tachycardia and cardiac arrhythmias
17. S_3 gallop and decreased heart sounds
18. Murmur, if valve disease present

SUPPORTING TEST FINDINGS

Laboratory Tests

1. Arterial blood gases (ABGs)
   Abnormality: Early stages: Increased pH
      Decreased PaO_2
      Decreased $PaCO_2$
   Late stages: Decreased pH
      Decreased PaO_2
      Increased $PaCO_2$
2. Liver function tests
   Abnormality: Increased serum glutamic oxaloacetic transaminase
      Increased serum glutamic pyruvic transaminase
3. Renal function tests
   Abnormality: Increased blood urea nitrogen
      Increased serum creatinine
      Decreased urine sodium
      Increased urine osmolarity
4. Serum electrolytes
   Abnormality: Varied electrolyte imbalances related to sodium or fluid intake or diuretic therapy
5. Serum cardiac enzymes
   Abnormality: Increased creatine kinase (CK) and myocardial band isoenzyme of CK (if AMI precipitated it)
      Increased lactic dehydrogenase
6. Serum drug levels (for those patients taking drugs that accumulate in the system)
   Abnormality: Nontherapeutic levels of digoxin, aminophylline, lidocaine, or quinidine

Diagnostic Tests

1. Chest X-ray
   Abnormality: Alveolar flooding (white out) is seen
      Enlarged cardiac silhouette

Pulmonary venous congestion
Interstitial edema
2. Hemodynamic monitoring
    Abnormality: Increased pulmonary capillary wedge pressure (PCWP)
        Decreased cardiac output (CO)
        Increased CVP
        Increased right atrial pressure
3. Pulmonary function tests
    Abnormality: Decreased functional residual capacity
        Decreased compliance
4. Electrocardiogram
    Abnormality: Signs of ischemia, injury, or infarction
        Signs of previous pathology (i.e., left atrial or ventricular enlargement)

Planning/Intervention

COLLABORATIVE MANAGEMENT

Procedures

1. Institute measures to decrease venous return to the heart and lungs.
    a. Elevate the patient's head and chest.
    b. Administer diuretics as ordered for fluid overload.
    c. May apply rotating tourniquets, an old treatment, designed to decrease venous return to the heart, that involved applying a tourniquet to three of the four extremities and rotating the tourniquets every 15 minutes. This therapy has been replaced with drugs that decrease venous return.
    d. Assist with phlebotomy, a treatment that involves removing some of the patient's blood to decrease fluid overload. It is used when the patient is in imminent danger of death from the pulmonary edema.
2. Improve gas exchange within the lungs.
    a. Institute oxygen therapy.
    b. As needed, assist with intubation and initiating mechanical ventilation and positive end-expiratory pressure, if the pulmonary edema is refractory to other therapies.

3. Improve CO.
   a. Administer digitalis, as ordered.
   b. Administer antiarrhythmics, followed by cardioversion if drugs are ineffective, to control supraventricular arrhythmias and ventricular tachycardia.
4. Treat complications.

Drug Therapy

1. Opioid analgesics
   Example: morphine (Duramorph)
   Action: Induces vasodilation
       Decreases venous return to the heart
       Reduces pain
       Decreases anxiety
       Decreases myocardial oxygen demand
   Caution: Can cause bradycardia, hypotension, and decreased respirations
2. Vasodilators
   Examples: nitroglycerin (Tridil)
       sodium nitroprusside (Nipride)
   Action: Lower systemic vascular resistance thus decreasing afterload
       Improve left ventricular function: increase venous capacity, decrease preload
   Caution: Can cause headache, dizziness, and hypotension
       Intravenous (IV) nitroprusside may be light brown and must be protected from light
       IV nitroglycerin must be mixed in a glass bottle and administered with special tubing
3. Antiarrhythmics
   Examples: lidocaine (Xylocaine)
       quinidine (Quinidex)
       procainamide (Pronestyl)
   Action: Increase electrical stimulation threshold in the ventricular conduction system
       Control supraventricular and ventricular arrhythmias
   Caution: Can cause drowsiness, confusion, seizures, and nausea and vomiting
       Lidocaine may result in cardiac arrest
       Lidocaine and quinidine may accumulate and cause toxicity; monitor blood levels

4. Inotropic agents
    Examples: digoxin (Lanoxin)
        dopamine (Intropin)
        dobutamine (Dobutrex)
        amrinone (Inocor)
    Action: Increases CO
        Increases cardiac contractility
        Reduces preload
        Reduces PCWP
        May increase myocardial oxygen consumption
    Caution: Use cautiously with AMI
        Can cause arrhythmias, tachycardia, and hypotension or hypertension
5. Diuretic therapy
    Example: furosemide (Lasix)
        bumetanide (Bumex)
    Action: Increases venous capacity
        Reduces venous return
        Reduces circulatory volume
        Increases urine output
    Caution: Can cause hypotension, dehydration, and hypokalemia
6. Bronchodilator
    Example: aminophylline (Theophylline)
    Action: Dilates bronchioles
        Increases urine output
        Produces positive inotropic effects
    Caution: Can cause nervousness, anxiety, tachycardia, nausea, vomiting, and tremors
        Monitor blood levels to determine therapeutic dosage levels

NURSING MANAGEMENT

Monitoring and Managing Clinical Problems

1. Fluid Volume Excess—Monitor for fluid overload and promote fluid balance
    a. Assess hemodynamic parameters frequently and report abnormalities.
    b. Monitor intake and output hourly.
    c. Promote fluid restriction.
    d. Restrict sodium intake.

e. Monitor and record daily weights.

f. Assess for distended neck veins every 4 hours.

g. Assess for peripheral edema.

h. Assess for increasing crackles in the lungs.

i. Assess for new onset of an S_3 every 4 hours.

j. Monitor laboratory values for electrolyte imbalances.

k. Administer diuretics, as ordered, and monitor patient response.

2. Cardiac Output: decreased — Monitor for and treat arrhythmias

a. Continuously monitor cardiac rhythm.

b. Monitor serial serum electrolytes, especially serum potassium and magnesium.

c. Administer ordered antiarrhythmics and observe patient response.

d. Have emergency resuscitation equipment nearby and be prepared for cardioversion, if necessary.

e. Treat life-threatening arrhythmias, as ordered.

f. Administer oxygen, as ordered, to prevent myocardial ischemia.

3. Breathing Pattern: ineffective — Monitor for and promote improved ventilation

a. Administer oxygen therapy, as ordered.

b. Auscultate lung sounds every 4 hours and report abnormal findings.

c. Elevate the head of bed to semi-Fowler's or high Fowler's position.

d. Encourage incentive spirometry.

e. Turn the patient every 2 hours.

f. Assess for signs of hypoxemia (confusion, cyanosis, and anxiety).

g. Monitor serial ABGs and report abnormal findings.

h. Administer ordered inotropic agents and monitor patient response.

i. Organize care to allow for rest periods.

4. Recognize and treat complications.

a. Acute respiratory distress

1) Elevate head of bed and lower legs, if possible.

2) Give medications, as ordered.

3) Administer supplemental oxygen.

4) Prepare for intubation and mechanical ventilation, if necessary.

Mnemonic for Treating Pulmonary Edema

M = Morphine
O = Oxygen
S = Sit up
T = Tourniquets (mechanical or chemical, such as nitroglycerin, used to decrease venous return)
D = Diuretics
A = Aminophylline
M = Monitor
P = Provide breathing treatments

b. Digitalis toxicity
   1) Monitor serial serum digoxin levels.
   2) Recognize signs of toxicity (abdominal pain, anorexia, nausea, vomiting, visual disturbances, bradycardia, and other arrhythmias).
   3) Count apical pulse for 1 minute before administration. If the pulse is less than 60 bpm, do not give the drug. Notify the physician of the pulse rate and ask whether or not to administer the digitalis.
c. Fluid/Electrolyte imbalances
   1) Monitor hourly intake and output.
   2) Weigh daily.
   3) Promote fluid restriction.
   4) Administer diuretic therapy and assess for hypovolemia, fatigue, nausea, vomiting, headache, dry mouth, muscle cramps, or dizziness; report positive findings.
   5) Perform sodium restriction.
   6) Monitor serial serum electrolytes, particularly sodium and potassium, for abnormalities, and report any to the physician.
d. Oxygen toxicity caused by too high a percentage of inspired oxygen for prolonged periods
   1) Monitor serial ABGs frequently and decrease FiO_2 to <50% as quickly as possible.
   2) Apply pulse oximeter continuously to maintain oxygen saturation greater than 90%.
   3) Recognize early signs of oxygen toxicity (retrosternal pain, paresthesias, nausea, vomiting, fa-

tigue, dyspnea, coughing, anorexia, and rest-lessness).

Monitoring, Managing, and Preventing of Life-Threatening Emergencies

1. Acute pulmonary edema is, in and of itself, a life-threatening emergency.
   a. Progressive deterioration of cardiac function is currently treated with heart transplantation.
   b. Serious cardiac arrhythmias are treated with antiarrhythmics and synchronized or unsynchronized cardioversion, as needed.
2. Cardiogenic shock
   a. Monitor for hemodynamic instability and promote hemodynamic stability.
      1) Continuously monitor hemodynamic parameters to evaluate the cardiovascular response to treatment.
      2) Titrate fluids and inotropes to maintain a systolic blood pressure of at least 80 mm Hg.
      3) Position the patient in modified Trendelenburg (elevation of the legs at 45 degrees) position.
      4) Continuously monitor blood pressure to determine the cardiovascular response to treatment.
      5) Monitor cardiac rhythm for tachycardia and life-threatening ventricular arrhythmias (ventricular tachycardia and/or fibrillation).
   b. Monitor for and promote adequate oxygenation.
      1) Administer supplemental oxygen, as ordered.
      2) Obtain specimens and monitor results of serial ABGs and hemoglobin, and report abnormalities.
      3) Monitor capillary refill and monitor skin color to assess peripheral perfusion.
      4) Maintain a patent airway and adequate ventilation. Administer supplemental oxygen to ensure that sufficient oxygen is delivered to the lungs.
   c. Monitor for altered organ and tissue perfusion.
      1) Insert indwelling urinary catheter and monitor for decreased urine output, increased renal function tests, and signs of acute renal failure. Continuously monitor urinary output via catheter to evaluate renal function.

2) Monitor ABGs for a falling arterial oxygen concentration possibly indicating adult respiratory distress syndrome.

3) Auscultate bowel sounds for decreased or absent sounds, possibly indicating gastroparesis and observe nasogastric tube drainage for bright red or coffee ground material, possibly indicating stress ulceration.

4) Check patient's temperature every 4 hours to monitor for hypothermia or hyperthermia.

5) Assess patient for decreased alertness and attention span, drowsiness, or excessive sleeping indicating downward changes in the level of consciousness.

  d. Provide nutrition via enteral or parenteral nutritional support to prevent a negative nitrogen balance.

3. Cardiopulmonary arrest
  a. Call for help.
  b. Begin cardiopulmonary resuscitation.
  c. Follow with advanced cardiac life support.

Cardiac Tamponade

Cardiac tamponade is a life-threatening condition that results from a collection of air, fluid, or blood in the pericardial cavity causing compression of the heart, obstruction of venous return, and decreased cardiac output (CO). The pericardial cavity is the space between the serous membranes of the pericardial sac and epicardium. It normally holds 20–30 mL of fluid. The pericardial sac is a fixed, fibroserous, minimally distensible sac surrounding the heart and great vessels.

Etiology/Pathophysiology

1. Traumatic causes of cardiac tamponade include:
    a. Cardiac perforation from any catheter placed within the heart
    b. Penetrating chest wounds
    c. Blunt trauma to the anterior chest wall
2. Medical causes of cardiac tamponade include:
    a. Various neoplastic syndromes resulting in pericardial effusion
    b. Clogged mediastinal or chest tubes following cardiac surgery
    c. Infection
    d. Inflammation/pericarditis
    e. Ruptured aortic aneurysm with bleeding into the pericardial cavity
    f. Acute myocardial infarction (AMI)
    g. Chronic renal failure
3. The speed of air, blood, or fluid accumulation determines the degree of decline in cardiac performance
    a. The slower the accumulation, the longer the increased pressure can be tolerated and the larger the amount of fluid can be accommodated. Several hundred milliliters of accumulation may be tolerated before signs and symptoms occur.
    b. A rapid increase of an additional 50–100 mL or more can produce signs and symptoms.

Beck's Triad

Classic Symptoms of Cardiac Tamponade
Systemic hypotension
Muffled heart sounds
Neck vein distention

Assessment/Analysis

ASSESSMENT FINDINGS
Subjective

1. Midthoracic chest pain
2. Dyspnea and shortness of breath

3. Feelings of apprehension and restlessness

Objective

1. Evidence of precordial trauma or history or predisposing medical condition
2. Decreased urine output
3. Cough
4. Weak, tachycardiac pulse
5. Cool, pale, diaphoretic skin
6. Pulsus paradoxus of greater than 10–15 mm Hg during inspiration
7. With slow development of tamponade, pericardium has a chance to dilate slowly. 1,000–2,500 mL of fluid may be present. This causes signs and symptoms that resemble right-sided heart failure and include:
   a. Dyspnea
   b. Orthopnea
   c. Tachycardia
   d. Edema
   e. Hepatic engorgement
   f. Positive hepatojugular reflex — Distended veins in the neck
8. With fast development of tamponade, the signs and symptoms resemble cardiogenic shock and include:
   a. A fall in CO
   b. Electrical alternans (alternating large and small QRS complexes or altered direction of complexes)
   c. Distended neck veins
   d. Dependent edema
   e. Arterial hypotension
   f. Faint heart sounds

SUPPORTING TEST FINDINGS

Laboratory Tests

1. Culture and sensitivity of pericardial fluid
   Abnormality: Organisms present in the pericardial fluid when infection is the cause

Diagnostic Tests

1. Echocardiogram
   Abnormality: Fluid accumulation in the pericardial sac

2. Hemodynamic monitoring
   Abnormality: central venous pressure >15 mm Hg
      pulmonary artery pressure >32/13 mm/Hg
      pulmonary capillary wedge pressure (PCWP) >12 mm/Hg
      PCWP = right atrial pressure
      CO <4 L/min
3. Specific radiographic tests including: Computed tomography scan, carbon dioxide angiography, and chest X-ray
   Abnormality: Enlargement of heart silhouette with fluid accumulation
4. Electrocardiogram (ECG)
   Abnormality: ST-T wave changes and/or electrical alternans may occur, but this is a nonspecific finding.
      Low voltage complexes in the precordial leads of an ECG
      Recurrent arrhythmias after AMI
      Electromechanical dissociation

Planning/Intervention

COLLABORATIVE MANAGEMENT

Procedures

1. Identify symptoms and assist with differential diagnosis of cardiac tamponade, tension pneumothorax, right ventricular failure, and right ventricular myocardial infarction.
   a. Assist with hemodynamic catheter insertion and monitoring.
   b. Obtain echocardiogram, as ordered.
   c. Accompany patient for definitive X-ray studies.
   d. Obtain blood specimens for ordered laboratory studies.
   e. Monitor serial ECGs.
2. Once identified, assist with evacuation of the tamponade.
   a. Assist with pericardiocentesis — removal of as little as 20–50 mL of fluid may improve CO. A pericardial catheter may then be inserted and connected to a low-suction drainage container for a longer period (hours or days).

b. Prepare patient for a pericardial window — an opening into the pericardium that allows for fluid drainage into the pleural space.
c. Prepare patient for thoracotomy to identify and repair the source of bleeding.
3. Monitor for recurrence of the tamponade.

Drug Therapy

1. Oxygen
   Example: oxygen
   Action: Increases oxygen content in the lungs
   Helps to deliver adequate amounts of oxygen to the cells
   Caution: High concentrations for a long time results in oxygen toxicity
2. Inotropic agents
   Examples: isoproterenol (Isuprel)
   dobutamine (Dobutrex)
   Action: Improve cardiac contractility
   Increase CO by increasing stroke volume, and decreasing systemic vascular resistance
   Heart rate is also increased, which is undesirable in cardiac tamponade
   Caution: Can cause tachycardia, increased myocardial oxygen demand, ventricular arrhythmias, and hypertension
3. Diuretics
   Examples: furosemide (Lasix)
   bumetanide (Bumex)
   Action: Increase urine output by increasing the excretion of sodium and chloride in the loop of Henle, thus decreasing fluid overload and treating oliguria
   Caution: Can cause hypokalemia and dehydration

NURSING MANAGEMENT

Monitoring and Managing Clinical Problems

1. Tissue Perfusion, altered, peripheral, high risk for — Monitor for response to treatment and promote increased perfusion
   a. Monitor for changes in hemodynamic parameters

every 2–4 hours. Report findings consistent with worsening cardiac tamponade.
  b. Maintain the patient in Fowler's position.
  c. Administer ordered oxygen, inotropic agents, and diuretics.
  d. Monitor peripheral pulses to check perfusion.
  e. Maintain at least two patent intravenous lines.
  f. Monitor hourly intake and output.
  g. Maintain patency of chest tubes patent with gentle milking action, especially with mediastinal tubes. Report a sudden decrease in chest-tube drainage.
  h. Monitor ECGs for abnormalities and report abnormal findings.

2. Cardiac Output: decreased, high risk for — Promote normal cardiac functioning
  a. For stable patients — Assist with pericardiocentesis.
    1) Catheter may be secured and left in place because of the chance of recurrence.
    2) Results may be falsely negative if the needle is obstructed by debris (cells, tissue, or blood clots) in the fluid.
    3) To determine whether blood obtained is pericardial or intracardial, test for clotting. Pericardial blood should not clot.
  b. For unstable patients — Prepare the patient for immediate thoracotomy.

3. Tissue Perfusion, altered, cardiac, high risk for
  a. Maintain chest tube patency
  b. Monitor for recurrence of cardiac tamponade

4. Infection: high risk for
  a. Monitor for infection.
  b. Institute ordered treatment should infection occur.

5. Injury: high risk for
  a. Avoid the use of anticoagulants, thrombolytics, and steroids in cases where bleeding caused the cardiac tamponade. These drugs will increase the chance of bleeding into the pericardial sac.
  b. Monitor for recurrence.

Monitoring, Managing, and Preventing Life-Threatening Emergencies

1. Cardiac tamponade is a life-threatening emergency in

and of itself and should be recognized promptly and treated immediately.

2. Hypovolemic shock
   a. Monitor for hemodynamic instability.
      1) Hemodynamic monitoring is continuous.
      2) Titrate fluids and inotropic agents to maintain a systolic blood pressure of at least 80 mm Hg.
      3) Position the patient in modified Trendelenburg position (elevation of the legs at 45 degrees).
   b. Promote adequate oxygenation.
      1) Administer supplemental oxygen, as ordered.
      2) Obtain blood specimens and monitor results of serial arterial blood gases (ABGs) and hemoglobin, and report abnormalities.
      3) Monitor capillary refill and monitor skin color to assess peripheral perfusion.
   c. Monitor for altered organ and tissue perfusion.
      1) Monitor for decreased urine output and elevated renal function tests, possibly indicating acute renal failure.
      2) Monitor for a falling arterial oxygen concentration, possibly indicating adult respiratory distress syndrome.
      3) Auscultate for decreased or absent bowel sounds, suggesting gastroparesis, and observe for bright red or coffee-ground drainage from the nasogastric tube, possibly indicating stress ulceration.
      4) Check temperature every 4 hours to monitor for hypothermia or hyperthermia.
      5) Assess patient for decreased alertness and attention span, drowsiness, or excessive sleeping, indicating downward changes in the level of consciousness.
   d. Monitor for loss of fluid volume from the vasculature.
      1) Administer ordered fluid replacement.
      2) Maintain accurate intake and output measurements hourly.
      3) Continuously monitor blood pressure.
      4) Monitor skin turgor for signs of dehydration.
      5) Monitor for onset of an S_3 heart sound, peripheral edema, and moist crackles in the lungs indicating fluid volume overload.

      6) Closely monitor pertinent laboratory data (serum electrolytes, urine studies) to assess hydration status.

3. Pulmonary emboli (Air)
   a. Monitor for signs of respiratory distress.
      1) Observe for dyspnea and tachypnea.
      2) Check nailbeds for pallor or cyanosis.
      3) Observe for anxiety, apprehension, and restlessness.
      4) Be prepared for mechanical ventilation if necessary.
      5) Apply pulse oximeter and continuously monitor oxygen saturation.
      6) Obtain blood specimens and monitor serial ABGs.
   b. Promote activities to improve ventilation.
      1) Encourage coughing and deep breathing.
      2) Observe color and consistency of expectorated secretions. Hemoptysis may occur.
      3) Administer ordered oxygen.
      4) Observe for respiratory distress with patient care activities; interrupt care if it occurs; and space activities to prevent recurrence of respiratory distress.
      5) Elevate the head of the bed.
      6) Auscultate the lungs frequently for abnormalities and report findings.
      7) Assist with incentive spirometry.

4. Tension pneumothorax and mediastinal shift
   a. Observe for and immediately report signs of tension pneumothorax.
   b. Assist with immediate needle decompression using a 14- to 16-gauge needle at the second intercostal space, midclavicular line on affected side.
   c. Assist with chest-tube insertion.
   d. Monitor chest drainage color, consistency, and amount. Report signs of hemorrhage.
   e. Monitor chest drainage for air leaks. These will either close within the first few days after injury or require surgical repair.
   f. Assess breath sounds frequently for reexpansion.
   g. Monitor serial ABGs and serial chest X-ray reports to determine successful reexpansion.

5. Cardiopulmonary arrest
   a. Call for help.
   b. Begin cardiopulmonary resuscitation.
   c. Follow with advanced cardiac life support.

Cardiovascular Trauma

Cardiovascular trauma is a blunt or penetrating injury to the heart or great vessels. Any patient with cardiac trauma should be assumed to have traumatic injury to the rest of the organs in the thorax until proven otherwise.

Etiology/Pathophysiology

1. The types of trauma to the heart include:
   a. Hemopericardium — Bleeding into the pericardial sac that may or may not be accompanied by cardiac tamponade
   b. Cardiac tamponade — Excessive fluid accumulation in the pericardium, producing pressure on the heart. The fluid is most often blood from myocardial rupture or aortic rupture. (See Cardiac Tamponade.)
   c. Penetrating wounds — Injuries caused by knives, bullets, or any other foreign object
   d. Myocardial contusion — A bruise to the muscular layer of the heart caused by blunt trauma
      1) The right ventricle is more often contused than the left because of its anatomic location.
      2) A contused myocardium has diminished contractile ability and compliance, thus decreasing cardiac output (CO).
      3) Decreased CO begins in the right side first and then decreases on the left side.
      4) A contusion can result in perfusion abnormalities in the microvasculature of the myocardium.
2. The types of trauma to the great vessels include:
   a. Partial or complete rupture of the vessels — Resulting in a hemothorax
      1) Four major locations of vessel rupture:
         a) Distal to and left of the subclavian artery
         b) Ascending aorta where it exits the pericardial sac
         c) Descending aorta at entry to diaphragm
         d) Avulsion of the innominate artery from the aortic arch
   b. Traumatic aneurysm of the aorta — Rupture of the inner two layers of the vessel with an outpouching of the outer layer
      1) Long-term survival rate for traumatic rupture of the aorta ranges from 6–8%
      2) Most patients die at the accident or injury scene. Those who reach the hospital frequently die within 6 hours.

3. Injuries to the heart and great vessels — May be caused by penetrating or blunt trauma
   a. Penetrating injuries are wounds caused by foreign objects entering the heart or great vessels.
   b. Blunt injuries are injuries that are transmitted to the organs from injury to the chest wall or injuries that occur as a result of shearing force involved in acceleration/deceleration (high-speed impact) injuries.

Assessment/Analysis

ASSESSMENT FINDINGS

Subjective

1. Mechanism of injury consistent with cardiothoracic trauma
   a. History of penetrating injury
   b. History or suspicion of acceleration-deceleration injury
   c. History or suspicion of blunt trauma
2. A history of pre-existing cardiac disease makes the diagnosis of myocardial contusion difficult if not impossible
3. Feelings of apprehension

Objective

1. Myocardial contusion

Signs and Symptoms of Myocardial Contusion as Related to Severity of Injury		
Mild Injury	*Moderate Injury*	*Severe Injury*
Injury to the skin over the sternum	Chest pain that may be refractory to coronary vasodilators	Thready pulse and decreased blood pressure
Pericardial friction rub	Sinus tachycardia (heart rate >100 bpm)	Recurrent ventricular tachycardia and fibrillation

Continued

Signs and Symptoms of Myocardial Contusion as Related to Severity of Injury — *Continued*

Mild Injury	*Moderate Injury*	*Severe Injury*
Benign arrhythmias	Murmur signifying valvular regurgitation	Decreased level of consciousness
Nonspecific ST-T wave changes	Atrial and ventricular arrhythmias	Decreased urine output
	New conduction defects such as bundle branch blocks	Cyanosis and/or pallor
	Dependent edema	
	Cardiopulmonary arrest	

2. Aorta injury
   a. Chest pain radiating to the back
   b. Respiratory distress
   c. Dysphagia
   d. Enlarged neck and hoarseness
   e. Harsh systolic murmur
   f. Higher pulse amplitude and blood pressure in the upper extremities
3. Great vessel injury
   a. Extremity ischemia
   b. Bruising of the neck and upper chest
   c. Neurologic deficit from interruption of blood supply to the spinal cord
   d. Diminished or absent pulse in injured arm
   e. Diminished or absent carotid pulses. Bruits may be present.
   f. Precordial murmur
4. Rupture of the aorta and/or great vessels
   a. Respiratory distress progressing to apnea
   b. Neurologic deficits (weakness or paralysis of upper

and/or lower extremities) may be seen if blood supply to the spinal cord is impaired.
  c. Hypotension with rapidly falling blood pressure and rising pulse, leading to rapid profound shock
  d. Respiratory distress, diminished breath sounds over the affected area, decreased PaO_2, and jugular vein distension, indicating hemothorax or pneumothorax
  e. Systemic hypotension, muffled heart sounds, and neck vein distention, indicating cardiac tamponade
  f. Diminished or absent carotid or brachial pulses
  g. Rapid patient deterioration to death

SUPPORTING TEST FINDINGS

Laboratory Tests

1. Hematocrit and Hemoglobin
   Abnormality: Nonspecific for trauma
      Decreased — May indicate hemorrhage-induced hypovolemia
      Normal — May indicate no hemorrhage
2. White blood cell (WBC) count and differential
   Abnormality: Nonspecific for trauma
      Increased — May indicate sepsis present
      Normal — May indicate no infection
3. Arterial blood gases
   Abnormality: Increased — Respiratory alkalosis (early shock)
      Decreased — Metabolic acidosis (late shock)
4. Cardiac enzymes
   Abnormality: Increased myocardial band isoenzyme of creatinekinase (CPK-MB) for the first 3 days
5. Blood chemistries
   Abnormality: Nonspecific for trauma
      Glucose increased in early shock
      Blood urea nitrogen and creatinine increased with renal failure
      Sodium increased in early shock
      Potassium increased in all stages but early shock; decreased in early shock
      Calcium increased with lactic acidosis
6. Platelet count

Abnormality: Increased following traumatic injury or surgery

Diagnostic Tests

1. Chest X-ray
   Abnormality: Widening mediastinum >8 cm on chest X-ray before repair of aortic injury
2. Echocardiography
   Abnormality: Structural injury to the heart chambers or valves
3. Aortography
   Abnormality: Evidence of false aneurysm
4. Angiography
   Abnormality: Dye markings reflecting a vessel aneurysm or tear
5. Radioisotope scan
   Abnormality: Myocardial tissue damage
6. Electrocardiogram (ECG)
   Abnormality: Atrial and/or ventricular arrhythmias
7. Hemodynamic monitoring
   Abnormality: CO <4 L/min
   Pulmonary artery pressure (PAP) <20/8 mm Hg
   Pulmonary mean pressure <10 mm Hg
   Pulmonary capillary wedge pressure (PCWP) <8 mm Hg
   Central venous pressure <2 mm Hg
8. Continuous blood pressure monitoring via arterial line or automatic cuff
   Abnormality: Systolic blood pressure <100 mm Hg
9. Pulmonary function tests
   Abnormality: Decreased static compliance to <50 cm H_2O
   Increased dead space

Planning/Intervention

COLLABORATIVE MANAGEMENT

Procedures

1. Control hemorrhage
   a. Prepare patient for surgical intervention for vessel injury or rupture

    1) Immediate thoracotomy and cross-clamping of the aorta to maintain cerebral perfusion with aortic transection

    2) Emergency surgery to determine the amount of injury and to repair the injury

  b. Monitor serial chest X-rays to monitor small hemothorax.

  c. Assist with chest-tube placement for moderate-to-large hemothorax.

  d. Apply medical antishock trousers to increase organ perfusion. (Note: This procedure is controversial.)

  e. Type and crossmatch for transfusion therapy as ordered. In extreme emergencies, untyped and uncrossmatched blood (O negative) or type-specific, but uncrossmatched, blood may be given.

2. Provide fluid replacement with crystalloids, colloids, and blood products including autotransfusion to replace lost circulating volume, as ordered.

3. Monitor serial ECGs to identify cardiac injury by monitoring for ST-T wave changes, QRS abnormalities, and conduction defects.

Drug Therapy

1. Volume expanders

  Examples: Crystalloids — Should be used in the early phases of fluid replacement; Ringer's, Ringer's lactate (Plain Ringer's is used if the patient has a chance of returning to aerobic metabolism) and 0.9% normal saline solution are commonly used

    Colloids — such as albumin and plasma substitutes (dextran, hetastarch) may be used but are not recommended for trauma

    Blood or blood products — Packed red blood cells, whole blood, autotransfusion, and synthetic blood products may be used

  Action: Replaces lost intravascular volume

  Caution: Can cause hypervolemia and pulmonary edema; transfusion reactions may occur with blood products

2. Inotropic agents

  Example: dopamine (Intropin)

    dobutamine (Dobutrex)

  Action: Improves myocardial contractility

Increases CO

Assists with hypotension

Caution: Increases myocardial oxygen consumption

May worsen hypokalemia and arrhythmias

3. Diuretics

Examples: furosemide (Lasix)

bumetanide (Bumex)

Action: Increases urine output by increasing sodium and chloride excretion in the loop of Henle

Caution: Can cause hypokalemia and dehydration

4. Vasodilators

Examples: nitroprusside (Nipride)

Action: Decreases preload and afterload in aortic rupture to prevent complete disruption

Caution: Can cause hypotension and cyanate toxicity

5. Steroids

Examples: hydrocortisone (Solu-Cortef)

cortisone (Cortone)

Action: Inhibits the inflammatory response to trauma

Caution: Causes hypokalemia, hypernatremia, nausea, and petechiae

6. Antibiotics

Examples: cephalosporins

ticarcillin (Timentin)

ceftazidime (Fortaz)

aminoglycosides

gentamycin (Garamycin)

tobramycin (Nebcin)

Action: Bacteriocidal; broad-spectrum antibiotics that kill aerobic and anaerobic gram-negative and gram-positive bacteria.

Before the source is identified, at least a two-drug combination should be given.

When the source is identified, therapy may be tailored to the cause.

Caution: Can cause renal failure, allergic reaction, and ototoxicity

7. Antiarrhythmics

Examples: lidocaine (Xylocaine)

bretylium (Bretylol)

Action: Increases the electrical stimulation threshold in the ventricular conduction system; used to treat life-threatening arrhythmias

Caution: Can cause seizures and postural hypotension
8. Analgesics
Examples: morphine (Duramorph)
   meperidine (Demerol)
   hydromorphone (Dilaudid)
Action: Depresses pain impulse transmission to relieve the pain associated with trauma
Caution: Can cause sedation and respiratory depression

NURSING MANAGEMENT

Monitoring and Managing Clinical Problems

1. Myocardial contusion nursing care is similar to that of patients with acute myocardial infarction. (See Acute Myocardial Infarction.)
2. Fluid Volume Excess or Deficit: high risk for—Monitor for hemodynamic instability from vascular injury and promote hemodynamic stability.
   a. Monitor for signs and symptoms of vascular injury.
      1) Frequently check presence and amplitude of peripheral pulses in the arms and legs. Report variations in amplitude or absence of pulses.
      2) Measure blood pressure in the arms and legs frequently using an automatic blood pressure cuff. Report blood pressure differences of >20 mm Hg.
      3) Monitor for signs of occult or overt blood loss. Also observe the area of trauma for swelling.
      4) Reassess the patient frequently, paying special attention to even minor changes. One third of all patients with ruptured aortas have no signs of chest trauma on first examination.
      5) Check skin for pallor and bruising.
   b. Promote hemodynamic stability.
      1) Control obvious bleeding with pressure. Prepare the patient for surgery if the bleeding cannot be controlled.
      2) Monitor hemodynamic parameters to determine adequacy of CO. Report CO of <4 L/min.
      3) Administer blood products as ordered. Observe for reaction to the blood products (e.g., chills, fever, rash).
      4) Administer crystalloids as ordered. Observe for

signs and symptoms of fluid overload (e.g., moist lung sounds, S_3, edema).

5) Accurately measure intake and output to determine fluid volume status. Measure urine output every hour to ensure adequate renal function. Report output <30 mL/h.

6) Assist with chest-tube insertion for hemothorax, measure drainage, and replace blood loss.

7) Perform frequent neurologic checks to assess cerebral perfusion.

3. Cardiac Output: altered, high risk for — Recognize complications of ineffective cardiac function from cardiac trauma.

   a. Monitor for signs and symptoms of injury to the heart.

     1) Auscultate heart sounds, paying particular attention to the development of new murmurs.

     2) Monitor cardiac rhythm strips continuously and note presence of conduction defects and arrhythmias.

     3) Administer antiarrhythmics for ventricular arrhythmias.

     4) Observe for signs and symptoms of decreased CO (e.g., neck vein distension, dyspnea, pallor, dusky nailbeds with increased capillary refill time, activity intolerance).

   b. Promote rest to facilitate return of cardiac function, then follow with a gradual increase in self-care activities.

     1) Allow activity levels consistent with level of heart injury.

     2) Assist patient with activities of daily living, as needed.

     3) Discontinue activities that cause distress (e.g., increased heart rate, systolic blood pressure that rises 20 mm Hg above baseline, tachypnea) and allow the patient to rest.

     4) Schedule daily care throughout the day to allow for rest periods between activities.

     5) Institute cardiac rehabilitation protocol for activity management.

4. Infection: high risk for — Recognize potential complication of infection following penetrating trauma.

  a. Monitor for signs and symptoms of infection.
      1) Check WBC counts daily and more often if elevated. Report elevations.
      2) Monitor temperature every 4 hours and more often if fever develops. Report elevations.
      3) Observe wound drainage for odor or appearance of purulent drainage and report any noted changes.
      4) Observe the wounds for evidence of healing or infection.
  b. Promote activities to decrease risk of nosocomial infection.
      1) Use sterile technique when changing dressings.
      2) Administer ordered antibiotics.
      3) Obtain a specimen of suspicious wound drainage for culture and sensitivity testing.
      4) Wash hands frequently to prevent crosscontamination.

Monitoring, Managing, and Preventing Life-Threatening Emergencies

1. Cardiopulmonary Failure — May occur if the injury involves more than 40% of the ventricular surface.
  a. Report hemodynamic monitoring abnormalities consistent with cardiogenic shock, such as:
      1) Tachycardia
      2) Hypotension
      3) CO <4 L/min
      4) PAP >25/12 mm Hg
      5) PCWP >12 mm Hg
      6) Systemic vascular resistance >1,200 dynes per centimeter
  b. Titrate medications and fluids to correct abnormalities.
  c. Monitor lung function and report decreases in compliance (static compliance <50 cm H_2O).
  d. Monitor lung function and report evidence of ventilation-perfusion mismatch — Falling arterial oxygen content with increasing percentages of oxygen delivery.
      1) Continuously monitor SvO_2 and report decreases.
      2) Monitor arterial as well as mixed venous blood gases and report abnormalities.

   e. Monitor cardiac rhythm strips for life-threatening ventricular arrhythmias and treat with antiarrhythmics, as needed.
2. False aneurysm of the aorta—The inner two layers of the vessel tear, leaving only the outer layer intact. This prolongs survival time, but death will result if it is left unrepaired.
   a. Accompany patient to X-ray for diagnostic studies.
   b. Observe for signs and symptoms of rupture (e.g., rapid, profound shock as evidenced by hypotension; decreased sensorium; tachycardia; tachypnea; decreased urine output; moist, pale skin progressing to unconsciousness; anuria; apnea; and asystole).
   c. Prepare the patient for emergency surgery to repair the defect. Understand that most patients with ruptured aortic aneurysms die either before or during surgery.
3. Hemothorax—Can be caused by blunt or penetrating trauma.
   a. Signs and symptoms vary according to the amount of blood accumulated.

Small	*Moderate*	*Large*
<350 mL	*350–1500 mL*	*>1500 mL*
Asymptomatic	Shortness of breath	Chest tightness
	Dullness over the affected site on percussion	Severe chest pain that may radiate to the chest, shoulder, and upper abdomen
		Cyanosis
		Decreased PaO_2
		Profound shock leading to cardiopulmonary compromise
		Syncope

Continued

Small *<350 mL*	Moderate *350–1500 mL*	Large *>1500 mL*
		Tracheal deviation toward the unaffected side
		Dullness over the affected site on percussion
		Decreased or absent breath sounds on the affected side

    b. Prepare for chest-tube insertion. Use chest-tube drainage setup with autotransfusion unit attached.

    c. Prepare for blood replacement. May replace blood with crystalloid, banked blood products, colloids, or autotransfusion.

    d. Prepare patient for emergency surgery to repair injury.

4. Cardiopulmonary arrest

    a. Call for help.

    b. Begin cardiopulmonary resuscitation.

    c. Follow with advanced cardiac life support.

Hypertensive Crisis

A hypertensive crisis is an increase in diastolic blood pressure greater than 120 mm Hg with clinical manifestations of specific organ damage. This hypertensive state must be reduced within hours to prevent severe organ damage or death.

Etiology/Pathophysiology

1. Etiology
   a. It is sometimes difficult to determine if hypertension is the primary problem (essential hypertension) or a secondary illness
   b. Precipitating/associated illnesses
      1) Renal disease
         a) Acute glomerulonephritis
         b) Renovascular hypertension
         c) Renal tumors
      2) Cardiovascular disorders
         a) Acute myocardial infarction
         b) Acute congestive left-sided heart failure
         c) Pulmonary edema
         d) Dissecting aortic aneurysm
      3) Endocrine disorders
         a) Pheochromocytoma
         b) Cushing's syndrome
      4) Neurologic disorders
         a) Head injury
         b) Spinal injury with subsequent complication of autonomic dysreflexia
         c) Cerebrovascular accident (CVA)
         d) Subarachnoid hemorrhage
      5) Drug ingestion (e.g., cocaine)
2. Pathophysiology
   a. Most patients with hypertensive crisis have essential hypertension as well as a secondary illness.
   b. Generally, there is chronic vasoconstriction of the arteries, resulting in a thickened, less compliant arterial wall. This lack of elasticity, coupled with an atherosclerotic decrease in diameter of the vessel, causes an increase in the resistance to blood flow (increased peripheral or systemic resistance).
   c. Without treatment, extremely high blood pressure can lead to an acute myocardial infarction (MI), ruptured aortic aneurysm, CVA, or other vital organ failure.
   d. What differentiates a hypertensive crisis from essential hypertension is a sudden elevation in the blood pressure to greater than 250/120 mm Hg. However,

this varies with the individual; the chronic hypertensive patient may tolerate higher pressures without demonstrating additional physical findings.

Assessment/Analysis

ASSESSMENT FINDINGS

Subjective

1. Headache
2. Chest pain
3. Anxiety
4. Nausea
5. Abdominal pain
6. Visual difficulty
7. Numbness, tingling

Objective

1. Neck vein distention
2. Decrease in level of consciousness
3. Deterioration in speech, ability to complete simple written tasks, and motor/strength abilities
4. Nailbed discoloration: Distal portion of nail dark pink, red, or brown; proximal portion of nail pink or white
5. Ascites
6. Peripheral edema
7. Pupillary changes determined by etiology for hypertension
8. Ophthalmoscopic alterations
   a. Papilledema
   b. Siegrist's streaks: Colored spots, forming a chain, which follow alongside the choroidal artery
   c. Elschnig's spots: White discolorations of the retina, caused by edema associated with a detachment of the retina
9. Enlarged point of maximal impulse (ventricular hypertrophy)
10. Enlarged kidneys
11. Moist lung sounds (crackles)
12. S_3, S_4 heart sounds

13. Abdominal masses
14. Abdominal bruit (indicating dissecting aortic aneurysm or renal artery stenosis)

SUPPORTING TEST FINDINGS

Laboratory Tests

1. Serum creatinine
   Abnormality: Increased with renal disease
   Caution: Often elevated during initial antihypertensive therapy in the chronic renal insufficiency patient
2. Blood urea nitrogen (BUN)
   Abnormality: Increased with renal disease
3. Plasma catecholamine level
   Abnormality: Increased with pheochromocytoma and acute pulmonary edema
   Caution: Must be drawn from an indwelling intravenous (IV) line and handled correctly by laboratory personnel
       Must also be drawn while blood pressure high
4. Urine vanillylmandelic acid
   Abnormality: Increased with pheochromocytoma
   Caution: False-positive results may occur when patient is NPO at time of test, or due to ingestion of caffeine and a variety of different foods, drugs, and exercise
       False-negative results may occur with use of contrast dyes, as with intravenous pyelograms
       Container for 24-hour urine must contain proper preservative
       All urine must be saved within the 24 hours
5. Fasting blood glucose
   Abnormality: Increased with pheochromocytoma
6. Serum drug levels
   Abnormality: Positive in persons who have used cocaine and phencyclidine
7. Complete blood count
   Abnormality: Increased red blood cell (RBC) count and hemoglobin due to hemoconcentration from fluid depletion of pheochromocytoma
8. Serum lactate level
   Abnormality: Increases with anaerobic metabolism

May be seen with too rapid a decline in blood pressure

Diagnostic Tests

1. Arterial blood pressure
   Abnormality: Increased systolic and diastolic
2. Computed tomography scan and magnetic resonance imaging
   Abnormality: Adrenal tumor
   Lesion of brain
3. Electrocardiography
   Abnormality: Left ventricular hypertrophy, tachycardia, and arrhythmias
4. Chest X-ray
   Abnormality: Left ventricular enlargement with left-sided heart failure
   Patchy infiltrates indicating pulmonary edema
5. Digital subtraction angiography
   Abnormality: Aneurysms
   Arterial stenosis/occlusion
   Pheochromocytoma
   Pulmonary edema

Planning/Intervention

COLLABORATIVE MANAGEMENT

Procedures

1. Reduce/monitor deleterious effects of hypertension
   a. Assist with insertion of central IV line.
   b. Assist with insertion of arterial line and maintain continuous blood pressure monitoring.
   c. Initiate cardiac monitoring to observe for arrhythmias.
   d. Administer ordered antihypertensives and diuretics.
   e. Obtain blood specimens for ordered laboratory studies and prepare patient for ordered diagnostic studies.
   f. Monitor and report vital and neurologic vital signs.
   g. Maintain bed rest.
   h. Check peripheral pulses every 4 hours.

   i. Prepare patient for hemodialysis or continuous arteri-
       ovenous hemodiafiltration and monitor patient during
       procedure.

Drug Therapy

1. Inotropic agents
    Examples: sodium nitroprusside (Nipride)
         nitroglycerin (Nitrostat)
         diazoxide (Hyperstat)
    Action: Relaxes the smooth muscles of the venules and
    arterioles
    Caution: Nitroprusside decreases cerebral perfusion
         Nitroglycerin may cause circulatory collapse or
    anaphylaxis.
         Diazoxide causes reflex tachycardia and increased
    cardiac output (CO).
2. Autonomic nervous system agents
    Example: trimethaphan camsylate (Arfonad)
    Action: Blocks nerve transmission to sympathetic and au-
    tonomic systems, resulting in vasodilation and in-
    creased peripheral circulation
         Pressure returns to baseline 30 minutes after
    infusion
    Caution: May cause respiratory depression or even arrest
    after bolus
         Monitor blood pressure continuously with arterial
    line.
3. Alpha-adrenergic blocking agents
    Example: phentolamine (Regitine)
    Action: Acts on smooth muscles of vessles and blocks
    alpha-receptor sites
         Useful in pheochromocytoma
    Caution: May cause shock, reflex tachycardia, ischemia,
    or MI in susceptible patients
         May exacerbate gastrointestinal irritation and peptic
    ulcer disease
4. Beta-adrenergic blocking agents
    Example: propranolol (Inderal)
    Action: Reduces heart rate, irritability, and CO (causing
    decreased blood pressure)
         Useful with aortic dissection patient

Caution: Diuretic needed for retention of sodium and fluid
May cause false elevation laboratory test findings, such as serum potassium, lactic dehydrogenase, and BUN
May cause hyperglycemia
Compounds sinus bradycardia and heart block

5. Calcium channel blockers
Examples: nicardipine (Cardene)
nifedipine (Procardia)
verapamil (Isoptin)
Action: Block calcium influx into cardiac and smooth muscle cells
Decrease systemic vascular resistance and increase CO
Reduce oxygen requirements for cardiac muscle and prevent coronary artery spasm
Caution: Hypotensive effect can cause reflex tachycardia; or may cause extreme bradycardia and asystole; administer verapamil slow IV injection over at least 2 minutes

6. Angiotensin converting enzyme inhibitors
Examples: captopril (Capoten)
enalapril/enalaprilat (Vasotec)
Action: Prevents the production of angiotensin II, a strong vasoconstrictor
Decreases preload and afterload
Caution: Avoid use in the renal patient
Do not use captopril in patients with a collagen-vascular disorder

7. Diuretics
Example: furosemide (Lasix)
Action: Acts rapidly on primarily the loop of Henle, reabsorbing sodium and chloride, producing diuresis and decreasing blood pressure
Caution: Monitor serum potassium levels regularly
High doses may cause ototoxicity
Monitor patient's vital signs and cardiac monitor for hypotension and cardiac irregularities

NURSING MANAGEMENT
Monitoring and Managing Clinical Problems
1. Injury: high risk for — To heart, brain, and kidneys

a. Monitor organ function.
   1) Monitor vital signs every hour or as needed. Monitor right and left arm blood pressures.
   2) Monitor arterial line pressure—Compare with cuff pressure at least once every 8 hours.
   3) Monitor neurologic signs and fine motor skills every hour, or as indicated; report any changes immediately.
   4) Assess cranial nerves on routine basis.
   5) Monitor hourly urinary output; note odor and clarity.
   6) Monitor cardiac monitor for rate, rhythm, and the presence of any arrhythmias; compare findings with 12 lead electrocardiogram reports
   7) Assess patient for chest pain, rating pain on scale of 1–10, with 10 being the most severe.
   8) Assess patient's overall cardiovascular status, reporting the presence of extra heart sounds, and bruits.
   9) Palpate peripheral pulses and report any significant changes.
   10) Assess patient's reaction to pharmacologic intervention.
   11) Auscultate lungs for presence of abnormal and adventitious sounds.
   12) Assess for any nausea, fatigue, or muscle spasms during antihypertensive therapy.
   13) Obtain specimens and monitor results of laboratory studies for elevated serum enzymes, BUN, serum creatinine, and serum lactate levels.
b. Promote target organ homeostasis.
   1) Administer ordered antihypertensive medications. Note therapeutic response and any adverse reactions to the drugs.
   2) Assess level of consciousness on continual basis. Investigate any change in speech or behavior immediately.
   3) Infuse antihypertensive medications with a volume infusion pump to ensure consistent blood levels.
   4) Titrate medication dosage and check blood pressure every 15 minutes, or as needed, to avoid a

rapid decrease in blood pressure.

5) Relieve any chest pain by administering ordered pain medications. Note therapeutic response and any adverse reactions.

6) Report any complaints of nausea, fatigue, or muscle cramps.

7) Promote relaxation, reduce anxiety, fear, and stress; decrease environmental stimulation.

8) Once patient's blood pressure has reached acceptable range, begin weaning IV antihypertensive and instituting oral medication, as ordered.

c. Recognize complications associated with organ function.

   1) Antihypertensive medications could cause ischemia to the major organs of the body. Note the following:

     a) Increased cardiac arrhythmias and heart rate

     b) Decreased level of consciousness, change in behavior

     c) Decreased urinary output

Monitoring, Managing, and Preventing Life-Threatening Emergencies

1. Brainstem herniation syndrome—A protrusion of the brainstem from its normal compartment due to increased pressure within the compartment

  a. Monitor for change in behavior, deterioration in level of consciousness.

    1) Early signs—Difficulty concentrating, restlessness

    2) Late sign—Comatose

  b. Note any respiratory pattern change.

    1) Early sign—No change or possibly Cheyne-Stokes respirations

    2) Late sign—Shallow, grossly irregular respirations or possibly respiratory arrest

  c. Assess pupillary size and reaction.

    1) Early signs—Unilaterally sluggish to nonreactive and dilated pupils

    2) Late signs—Bilaterally fixed and dilated pupils

   d. Assess motor response.
     1) Early sign — Contralateral hemiparesis or possibly hemiplegia
     2) Mid-late signs — Ipsilateral rigidity, decorticate or decerebrate movements, or flaccidity with occasional decerebrate movement
   e. Assist physician with oculocephalic and oculovestibular tests.
2. Shock — Cardiogenic shock from MI or hypovolemic shock from rupture aortic aneurysm
   a. Monitor for hemodynamic instability.
     1) Continuously monitor hemodynamic parameters to evaluate response to treatment.
     2) Titrate fluids and inotropic agents to maintain a systolic blood pressure of at least 80 mm Hg.
     3) Position the patient in modified Trendelenburg position with the legs elevated at 45 degrees.
     4) Continuously monitor cardiac rhythm for tachycardia and life-threatening ventricular arrhythmias.
   b. Promote adequate oxygenation.
     1) Administer ordered supplemental oxygen, as indicated.
     2) Obtain specimens and monitor results of arterial blood gases and hemoglobin, and report significant changes.
     3) Monitor capillary refill and monitor skin color to assess peripheral perfusion.
   c. Monitor for altered organ and tissue perfusion.
     1) Monitor for decreased urine output and elevated renal function tests, possibly indicating acute renal failure.
     2) Monitor for a falling arterial oxygen concentration, possibly indicating adult respiratory distress syndrome.
     3) Auscultate for absent bowel sounds, possibly indicating gastroparesis, and note the presence of bright red or coffee-ground drainage from the nasogastric tube, possibly indicating stress ulceration.
     4) Monitor for decreased alertness and attention span, drowsiness, or excessive sleeping, indicating a deterioration in the level of consciousness.

3. Cardiopulmonary arrest
   a. Call for help.
   b. Begin cardiopulmonary resuscitation.
   c. Follow with advanced cardiac life support.
4. Pheochromocytoma
   a. Prepare patient for surgery.
5. Acute renal failure for acute tubular necrosis
   a. Administer ordered IV fluids to prevent complications of hypovolemia, infection, and nephrotoxic drug use.
   b. Regulate fluid intake to achieve fluid and electrolyte balance.
   c. Administer ordered buffering agents to achieve acid-base balance.
   d. Closely monitor neurologic vital signs and intervene quickly, as indicated, to preserve neurologic function.
   e. Manage nutrition.
      1) Restrict dietary protein intake to maintain anabolism while limiting load on kidneys; amount of protein will vary depending on patient's weight and activity level.
      2) Restrict dietary potassium.
      3) Restrict fluid intake.
      4) Provide sufficient calories to prevent catabolism.
      5) Administer ordered supplemental vitamins.
   f. Administer ordered blood transfusions to ensure optimal RBCs to tissue oxygenation.
   g. Initiate renal replacement therapy when indicated.
      1) BUN 100 mg/dL
      2) Serum creatinine >9 mg/dL; lower in patients with reduced muscle mass
      3) Signs of volume overload, pulmonary edema, pericarditis, hyperkalemia, uncontrollable acidosis, and central nervous system dysfunction
   h. Hemodialysis, continuous ultrafiltration, continuous renal replacement therapy, or peritoneal dialysis may be used.

Shock

Shock can be defined as a progressive syndrome that begins with failure of the circulatory system to adequately deliver oxygen and other nutrients to the cells of the body, or inability of the cells to use the oxygen and other nutrients delivered to them. Often insidious in onset, it may be difficult to recognize in early stages. It is a progressive syndrome that can be interrupted in some stages by therapeutic intervention. It is multicausal, although all types of shock produce impaired cellular metabolism resulting in cellular dysfunction and death. As cellular dysfunction and death increase, failure of tissues, individual organs, then organ systems occurs. Multiple system organ failure involving three or more systems almost always results in patient death.

Classification of Shock

Hypovolemic	Characterized by loss of circulating fluid volume, either blood or plasma
Cardiogenic	Failure of the heart to adequately pump blood throughout the vasculature as a result of major dysfunction of the left ventricle
Neurogenic	Generalized vasodilation and loss of vasomotor tone resulting in a massive increase in the vascular capacity, pooling of blood in the periphery, and decreased venous return to the heart
Anaphylactic	The result of an antigen-antibody reaction in which histamine or histamine-like substances are released; a histamine-induced dilation of the venous and arterial system plus a loss of fluid and protein into the tissue spaces from leaking capillaries results in decreased venous return to the heart and pooling of blood in the periphery
Septic	A generalized infection of the blood, usually by gram-negative bacteria, which results in fever, cellular dysfunction, marked vasodilation, peripheral pooling of blood, and decreased systemic vascular resistance

Etiology/Pathophysiology

1. Causes
   a. Decreased fluid volume from:
      1) External fluid losses — Hemorrhage, severe vomiting, severe diarrhea, dehydration
      2) Internal fluid losses — Third spacing as a result of ileus, intestinal obstruction, and burns
   b. Poor pumping ability of the heart from myocardial infarction, heart failure, cardiomyopathy, acute arrhythmias, acute pericardial tamponade, severe heart valve malfunction, massive pulmonary embolism, tension pneumothorax
   c. Impaired distribution with increased peripheral vasodilation from:
      1) Neurogenic causes — Spinal cord injuries, anesthetic paralysis, reflex vasodilation
      2) Anaphylactic causes — Adverse drug reactions, pollen hypersensitivity, hypersensitivity to insect stings, hypersensitivity to foreign proteins in the serum
      3) Septic causes — Gram-negative bacteria endotoxins (most common causative factor), gram-positive bacteria (toxic shock), fungi, viruses, rickettsiae
2. Stages
   a. Early stage (also called nonprogressive or compensated shock)
      1) Not severe and can be reversed
      2) Transient decrease in cardiac output (CO) and blood pressure, resulting in the sympathetic nervous system responses and renin-angiotensin-aldosterone responses to compensate and prevent further deterioration
      3) CO and arterial pressure return to normal and recovery occurs if shock does not become severe enough to enter the progressive phase.
      4) A loss of 10% of circulating volume initiates compensatory mechanism activation and results in maintenance of vital signs.
   b. Intermediate stage (also called progressive shock)

1) The body becomes unable to compensate for hemodynamic instability, resulting in cardiovascular deterioration. The progressive fall in arterial pressure decreases blood flow to the myocardium resulting in cellular dysfunction from insufficient oxygen and nutrients resulting in deterioration of cardiac function. The normal heart has massive reserves and can pump 300–400% more blood than needed, but if cardiogenic shock continues, eventually it will fail.

2) Ischemic cellular wastes cause agglutination or clotting in the small vessels, resulting in sluggish blood flow in the microvasculature and decreased flow of oxygen and nutrients to the cells.

3) Capillary hypoxia and lack of nutrients cause increased capillary permeability.

4) Endotoxin is released by gram-negative bacteria in the gut. Decreased blood flow to the intestine enhances endotoxin's formation and absorption. Endotoxin plays an important role in septic shock. It is also released in other forms of shock although its importance is unclear.

5) Generalized cellular deterioration results in:
   a) Diminished active transport of sodium and potassium through the cell membrane resulting in a buildup of sodium intracellularly and cellular swelling
   b) Depressed mitochondrial function that increased adenosine triphosphate production by anaerobic metabolism, causing excess lactic acid production and acidosis
   c) Release of hydrolases from the lysosomes, causing further cellular deterioration
   d) Depressed cellular metabolism of nutrients

6) Areas of necrosis develop within organs and organ failure occurs, especially in the liver, lungs, and heart.

c. Late stage (also called irreversible shock)
   1) Myocardial depression progresses secondary to pancreatic release of myocardial depressant factor. Cardiac deterioration is the most significant factor in progression.

2) The vasomotor center fails in late-stage shock, causing vasodilation that results in increased capillary permeability. This results in the movement of large amounts of fluids into the tissues (third spacing of fluid).

3) Shock becomes irreversible at a cellular level when the cells are depleted of high-energy phosphate compounds.

4) Tissue damage is extensive and is unable to be reversed by therapy, although improvement may be noted for a time.

5) When three or more organ systems fail, the patient will not survive. Organ failure becomes evident in most organ systems in late-stage shock. It is not responsive to treatment and leads to death.

Assessment/Analysis

ASSESSMENT FINDINGS

Subjective

1. The amount of subjective data that can be obtained will vary with the stage and type of shock.
2. Risk factors associated with traumatic injury and/or with infection
3. A mechanism of injury that could lead to shock
4. Patients may not be able to adequately describe what is happening to them in the early phase of shock, but they often express a feeling of impending doom without being able to pinpoint the cause of the feeling.

Objective

1. Level of consciousness ranges from inability to concentrate, restlessness, agitation, anxiety and/or confusion to bizarre behavior, lethargy, and/or apathy, to unconsciousness and unresponsiveness as shock progresses.
2. Pupils progress from normal and reactive to dilated and reactive, and eventually, to dilated with sluggish reaction.
3. Tachypnea—Initially rapid deep breathing that pro-

gresses to rapid, shallow breathing in the intermediate stage. In late-stage shock, rapid, shallow breathing with an irregular pattern is present.

4. Orthostatic symptoms — Initially no symptoms are present. Lightheadedness when sitting occurs in the intermediate stage and progresses to hemodynamic instability with position change in the late stage.

5. Decreasing urine output — Urine output is slightly decreased but within normal limits in early shock progressing to oliguria of less than 20 mL/h in the intermediate stage. Anuria and renal failure are seen in the late stage as renal function deteriorates.

6. Thirst — Occurs in the early stage of shock, becomes markedly increased in the intermediate stage, and severe in late shock (if the patient is oriented enough to report it)

7. Changes in core temperature — Core temperature is normal, but decreases with exposure to cold in all types of shock except septic. In sepsis, temperature increases.

8. Gastrointestinal bleeding from stress ulcer formation occurs in intermediate and late shock.

9. SaO_2 decreases as hypoxia from physiologic shunting occurs.

10. Pulse — Initial tachycardia from sympathetic stimulation may be seen progressing to tachycardia with arrhythmias and weak, rapid, thready peripheral pulses as shock worsens. In late-stage shock, an extremely slow and weak or absent pulse may be noted.

11. Edema progressing to anasarca can be seen in late-stage shock as fluid leaks into the tissues.

12. Skin is warm and flushed in the early stage of septic shock. In all other types, blood is shunted to the vital organs in the early stages, so skin becomes cool and pale. As all types progress, skin becomes cold and clammy, cyanosis may be seen, there is decreased capillary refill, and edema from fluid shifts is seen. Late-stage skin changes result in cold, mottled, ashen, or cyanotic skin.

13. Generalized muscle weakness and wasting occurs as blood is shunted to vital organs. Muscle aches may occur as lactic acid production increases in ischemic muscles.

14. Blood pressure varies with the stage. Initially systolic blood pressure is maintained or rises and diastolic blood pressure rises. This may result in decreased pulse pressure. Systolic blood pressure drops as shock progresses; diastolic rises as a result of vasoconstriction, causing a narrowing pulse pressure. Further progression results in frank hypotension with a widening pulse pressure. If shock is untreated, cardiovascular collapse results.

15. Lung sounds are initially clear, but may progress to crackles as shock progresses and adult respiratory distress syndrome (ARDS) ensues.

16. Bowel sounds become hypoactive as blood is shunted to other organs and progress to absent bowel sounds (paralytic ileus).

SUPPORTING TEST FINDINGS

Laboratory Tests

1. Hematocrit and hemoglobin
   Abnormality: Decreased in hemorrhage-induced hypovolemia
   Increased in other types of hypovolemia due to hemoconcentration
   Normal in all other types of shock

2. White blood cell (WBC) count and differential
   Abnormality: Increased in septic shock
   Normal in all other types of shock

3. Arterial blood gases (ABGs)
   Abnormality: Increased pH reflecting respiratory alkalosis in early shock
   Decreased pH reflecting metabolic acidosis in late shock

4. Serum lactate
   Abnormality: Increased in all types of progressive shock

5. Serum chemistries
   Abnormality: Increased serum glucose in early shock
   Increased blood urea nitrogen (BUN) and creatinine with renal failure
   Increased serum sodium in early shock
   Increased serum potassium in intermediate and late-stage shock

Increased serum calcium with lactic acidosis
Decreased serum potassium in early shock
Decreased serum calcium in early shock and with transfusions
6. Urinalysis
   Abnormality: Increased specific gravity
7. Cardiac enzymes
   Abnormality: Increased if cardiogenic shock follows acute myocardial infarction (AMI)
8. Blood culture
   Abnormality: Positive, usually for one organism in septic shock
9. Culture and sensitivity
   Abnormality: Positive results from a culture taken from the source of infection in septic shock

Diagnostic Tests

1. Hemodynamic monitoring
   Abnormality: CO <4 L/min; >8 L/min in the early (warm) phase of septic shock
   Pulmonary artery pressure (PAP) <17/4 mm Hg; >32/13 mm Hg in cardiogenic shock
   Pulmonary capillary wedge pressure <8 mm Hg; >12 mm Hg in cardiogenic shock
   Central venous pressure (CVP) <2 cm H_2O
   Systolic arterial blood pressure initially rises, systolic may be stable and diastolic may rise, systolic and diastolic may both fall, or no blood pressure may be present.
2. Chest X-ray
   Abnormality: Presence of thoracic trauma; infection; ARDS
3. Pulse oximetry and transcutaneous oxygen monitoring
   Abnormality: Oxygen saturation of less than 85%
4. Electrocardiogram (ECG)
   Abnormality: Evidence of myocardial injury or ischemia
5. Peritoneal lavage
   Abnormality: Frank blood or concentration of blood in lavage fluid to indicate intra-abdominal bleeding in hypovolemic shock
6. Angiography

Abnormality: Vessel tears or traumatic aneurysms in hypovolemic shock
7. Exploratory surgery
   Abnormality: Unrecognized internal injury in hypovolemic shock
8. Gastrointestinal endoscopy
   Abnormality: Gastritis and/or stress ulcers in hypovolemic shock
9. Spinal X-rays
   Abnormality: Spinal fractures and/or cord injury in neurogenic shock
10. Computed tomography scan or magnetic resonance imaging
    Abnormality: Spinal cord injury in neurogenic shock
11. Noninvasive cardiology studies (e.g., ECG, echocardiogram, or multiple gated acquisitions scan)
    Abnormality: Damage to the heart muscle and/or blood supply in cardiogenic shock
12. Invasive cardiology studies
    Abnormality: Damage to the heart muscle and/or blood supply in cardiogenic shock

Planning Intervention

COLLABORATIVE MANAGEMENT

Procedures

1. For all forms of shock
   a. Continuously monitor hemodynamic parameters to evaluate the cardiovascular response to treatment.
   b. Continuously monitor blood pressure to determine the cardiovascular response to treatment.
   c. Continuously monitor urinary output via catheter to evaluate renal function.
   d. Monitor cardiac rhythm for tachycardia and life-threatening ventricular arrhythmias (ventricular tachycardia and/or fibrillation).
   e. Maintain a patent airway and adequate ventilation. Use supplemental oxygen to ensure that sufficient oxygen is delivered to the lungs.

  f. Provide enteral nutrition or parenteral nutritional support to prevent a negative nitrogen balance.
2. For hypovolemic shock
   a. Apply pressure to control external hemorrhage.
   b. Apply medical antishock trousers (controversial) to assist with major organ perfusion.
   c. Prepare patient for exploratory surgery to ascertain the extent of injury and repair damage.
   d. In extreme emergencies, untyped and uncross-matched blood (O negative) or type-specific, un-crossmatched blood may be given.
   e. Replace calcium if large amounts of packed red blood cells (RBCs) are administered.
3. For cardiogenic shock
   a. Monitor mechanical assistive devices — intra-aortic balloon pump, external counterpulsation device, ventricular assist device — to assess left ventricular function.
   b. Prepare patient for surgery — coronary artery by-pass graft — to reperfuse the infarcted part of the left ventricle.

Drug Therapy

1. Volume expanders
   Examples: Crystalloids — Should be used in the early phases of fluid replacement for hypovolemic, neurogenic, and septic shock. Ringer's solution (if the patient has a chance of returning to aerobic metabolism), Ringer's lactate, and normal saline solution commonly used.
       Colloids — Such as albumin and plasma substitutes (dextran, hetastarch) may be used in hypovolemic, cardiogenic, and septic shock but are not recommended for trauma
       Blood or blood products — Packed RBCs, whole blood autotransfusion, and synthetic blood products may be used in severe hemorrhage with hypovolemic shock
   Action: Replace lost intravascular volume and blood components
   Caution: Can cause hypervolemia, pulmonary edema, or hepatitis

2. Sodium bicarbonate
   Action: Helps to reverse the metabolic acidosis that occurs as hypovolemic shock progresses
   Caution: Can cause metabolic alkalosis

3. Inotropic agents
   Example: dopamine (Intropin)
   norepinephrine (Levophed)
   dobutamine (Dobutrex)
   Action: Improves myocardial contractility; increases CO and arterial blood pressure; and organ perfusion in hypovolemic, cardiogenic, and septic shock
   Caution: Can increase myocardial oxygen consumption and demand, cause oliguria and vasoconstriction, and worsen hypokalemia and arrhythmias

4. Vasodilators
   Examples: Nitroglycerin (Trindil)
   nitroprusside (Nipride)
   chlorpromazine (Thorazine)
   phentolamine (Regitine)
   Action: Decreases preload and afterload and dilates the coronary arteries to improve myocardial oxygen supply in hypovolemic and cardiogenic shock
   Reverses vasoconstriction and improves tissue perfusion in septic shock
   Caution: Can cause hypotension; Nipride can cause cyanate toxicity

5. Diuretics
   Examples: furosemide (Lasix)
   bumetanide (Bumex)
   Action: Increases urine excretion by affecting water and electrolyte absorption within the glomerulus in hypovolemic shock
   Caution: Can cause hypokalemia and dehydration

6. Thrombolytics
   Examples: streptokinase (Streptase)
   tissue plasminogen activator (Activase)
   Action: In cardiogenic shock caused by AMI, can restore circulation to the ischemic portion of the left ventricle by dissolving the clot obstructing blood flow to the area
   Caution: Can cause uncontrolled bleeding and arrhythmias

7. Antihistamines
   Examples: epinephrine (Adrenalin)
      diphenhydramine (Benadryl)
   Action: Block the action of histamine, thus reversing bronchoconstriction, hypotension, and vasodilation in anaphylactic shock
   Caution: Can cause tachycardia, anxiety, and drowsiness
8. Steroids
   Example: hydrocortisone (Hydrocortone)
   Action: Stabilize capillary walls, thus decreasing fluid shifts out of the vasculature in anaphylactic shock
   Caution: Can cause hypokalemia, hypernatremia, nausea, and petechiae
9. Bronchodilators
   Example: aminophylline (theophylline)
   Action: Relieves bronchoconstriction in anaphylactic shock and is longer acting than epinephrine
   Caution: Can cause tachycardia and anxiety
      May reach toxic blood levels
10. Vagolytics
    Example: atropine sulfate
    Action: Counteracts the bradycardic effects of the vagus nerve on the heart, thus producing increased heart rate in neurogenic shock
    Caution: Can cause dry mouth, tachycardia, and urinary retention
11. Antibiotics
    Examples: cephalosporins
       ticarcillin (Timentin)
       ceftazidime (Fortaz)
    aminoglycosides
       gentamycin (Garamycin)
       tobramycin (Nebcin)
    Action: Bacteriocidal to gram-positive and gram-negative aerobic and anaerobic bacteria in septic shock
    Caution: May cause allergic reaction, nephrotoxicity, and ototoxicity
       Before the source is identified, at least a two-drug combination should be given
       When the source is identified, therapy may be tailored to the cause

Experimental Therapies for Septic Shock

Several drugs are thought to interrupt the septic process and are being used experimentally to treat septic shock. Below is how these drugs are thought to work.

Naloxone	Interacts with the endogenous opiate system
Monoclonal antibodies	Interact with endotoxin or tumor necrosis factor
Nonsteroidal anti-inflammatory drugs	Inhibit prostaglandin formation
Allopurinol	Inhibits production of toxic oxygen free radicals
Human endotoxin antiserum	Causes production of antibodies to endotoxin
Prostacyclin and PGE$_2$ analogs	Cause vasodilation and increased peripheral tissue perfusion

NURSING MANAGEMENT

Monitoring and Managing Clinical Problems

1. Fluid Volume Excess or Deficit: high risk for — Monitor for hemodynamic instability and promote hemodynamic stability.
   a. Assist with insertion of central lines and continuously monitor hemodynamic parameters.
   b. Titrate fluids and inotropic agents to maintain a systolic blood pressure of at least 80 mm Hg.
   c. Position the patient in modified Trendelenburg position (elevation of the legs at 45 degrees).
2. Gas Exchange: impaired: high risk for — Monitor and promote adequate oxygenation.
   a. Administer ordered supplemental oxygen.
   b. Obtain specimens for and monitor results of serial ABGs and hemoglobin, and report abnormalities.
   c. Monitor capillary refill and skin color to assess peripheral perfusion.

3. Tissue Perfusion, altered, peripheral, high risk for—
   Monitor for altered organ and tissue perfusion.
   a. Monitor for decreased urine output and elevated renal
      function tests, possibly indicating acute renal failure.
   b. Monitor for a falling arterial oxygen concentration,
      possibly indicating ARDS.
   c. Auscultate abdomen for decreased or absent bowel
      sounds, possibly indicating gastroparesis, and ob-
      serve for bright-red or coffee-ground drainage from
      nasogastric tube suggesting stress ulceration.
   d. Check temperature every 4 hours for hypothermia or
      hyperthermia.
   e. Monitor for decreased alertness and attention span,
      drowsiness, or excessive sleeping indicating down-
      ward changes in the level of consciousness.
4. Fluid Volume Deficit—Monitor for and prevent loss of
   fluid volume from the vasculature in hypovolemic shock.
   a. Provide ordered fluid replacement.
   b. Maintain accurate intake and output measurements
      hourly.
   c. Monitor blood pressure continuously.
   d. Monitor skin and mucous membranes for signs of
      dehydration.
   e. Monitor for onset of an S_3 heart sound, peripheral
      edema, and moist crackles in the lungs indicating fluid
      volume overload.
   f. Closely monitor pertinent laboratory data (serum
      electrolytes, urine studies) to assess hydration status.
5. Protection: altered—Monitor for and prevent complications of massive blood transfusions in hypovolemic
   shock.
   a. Monitor for coagulopathy.
      1) Can be due to the absence of functioning platelets
         and factors V and VIII in stored blood, hemodilu-
         tion, or possibly hypotension.
      2) Monitor platelet count, fibrinogen level, and bleed-
         ing time.
      3) Be prepared to administer fresh frozen plasma and
         platelet packs after patient's receiving 15–20 U of
         blood, if ordered.
   b. Monitor for hyperkalemia/hypokalemia.
      1) Hyperkalemia is due to leakage of intracellular po-

tassium into the plasma; each unit of blood may reach a potassium level of 30 mEq/L after 3 weeks of storage.

2) Hypokalemia may result due to the alkalosis that occurs when citrate in blood is metabolized into bicarbonate.

3) Identify patients at risk for developing hyperkalemia (patients with compromised renal function, shock and/or acidosis).

4) Monitor serial serum potassium levels and report abnormalities.

5) Monitor for cardiac arrhythmias that may result from altered serum potassium levels.

c. Monitor for hypocalcemia (rare).

1) Can be due to the addition of citrate to stored blood, which binds calcium and prevents clotting.

2) Assess for patients at risk for developing hypocalcemia (patients with severe liver disease and those receiving one unit of blood or more every 5 minutes).

3) Monitor for decreased serial ionized calcium levels and for prolongation of the QT interval.

4) Administer supplemental calcium, as ordered (rarely needed and should be administered only in cases of proven hypocalcemia).

d. Monitor for acid-base alterations.

1) Assess for metabolic acidosis in the acute phase. Patients requiring massive blood transfusions are in a low-flow shock state and develop a metabolic acidosis due to an increased lactic acid production.

2) Stored blood's pH decreases over time due to an increase in lactic acid and a fall in plasma bicarbonate level; may carry an acid load of 30–40 mEq/L per unit.

3) Assess for metabolic alkalosis as the patient stabilizes. As tissue perfusion is restored, the citrate in blood and the lactate in resuscitation fluids are metabolized to bicarbonate, causing a metabolic alkalosis. If perfusion and an aerobic metabolism are not restored, acidosis may develop.

4) Monitor serial arterial blood pH and venous CO_2 for acidosis/alkalosis.

e. Monitor for alterations in hemoglobin function.
   1) Levels of 2,3-diphosphoglycerate (2,3-DPG) in banked blood decline to 40% of initial levels after 3 weeks of storage. The low levels of 2,3-DPG result in a tighter binding of oxygen to hemoglobin and impaired tissue oxygenation (shift in the oxyhemoglobin dissociation curve to the left). RBCs rapidly regenerate 2,3-DPG within 24 hours of transfusion, depending on the patient's metabolic state.
   2) Assess for alkalosis, hypothermia, and hypoxemia. Alkalosis and hypothermia combined with low levels of 2,3-DPG enhance the binding of oxygen to hemoglobin, causing hypoxemia.
   3) Assess for acidosis, which enhances the release of oxygen from hemoglobin.
   4) Be prepared to use cryopreserved blood or blood that is less than 14 days old to ensure an adequate supply of 2,3-DPG, if clinically indicated.
f. Monitor for hypothermia from the rapid administration of cold, stored blood.
   1) Assess for the adverse effects of hypothermia.
      a) Arrhythmias
      b) Decreased CO
      c) Decreased metabolism of citrate and lactate
      d) Tighter binding of oxygen to hemoglobin
      e) Impaired hemostasis
   2) Monitor patient's core temperature continuously.
   3) Administer blood through a heating coil, when possible.
g. Monitor for ammonia intoxication from increased ammonia content in stored blood.
   1) Identify patients at risk for developing ammonia intoxication like those with severe liver disease.
   2) Monitor for signs and symptoms of hepatic encephalopathy/coma.
      a) Changes in the level of consciousness
      b) Behavioral changes
      c) Increased liver function tests
h. Monitor for microaggregates from the formation of blood clots and other cellular debris with increased storage time of blood.
   1) Use blood filters when administering blood to help

to reduce the number of microaggregates that reach the lung.

2) Administer all blood with a standard blood filter of 170–260 µm pore size to remove large clots and debris. Change blood filter after every 2 U of blood or packed RBCs.

3) When possible, use a microaggregate blood filter of 20–40 µm pore size to remove smaller clots and debris.

4) Always prime blood administration lines with normal saline solution.

5) Use normal saline solution in the intravenous (IV) line designated for blood transfusion.

i. Monitor for hemolytic transfusion reactions from ABO incompatibility.

1) Usually results from misidentification of the patient or the mismatching of blood, and results in intravascular hemolysis.

2) Monitor patient for hypotension, chest pain, back pain, chills, fever, pain at the infusion site, shock, nausea, acute renal failure, and bleeding.

3) Prevent this reaction by carefully labeling all blood specimens sent to the laboratory and by following hospital policy regarding the administration of blood.

j. Monitor for febrile transfusion reactions from the administration of platelets or leukocytes to which the patient has antibodies.

1) Monitor for fever, chills, and dyspnea.

2) Prevent reaction by administering washed RBCs or leukocyte-poor blood and premedication with antipyretics in patients with history of reaction.

k. Monitor for allergic transfusion reactions from hypersensitivity to a substance in the donor's plasma.

1) Monitor patient for signs and symptoms of urticaria progressing to an anaphylactic reaction.

2) Prevent reaction by administration of antihistamines and washed blood products in patients with history of reaction.

l. Monitor for transmission of infections from blood transfusion.

1) Human immunodeficiency virus (HIV [acquired

immunodeficiency syndrome]), HIV-II, human T-cell lymphomavirus (HTLV)-I, HTLV-II, hepatitis B and C, bacteria (gram-negative bacteria), cyto-megalovirus, Epstein-Barr virus, syphilis, malaria, and parasites can be transmitted by blood trans-fusion.

   2) Prevent infection by aseptic administration of blood, proper blood bank storage, adequate blood bank screening for infections, and proper blood bank treatment of blood products.

   3) Current estimate of getting HIV from blood transfu-sion is 1:40,000 to 1:200,000.

   4) Posttransfusion incidence of hepatitis ranges from 1–10%.

6. Cardiac Output: decreased — Monitor and promote ade-quate CO in cardiogenic shock.

   a. Continuously monitor hemodynamic parameters.

   b. Monitor ventricular assistive devices to assess pa-tient's response.

   c. Titrate drug therapy to improve CO.

   d. Restrict patient activity to decrease energy ex-penditure.

7. Tissue Perfusion, altered: peripheral, high risk for —

Ventricular Assist Devices

Type of Device	Advantages	Disadvantages
Centrifugally driven	Less expensive Most frequently used device Right, left, or biventricular support	Nonpulsatile flow Must have intra-aortic balloon pump to produce flow Machine is external High potential for infection Anticoagulation needed Hemolysis may occur with high flows

Ventricular Assist Devices — *Continued*

Type of Device	*Advantages*	*Disadvantages*
Pneumatically driven	Pulsatile flow Synchronous, asynchronous, or volume modes Right, left, or biventricular support	Machine is external High potential for infection
Electromagnetically driven	Pulsatile flow Machine is implanted internally Pumps synchronously with patient's heart Reduces afterload	Used only in left ventricular failure Machine is implanted

Monitor for and prevent failure of the vasomotor center in neurogenic shock resulting in massive vasodilation.

a. Reduce vagal stimulation by reducing patient straining with stool softeners.

b. Observe for bradycardia and treat with atropine, if necessary.

c. Monitor for hypothermia and apply extra blankets or external warming devices, as needed.

d. Administer ordered vagolytic drugs.

e. Continuously monitor blood pressure and report abnormalities.

8. Protection: altered — Monitor for and interrupt antigen-antibody reaction in anaphylactic shock.

a. Prevent further contact with the antigen.

b. Administer drugs to counteract the effects of the antigen.

c. Monitor closely for respiratory distress and intervene promptly.

9. Infection: high risk for — Monitor for and promote treatment of sepsis in septic shock.

a. Administer ordered antibiotics.
b. Obtain specimens for culture and sensitivity of all potential infection sites.
c. Monitor serial WBC counts and serum peak and trough levels of antibiotics for effectiveness of treatment.
d. Monitor temperature every 4 hours and treat, as needed, with medications or external cooling devices.

Monitoring, Managing, and Preventing Life-Threatening Emergencies

1. Shock, in and of itself, is a life-threatening emergency.
2. Respiratory failure
   a. Monitor for and prevent increasing respiratory distress leading to increasing hypoxemia.
      1) Monitor serial ABGs and report abnormalities.
      2) Monitor serial chest X-ray reports.
      3) Auscultate lungs frequently for decreased breath sounds, crackles, and/or rhonchi.
      4) Apply pulse oximeter and continuously measure oxygen saturation.
      5) Administer ordered bronchodilators.
      6) Monitor for air hunger, tachypnea, restlessness, and confusion indicating increasing respiratory distress.
   b. Prepare for immediate intubation, if necessary.
   c. Monitor for effective ventilation while patient is on mechanical ventilator.
      1) Reassess lung sounds frequently.
      2) Suction, as needed, to remove sputum and promote a clear airway.
      3) Measure lung compliance frequently and report decreases.
      4) Measure pulmonary peak pressures and report increases.
      5) Sedate the patient, as needed, to control ventilator fighting. Administration of paralytics also may be necessary.
      6) Monitor serial ABGs for effectiveness of mechanical ventilation. Indications for positive end-expiratory pressure (PEEP) include the following:
         a) PaO_2 <60 mm/Hg on an FiO_2 >50%
         b) pH <7.25

       c) $Paco_2$ >45 mm Hg

   7) Decrease Fio_2 to <50% as quickly as possible to prevent oxygen toxicity.

   8) PEEP holds alveoli open, thus increasing functional residual capacity, decreasing shunting, and decreasing hypoxemia. But, PEEP can:

       a) Decrease CO

       b) Increase the chance of oxygen toxicity

       c) Cause fluid overload

3. Multisystem organ failure

  a. Monitor patients at risk and recognize onset during the early phases.

    1) Assess for risk factors.

    2) Be alert for early warning signals.

      a) Increased or decreased temperature

      b) Increasing heart rate

      c) Tachypnea (increased respiratory rate)

      d) Increased or decreased WBC count

      e) Subtle changes in sensorium

    3) Report findings consistent with the development of multisystem organ failure.

  b. Prevent organ injury.

    1) Provide ventilatory support through intubation and mechanical ventilation.

    2) Institute measures to control body temperature to adjust for hyperthermia or hypothermia.

    3) Reverse acidosis.

    4) Monitor for progression of disorder.

      a) Monitor for subtle changes in assessment findings that may indicate deterioration from the hyperdynamic phase to the hypodynamic phase.

      b) Measure hemodynamic parameters frequently and report changes.

      c) Assess the patient frequently, paying particular attention to serial findings to identify deterioration in previously uninvolved organ systems.

      d) Analyze changes in laboratory values to determine deterioration of multiple organs.

      e) Monitor patient's responses to medications and treatments, and report significant findings.

  c. Provide supportive care.

    1) Control the infection.

a) Obtain a specimen of all secretions for culture and sensitivity testing.
b) Prepare the patient for surgical intervention to remove sources of infection.
c) Promote an aseptic environment to prevent nosocomial infections.
   1] Use aseptic technique when providing care.
   2] Monitor invasive tube sites for signs and symptoms of infection.
   3] Wash hands frequently.
   4] Monitor serial WBCs for signs of infection.
   5] Obtain specimen of suspicious secretions for culture and sensitivity testing.
   6] Immediately report signs and symptoms of infection.
   7] Monitor the patient's temperature every 4 hours and more frequently if fever develops.
   8] Administer ordered medications to prevent or fight infection, and monitor patient's response to them.

2) Arrest and reverse the progress of the syndrome.
   a) Prevent translocation of bacteria from the gut with enteral feeding of glutamine, an immuno-nutrient that maintains gut integrity and stimulates the immune system.
   b) Prepare for continuous arteriovenous hemo-diafiltration, which has been used successfully in trauma patients.
   c) Recognize complications, such as:
      1] Skin breakdown
         a] Use pressure-relieving devices (e.g., pads, mattresses, specialty beds) to prevent breakdown.
         b] Turn the patient every 2 hours, if possible.
         c] Assess the skin every 4 hours to identify and intervene in the early stages of breakdown.
         d] Consult the enterostomal therapy nurse for definitive treatment of skin breakdown.
      2] Third spacing of fluid

a] Assess the patient every 4 hours for edema, ascites, or anasarca.

b] Weigh the patient daily and report significant increases.

c] Accurately measure intake and output, and report significant disparities.

d] Monitor lung sounds every 4 hours and report changes.

e] Administer ordered diuretics to increase urine output.

  3) Provide metabolic support.

a) Measure oxygen consumption with increased oxygen flow rate until lactic acid level returns to normal.

b) Provide adequate nutrition. Enteral route is preferred over parenteral using a formula that is high in protein and has medium-chain triglycerides for lipids.

4. Acute tubular necrosis

a. Prevent complications related to continued hypotension, infection, and use of nephrotoxic agents.

  1) Administer ordered IV fluids and medications.

  2) Regulate fluid intake to achieve fluid and electrolyte balance.

  3) Administer ordered buffering agents to regulate acid-base balance.

  4) Preserve neurologic function by closely observing for decreasing level of consciousness.

b. Manage nutritional status.

  1) Restrict protein intake to maintain anabolism while limiting load on kidneys; amount varies depending on patient's weight and activity level and whether or not patient is on dialysis; protein needs to be high biologic value.

  2) Restrict dietary potassium intake.

  3) Restrict fluid intake.

  4) Provide adequate calories to prevent catabolism.

  5) Administer ordered supplemental vitamins.

c. Maintain adequate level of RBCs for optimum tissue oxygenation through transfusion, as ordered.

d. Prepare to initiate renal replacement therapy for any of the following:

1) BUN >100 mg/dL
2) Serum creatinine >5–9 mg/dL or at lower serum creatinine levels for patients with reduced muscle mass, such as the elderly
3) Volume overload and signs of pulmonary edema
4) Pericarditis
5) Hyperkalemia that has not responded adequately to other treatment modalities
6) Uncontrollable acidosis
7) Central nervous system dysfunction related to uremia (e.g., encephalopathy or seizures)

e. Institute ordered renal replacement therapy.
   1) Hemodialysis
   2) Continuous ultrafiltration or continuous renal replacement therapy
   3) Peritoneal dialysis

5. Disseminated intravascular coagulopathy
   a. Assist with treatment of the underlying cause, such as surgical debridement of necrotic tissue/abscess or antibiotic treatment of pathogenic organisms.
      1) Sepsis—Administer IV fluids and antibiotics.
      2) Shock—Administer IV fluids, inotropic agents, and vasopressors.
   b. Administer heparin therapy, blood component therapy, and antithrombin therapy to stop the vicious cycle of thrombosis-hemorrhage.
   c. Maintain the patient on strict bed rest.
   d. Administer ordered medications to correct hemostatic deficiencies that compromise the clotting mechanisms.
   e. Administer ordered IV fluids to correct hypovolemia, hypotension, and tissue ischemia.
   f. Monitor vital signs for the following:
      1) Heart rate >100 bpm
      2) Systolic blood pressure <90 mm Hg
      3) CVP <5 mm Hg
      4) Mean arterial pressure <60 mm Hg
   g. Palpate pulses for adequate extremity perfusion.
   h. Monitor adequate oxygenation and acid-base status.
      1) Assess breath sounds every 4 hours and as needed.

2) Monitor for abnormal ABGs, dyspnea, cyanosis, and hypoxemia.
3) Administer ordered oxygen.
4) Apply pulse oximeter and continuously monitor arterial oxygen saturation.
5) Prevent atelectases by having the patient turn, cough, and deep breath every 2 hours.
6) Administer ordered bronchodilators and fluid replacement.
7) Monitor mental status for oxygenation problems.
8) Implement PEEP, sedation, and paralysis, as ordered.

i. Monitor for decreased urine output and increased specific gravity.
1) May indicate hypovolemia or renal microemboli.
2) May indicate fluid retention.

j. Monitor for fluid overload, which can lead to pulmonary edema or pleural effusion.
1) Assess heart and lung sounds for abnormalities every 4 hours.
2) Monitor CO and PAP every 4 hours.
3) Record hourly intake of IV and oral fluids, and hourly urine output.

k. Monitor and manage skin and mucous membranes for ischemia, bleeding, cyanosis, and lesions.
1) Perform frequent mouth care, since ischemia is common in the mouth.
2) Use a mild solution of peroxide for oral care.
3) Avoid mouthwashes containing alcohol.
4) Suction trachea, as needed, using low pressure to prevent damage to the tracheal mucosa.
5) Keep the skin moist and intact by applying lotions to the skin and lubricants to the lips.
6) Note extremity warmth, color, and pulses.
7) Check emesis, nasogastric drainage, and stool for occult blood.

l. Monitor and manage comfort level.
1) Reposition every 2 hours for comfort and proper alignment.
2) Rate pain level on a scale of 0–10 every 1–2 hours.
3) Administer pain medication promptly.

    4) Use noninvasive pain relief measures such as re-laxation techniques.

    5) Prepare patient for all treatments and procedures.

    6) Involve patient's family and friends in open discussions of emotional issues.

    7) Perform gentle range of motion exercises every 2 hours.

m. Monitor and manage nutrition.

    1) Maintain strict intake and output.

    2) Monitor hyperalimentation, if ordered.

    3) Avoid the use of hot fluids that will irritate the oral mucosa and cause gingival bleeding.

    4) Weigh daily and maintain body weight within 10% of normal weight.

    5) Assess bowel sounds for presence of paralytic ileus.

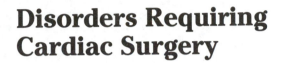

Disorders Requiring Cardiac Surgery

Cardiac surgery describes many different procedures to repair both congenital as well as acquired heart defects.

The major types of cardiac surgery include the following:

1. Coronary artery bypass graft surgery (CABG) is the most common type of open heart surgery performed for occlusion of the coronary artery. It involves bypassing the occluded coronary vessel with a venous graft attached proximal and distal to the occlusion. Multiple bypasses can be done during one surgical procedure. The graft is usually from the mammary artery or the saphenous vein. A surgical incision will be present in the leg if the saphenous vein is used.

2. Valve replacement is open heart surgery during which a defective valve is replaced by an artificial valve.

3. Commissurotomy is closed heart surgery during which the commissures of the valve leaflets are opened and the overall size of the valve opening enlarged. This surgical procedure provides palliative relief, and the patient will require valve replacement in the future.

4. Annuloplasty is closed heart surgery during which the patient's own valve ring is modified by suturing or adding a Carpentier ring to pull together the annulus (or opening) and promoting proper valve leaflet closure. This also offers palliative relief. The patient will require future valve replacement.

5. Automatic implantable cardiac defibrillator insertion requires a thoracotomy to implant a small generator, electrodes, and defibrillator patches onto the closed heart. Defibrillator patches are placed on the exterior surface of the heart in the area best suited for defibrillation of the individual. A subcutaneous pocket and tunnel are formed for the generator and electrodes. The device is tested before closure of the chest. These devices also may have the capability to pace the heart.

6. Permanent pacemaker insertion is closed heart surgery to insert a pacemaker battery and electrodes. Depending on where the electrode is attached to the cardiac muscle, the patient may or may not have a thoracotomy. In a transvenous approach, there is only a small incision for the pulse generator. A transmediastinal approach is common for epicardial pacemaker insertion. The pulse generator, or battery pack, is usually placed either in the subcutaneous tissue of the clavicular or upper epigastric area. There may be either one (unipolar) or two (bipolar) pacing leads. Permanent pacemakers often use only one lead. The electrodes on the pacing leads are placed either in contact with the endocardium of the right atrium and/or right ventricle, or may be attached to the left ventricular epicardium.

7. Maze surgery requires open heart surgery to treat atrial fibrillation. In this procedure, small incisions are placed in the right and left atria that act as circuit breakers to prevent atrial fibrillation.

Etiology/Pathophysiology of Cardiac Disorders Requiring Surgery

1. Coronary artery occlusion
   a. Can occur slowly over many years, without symptoms, until the patient decompensates when the heart is stressed. Angina occurs when the coronary muscle is ischemic.
   b. CABG redirects blood around the obstruction to the affected area, bypassing the occlusion and providing oxygen to the ischemic area.
2. Valvular defects
   a. Occur as a result of congenital defects, aftermath of rheumatic fever, syphilis, mitral valve prolapse, or infective endocarditis.
   b. Valve malfunction may be caused by either of the following:
      1) Stenosis — Valve becomes calcified; movement of the valve leaflets is compromised by the stiffness of the valve as well as by the fibrosis of the muscle support structures
      2) Regurgitation — Valve is incompetent, resulting in regurgitation, or blood backflow into the previous chamber (See Table, Assessing and Treating Valvular Disorder)
3. Ruptured papillary muscle after acute myocardial infarction (AMI): A complication of myocardial infarction (MI), in which the muscle that anchors the mitral valve malfunctions. There is massive mitral valve regurgitation and subsequent pulmonary edema. This is a medical emergency; without replacement of the mitral valve, death is imminent.

Assessment/Analysis

POSTOPERATIVE ASSESSMENT FINDINGS

Subjective

1. Blurred vision
2. Incisional pain, which must be differentiated from angina

Objective

1. Temperature will be hypothermic upon arrival at intensive care unit; elevation occurs approximately 4–8 hours after surgery.
2. Elevated systemic vascular resistance due to hypothermia and vasoconstriction

Nursing Alert

As temperature elevates to normal, systemic vascular resistance decreases with vasodilation and blood pressure drops.

3. Bloody mediastinal and/or chest-tube drainage
4. Elevated urine output first few hours postoperatively due to primary hemodilution and fluid shifts; may also be due to osmotic diuresis induced by mannitol administered intraoperatively
5. Cardiac arrhythmias, varying in origin
6. Midline chest incision
7. Leg incision(s) for saphenous vein graft (no incision noted for mammary artery graft)
8. Respirations supported on mechanical ventilator with endotracheal tube in place
9. Nasogastric tube to low suction
10. Level of consciousness varies — Should easily awaken. Decreased level of consciousness indicates possible hypoxemia, embolism to brain, drug overdose, poor cerebral perfusion.
11. Lung sounds vary with cardiopulmonary status.
12. Heart sounds vary with cardiopulmonary status; they are generally weaker than preoperative assessment.

SUPPORTING TEST FINDINGS

Laboratory Tests

1. Arterial blood gases (ABGs)
   Abnormality: Metabolic acidosis in immediate postoperative period due to "washout acidosis"; when patient taken off cardiopulmonary bypass machine, the lactic acid from poorly perfused areas washes into the circulation

2. Partial thromboplastin time (PTT), activated partial thromboplastin time (APTT)
   Abnormality: Increased; prolonged clotting time first few hours after surgery; results from heparin rebound (drug hidden then released from tissues) or from inadequate heparin reversal after bypass
3. Platelets
   Abnormality: Decreased; may be due to damage incurred while on heart-lung bypass machine
4. White blood cell count
   Abnormality: Increased for at least 48 hours postoperatively
5. Hemoglobin and hematocrit
   Abnormality: Decreased with postoperative bleeding
6. Serum cardiac enzymes/isoenzymes
   Abnormality: Increased if myocardial injury present
7. Blood glucose
   Abnormality: Increased postoperatively due to decreased insulin production and epinephrine discharge

Diagnostic Tests

1. Electrocardiography
   Abnormality: Identification of new MI
2. Cardiac monitoring
   Abnormality: Atrial arrhythmias including atrial fibrillation; sinus tachycardia, bradycardia; first-, second-, or third-degree heart block
   Ventricular arrhythmias including premature ventricular contractions, ventricular tachycardia, and ventricular fibrillation
3. Cardiac catheterization
   Abnormality: Dependent on area affected; coronary occlusion or valve dysfunction
   Abnormal pressures or blood gas analysis within heart chambers
4. Echocardiography—M-mode, two-dimensional, color Doppler
   Abnormality: Aberrant direction of blood flow through heart chambers
   Decreased oxygenation or valvular function
   Left ventricular wall motion abnormalities
   Pericardial effusions

5. Hemodynamic monitoring

Abnormality: Pulmonary artery pressure (PAP) >30 mm Hg

Pulmonary capillary wedge pressure (PCWP) >12 mm Hg

Cardiac output (CO) <4 L/min

Cardiac index <2.5 L/min per meter squared

Planning/Intervention

COLLABORATIVE MANAGEMENT

Procedures

1. Support and monitor CO.
   a. Administer oxygen via endotracheal tube and mechanical ventilation.
   b. Insert multiple intravenous (IV) lines.
      1) Administer ordered crystalloid and colloid solutions.
      2) Administer ordered blood products.
   c. Monitor chest-tube drainage and report abnormalities.
   d. Monitor arterial pressure line for stability and patency. Arterial line will be placed during surgery.
   e. Observe cardiac monitor for the following:
      1) Proper pacemaker function
      2) Change in rate, rhythm, or presence of arrhythmias
   f. Observe pulmonary artery catheter measurements and report significant changes.
   g. Monitor and report hourly intake and output.
   h. Maintain intra-aortic balloon pump.
2. Prevent damage to myocardium, kidneys, and lungs.
   a. Observe cardiac monitor for changes in rhythm or rate.
   b. Administer ordered analgesics and monitor patient response.
   c. Administer ordered antiarrhythmics and monitor patient response.
   d. Administer ordered beta$_2$-receptor antagonists and monitor patient response.

e. Maintain mechanical ventilator and endotracheal airway.
f. Protect integrity of mediastinal/chest tube.
g. Maintain intra-aortic balloon pump.
h. Administer ordered inotropic agents and monitor patient response.
i. Keep strict intake and output.
j. Observe for nasogastric tube patency.
k. Measure daily weights.
l. Observe and record hemodynamic parameters and report significant changes.

Drug Therapy

1. Antihypertensives/vasodilators
   Examples: sodium nitroprusside (Nipride)
   nitroglycerin (Nitro-bid)
   Action: Acts directly on vascular smooth muscles of arterial and venous vessels, causing dilation
   Decreases preload and afterload of heart
   Vasodilates coronary arteries and decreases coronary vascular resistance
   Caution: Use with extreme caution in the postcardiac surgery patient; patient status is dynamic; hypotension can create high probability of cardiovascular dysfunction
2. Inotropic agents
   Example: dopamine (Intropin)
   dobutamine (Dobutrex)
   Action: Increases CO and augments renal blood flow
   Caution: Dopamine may increase workload on heart
   Correct hypovolemia before administering either drug
3. Opioid analgesics
   Example: morphine sulfate (Duromorph)
   Action: Relieves severe pain, relaxes, and vasodilates
   Caution: Vasodilation can cause a hypotensive episode
   Administer cautiously; monitor patient's reaction
4. Blood products
   Example: Fresh frozen plasma
   Action: Stabilizes the clotting mechanism that has been altered by drugs (aspirin, heparin, nitroprusside) or by

the cardiopulmonary bypass machine; combats abnormal prothrombin time and PTT

Caution: Observe for febrile and allergic reaction due to development of antibodies

Example: Cryoprecipitate

Action: Increases fibrinogen levels

Caution: Observe for febrile and allergic reaction due to development of antibodies

Example: Platelets

Action: Increases platelet count; aids in restoring hemostasis and preventing bleeding

Caution: Observe for febrile and allergic reaction due to development of alloantibodies

5. Heparin antidote

Example: protamine sulfate

Action: An anticoagulant when used alone

Protamine's strong basic pH neutralizes acidic heparin to render both inactive

Caution: Protamine has longer half-life than heparin; must titrate dose to prevent anticoagulation

Can cause hemorrhage and subsequent shock; monitor vital signs and laboratory coagulation studies closely

6. Beta$_2$-receptor antagonist

Example: propranolol (Inderal)

Action: Decreases heart rate and myocardial irritability

Caution: Do not use in patients who are susceptible to congestive heart failure or slow heart rate

7. Inotropic agent

Example: isoproterenol (Isuprel)

Action: Stimulates myocardium in cardiac arrest

Caution: Do not use in cardiogenic shock secondary to AMI

Increases oxygen requirement of myocardial muscle

Causes ventricular arrhythmias

8. Antiarrhythmics

Example: lidocaine (Xylocaine)

Action: Anesthetic agent that decreases irritability of heart muscle, thus decreasing arrhythmias

Caution: Lidocaine toxicity can cause respiratory depression and arrest, as well as cardiac arrest

Do not use with slow heart rate or heart block

(See arrhythmias in the Rhythm Strip appendix.)

NURSING MANAGEMENT

Monitoring and Managing Clinical Problems

1. Fluid Volume Excess or Deficit
   a. Monitor fluid and electrolyte status.
      1) Monitor hourly intake and output.
      2) Monitor for abnormal PAP and PCWP hourly.
      3) Monitor for abnormal blood pressure or pulse continuously during the early postoperative hours.
      4) Obtain blood specimens and monitor serial serum electrolyte and blood glucose results; note and report significant changes.
      5) Observe cardiac monitor for changes in cardiac rhythm suggesting electrolyte imbalance.
      6) Monitor hemoglobin and hematocrit, as well as blood clotting studies immediately postoperatively and at regular intervals (4–8 hours, as indicated).
      7) Monitor chest-tube drainage amount and color hourly. Note/report any change in color and/or acute increase in amount.
   b. Promote fluid and electrolyte stability.
      1) Anticipate vasodilation upon patient rewarming. Administer crystalloid fluids as vascular space increases.
      2) Administer vasopressors to maintain effective hemodynamics parameters.
      3) Administer fluids and blood products as ordered, so that patient will have adequate CO, without stressing the suture site and thus increasing the possibility of bleeding.
      4) Administer additional potassium for hypokalemia.
      5) Obtain blood specimen for serum potassium if suspicious cardiac arrhythmias occur postoperatively.
      6) Notify doctor if chest-tube drainage >200 mL/h for more than 2 hours.
      7) Autotransfuse mediastinal drainage per protocol.
2. Cardiac Output: decreased
   a. Monitor/assess CO.

1) Note skin color, temperature.
2) Observe patient's level of consciousness.
3) Assess hourly urine output.
4) Monitor hemodynamic parameters, particularly CO and cardiac index.
5) Assess lungs for moist sounds, possibly indicating fluid overload or heart failure.
6) Assess heart for murmurs, S_3, and S_4.
7) Auscultate for presence or absence of bowel sounds.

b. Promote CO.
1) Administer ordered volume expander fluids.
2) Administer ordered antiarrhythmics to treat arrhythmias, as indicated.
3) Initiate temporary pacing, as indicated, by heart rate parameters.
4) Administer inotropic agents to maintain an adequate CO.
5) Administer vasodilator to lower peripheral vascular resistance.
6) Prepare for and maintain patient on intra-aortic balloon pump or ventricular assist device. Monitor results of therapy. Ensure proper timing of the balloon pump inflation/deflation as well as weaning.

3. Fluid Volume Deficit: high risk for (Actual Loss)— Postoperative bleeding
   a. Report significant changes in chest-tube output such as output >200 mL/h for more than 2 hours, sudden increase of >300 mL/h in a chest tube that previously has had only small amounts, or no drainage from previously patent tube.
   b. Report signs of cardiac tamponade, such as:
      1) Muffled heart sounds, softer than previous assessment
      2) Decreased blood pressure, CO
      3) Increased central venous pressure (CVP)
      4) Right- and left-sided intracardiac pressures elevated or similar
      5) Enlarged cardiac silhouette on chest X-ray
4. Cardiac Output: decreased, high risk for
   a. Arrhythmias

      1) Monitor blood gases for decreased oxygen, elevated carbon dioxide levels.

      2) Monitor electrolytes for imbalances.

      3) Initiate overdrive pacing for appropriate arrhythmias, as ordered.

  b. Improper intra-aortic balloon pump timing

      1) Use timing pin to inflate balloon at precise time for most beneficial augmentation.

      2) Monitor hemodynamics while adjusting timing pin to determine patient status.

  c. Pacemaker malfunction

      1) Monitor cardiac pattern continuously.

      2) Routinely check pacemaker function.

      3) Monitor pacemaker leads for microshock, leading to arrhythmias.

      4) Observe electrical safety standards with use of pacemaker, invasive lines.

5. Tissue Perfusion, altered: high risk for — Postperfusion syndrome: A failure of the heart to respond to the increased preload requirements postsurgery, causing decreased perfusion to the kidneys, liver, and brain

  a. Report decreased urinary output.

  b. Report decreased level of consciousness, confusion, or inappropriate behavior.

  c. Obtain blood specimens and monitor laboratory results for elevations of cardiac enzymes and isoenzymes, serum creatinine, and blood urea nitrogen.

Monitoring, Managing, and Preventing Life-Threatening Emergencies

1. Cardiac tamponade: Leakage of blood from the graft site, causing bleeding into the pericardial space, increasing pressure on the heart, and decreasing CO due to pump failure

  a. Recognize signs of fluid accumulation in pericardial space.

      1) Stabbing pain that worsens with movement or increased thoracic pressure

      2) Distended neck veins

      3) Dyspnea and cyanosis

        4) Restlessness, agitation
        5) Increased CVP
        6) Tachycardia
        7) Pericardial friction rub
        8) Muffled heart sounds
        9) Decreased blood pressure
        10) Pulsus paradoxus
   b. Check chest X-ray reports for widened mediastinum.
   c. Infuse IV colloids to aid in increasing CO.
   d. Prepare for and assist with immediate pericardiocentesis.
       1) Have emergency resuscitation equipment nearby.
       2) Monitor cardiac rhythm and immediately report elevations in PR or ST segments during pericardiocentesis. These elevations indicate the needle for aspiration is touching the myocardium.
       3) Upon aspiration of fluid, apply pressure to needle puncture site.
       4) Continuously monitor vital signs before, during, and after procedure.
       5) Observe for recurrent signs/symptoms of tamponade.
2. Severe hemorrhage leading to hypovolemic shock
   a. Monitor continuously for hemodynamic instability.
       1) Use continuous hemodynamic monitoring.
   b. Promote adequate oxygenation.
       1) Administer ordered supplemental oxygen, as indicated.
       2) Obtain specimens and monitor results of serial ABGs, hemoglobin, and hemocrit and report significant changes.
       3) Monitor capillary refill and monitor skin color to assess peripheral perfusion.
       4) Titrate fluids and inotropic agents to maintain a systolic blood pressure of at least 80 mm Hg.
       5) Position the patient in modified Trendelenburg position (elevation of the legs at 45 degrees).
   c. Monitor for altered organ and tissue perfusion.
       1) Monitor for decreased urine output and elevated renal function tests, possibly indicating acute renal failure.
       2) Monitor for a falling arterial oxygen concentration,

possibly indicating adult respiratory distress syndrome.
   3) Auscultate for decreased or absent bowel sounds suggesting gastroparesis, and note the presence of bright-red or coffee-ground drainage from the nasogastric tube, possibly indicating stress ulceration.
   4) Check temperature every 4 hours to monitor for hypothermia or hyperthermia.
   5) Monitor for decreased alertness and attention span, drowsiness, or excessive sleeping indicating downward changes in the level of consciousness.
   6) Monitor for loss of fluid volume from the vasculature.
      a) Administer ordered fluid replacement.
      b) Maintain accurate intake and output measurements hourly.
      c) Continuously monitor blood pressure.
3. Intra-aortic balloon rupture: The fracture of the balloon wall, with helium escaping into the bloodstream and immediate decrease in CO
   a. Have emergency resuscitation equipment nearby.
   b. Monitor intra-aortic balloon pump for abnormal pressure and absence of augmentation waveform.
   c. If CO drops, call for help.
   d. Continuously monitor hemodynamics and level of consciousness for evidence of deterioration.
   e. Administer ordered vasopressors and volume expanders, as indicated.
4. Cardiopulmonary arrest
   a. Call for help.
   b. Begin cardiopulmonary resuscitation.
   c. Follow with advanced cardiac life support.
5. Pulmonary embolism
   a. Monitor for signs of respiratory distress.
      1) Observe for dyspnea and tachypnea.
      2) Observe for anxiety, apprehension, and restlessness.
      3) Assess nailbeds for pallor or cyanosis.
      4) Assist with intubation and institute mechanical ventilation, if necessary.

    5) Apply pulse oximeter and continuously monitor oxygen saturation.

    6) Obtain specimens and monitor ABGs.

b. Promote activities to improve ventilation.

    1) Encourage coughing and deep breathing.

    2) Observe color and consistency of expectorated secretions. Hemoptysis (spitting or coughing blood) may occur.

    3) Administer ordered oxygen, as indicated.

    4) Observe for respiratory distress with patient care activities, interrupt care if it occurs, and space activities to prevent recurrence of respiratory distress.

    5) Elevate the head of the bed.

    6) Auscultate the lungs frequently for abnormalities and report significant findings.

c. Administer ordered anticoagulants and monitor for therapeutic and adverse effects.

    1) Observe injection sites, applying pressure until bleeding stops.

    2) Monitor nose and gums for bleeding during/following care.

    3) Monitor results of clotting studies to assess anticoagulation.

Assessing and Treating Valvular Disorders

Valve Dysfunction	Subjective Assessment Findings	Objective Assessment Findings	Treatment
Aortic stenosis	■ Anginal pain ■ Dyspnea ■ Syncope with exercise	■ Hypotension in advanced disease ■ Apical impulse forceful and displaced laterally and downward ■ Systolic thrill palpated at the base of the heart ■ Soft S_1; audible S_4; audible S_3 with left ventricular dilation and failure ■ Harsh midsystolic ejection murmur at the base of the heart	■ Digoxin* ■ Diuretics* ■ Sodium restriction* ■ Activity restriction* ■ Valve replacement*
Pulmonic stenosis	■ Exercise intolerance	■ Cardiac output unable to increase with exercise	■ Antibiotics* ■ Digoxin* ■ Diuretics*

Continued

Assessing and Treating Valvular Disorders—Continued

Valve Dysfunction	Subjective Assessment Findings	Objective Assessment Findings	Treatment
		■ Systolic thrill at second intercostal space, left sternal border ■ Harsh murmur at upper left sternal border	■ Sodium restriction ■ Valve commissurotomy or valvuloplasty*
Mitral stenosis	■ Dyspnea	■ Orthopnea ■ Paroxysmal nocturnal dyspnea ■ Cough ■ Dysphagia ■ Hoarseness ■ Soft, low-pitched, rumbling diastolic murmur ■ Opening snap (accentuated S_1)	■ Antibiotic prophylaxis ■ Digoxin* ■ Sodium restriction* ■ Activity restriction ■ Valvular commissurotomy or valve replacement*

Condition	Symptoms	Signs	Treatment

Tricuspid stenosis	- Fatigue
	- Exercise intolerance
		- In severe disease:
		  Resting tachycardia
		  Increased respirations
		  Narrowed pulse pressure
		  Neck vein distention with right ventricular dysfunction
		- Enlarged liver
		- Peripheral edema
		- Ascites
		- Jugular vein distention
		- Clear lungs
		- Rumbling diastolic murmur in the left lower sternal border
			- Antibiotic prophylaxis
			- Digoxin*
			- Diuretics*
			- Sodium restriction*
			- Valvular commissurotomy*

Aortic regurgitation (insufficiency)	- Dyspnea - Fatigue - Anginal pain	- Sweating - Warm, flushed appearance - Diastolic thrill palpated at the left lower sternal border	- Antibiotic prophylaxis - Digoxin* - Activity restriction* - Valve replacement*

Continued

Assessing and Treating Valvular Disorders — Continued

Valve Dysfunction	Subjective Assessment Findings	Objective Assessment Findings	Treatment
Pulmonic regurgitation (insufficiency)	■ Dyspnea ■ Fatigue	■ Apical pulse displaced laterally ■ Water-hammer pulse ■ Neck vein distention ■ Ascites ■ Weight gain ■ Peripheral edema ■ Enlarged liver ■ Diastolic murmur at the fifth intercostal space, left of the sternum	■ Antibiotic prophylaxis ■ Digoxin* ■ Sodium restriction* ■ Diuretics*
Mitral regurgitation (insufficiency)	■ Fatigue	■ Asymptomatic, in mild cases ■ Dyspnea, coughing, hoarseness ■ Enlarged liver ■ Embolization	■ Digoxin* ■ Vasodilators* ■ Sodium restriction ■ Activity restriction ■ Anticoagulants with atrial fibrillation

		■ Irregular pulse with atrial fibrillation ■ Apical pulse displaced laterally ■ Neck vein distention ■ Weak pulse ■ Tachycardia in acute cases ■ Split S_2 ■ S_3 in severe cases ■ Pansystolic murmur at heart apex, radiating to left midaxillary line ■ Lung congestion	■ Mitral valve replacement
Tricuspid regurgitation (insufficiency)	■ Dyspnea	■ Ascites ■ Neck vein distention ■ Enlarged liver ■ Systolic pulsations in neck ■ Irregular pulse with atrial fibrillation ■ Decreased bibasilar breath sounds	■ Digoxin* ■ Diuretics* ■ Sodium restriction* ■ Valve replacement, commissurotomy, or annuloplasty

Continued

Assessing and Treating Valvular Disorders— *Continued*

Valve Dysfunction	Subjective Assessment Findings	Objective Assessment Findings	Treatment
		■ Pansystolic murmur at the fourth intercostal space, left of the sternum, which increases on inspiration	

*Dependent on degree of congestive heart failure.

Arterial Peripheral Vascular Disorders Requiring Surgery

Arterial peripheral vascular disorders requiring surgical intervention describes those atherosclerotic disorders affecting arteries of the peripheral vascular system. Most commonly atherosclerosis causes occlusion of the vessel or weakens the vessel wall, causing an aneurysm, an outpouching of the arterial wall.

Etiology/Pathophysiology

1. Occlusive disorders
   a. Atherosclerosis is the buildup of fat and fibrous tissue within the lumen of the vessel. Buildup usually occurs at bifurcations or curves in the vessels, where pressure changes and injury to the inner lining most often occur. Eventually this injured tissue provides an opportune location for buildup of plaque.
   b. Risk factors associated with development of atherosclerosis
      1) Hypertension
      2) Diabetes mellitus
      3) Cigarette smoking
   c. Common areas of peripheral obstruction
      1) Carotid arteries
      2) Aorto-iliac junction
      3) Femoral-popliteal area
2. Aneurysms
   a. The outpouching is the result of the atherosclerotic process weakening the elasticity of the aorta. The aneurysm can further self-destruct by dissecting, or tearing, the length of the vessel.
   b. Common areas of weakened arterial walls
      1) Abdominal aorta
      2) Aortic arch
      3) Thoracic aorta
   c. Dissecting aneurysms are usually noted in the thoracic aorta, due to the high pressures being ejected from the heart. With dissection of the ascending thoracic aorta, the aortic valve may be damaged.
3. Major types of vascular surgeries/procedures
   a. Endarterectomy: Surgical removal of atherosclerotic deposits on the lining of the artery
   b. Bypass graft: Surgical detour of blood supply through an artificial graft, which is sewn above (superiorly) and below (inferiorly) to the obstructed/weakened area
   c. Graft: Surgical removal of the diseased or weakened vessel area and replacement with an artificial section
   d. Embolectomy, thrombectomy, or thromboembolec-

tomy: The surgical removal of an obstruction (either a blood clot, atherosclerotic plaque, or other substance) by use of a balloon or Fogarty catheter

e. Angioplasty: The widening of the inner lumen of the vessel by means of a balloon, inflated momentarily within the lumen

f. Arthrectomy: The use of a whirling blade to dislodge the atherosclerotic plaque during catheterization. This plaque is then sucked out through a portal drainage and emboli are avoided.

Assessment/Analysis

ASSESSMENT FINDINGS

Assessing for Common Peripheral Vascular Disorders

Type	Subjective Findings	Objective Findings
Peripheral vascular disease	■ Unilateral, cramping extremity pain, exacerbated by exercise and relieved by rest ■ Pain worsens in severity as tissue progresses from ischemic to necrotic ■ Pain depends on site of occlusion and presence of collateral circulation— calf, femoral, or popliteal; buttocks and upper thigh	■ Pale, shiny skin over affected extremity ■ Dependent rubor and edema as condition worsens ■ Line of demarcation in most severely affected area ■ Weak to absent peripheral pulses in affected extremity

Continued

Assessing for Common Peripheral Vascular Disorders — *Continued*

Type	Subjective Findings	Objective Findings
Aortic aneurysm	▪ May be asymptomatic ▪ Pain dependent on location and compression of adjacent structures ▪ Pain may increase in severity with rupture and lumbar nerve compression	▪ Palpable pulsatile mass in abdomen ▪ Weak to absent peripheral pulses bilaterally in lower extremities ▪ Abdominal bruit
Aortic dissection	▪ Pain reflecting point of dissection: neck, aortic arch; anterior chest, ascending aorta; low back, abdominal aorta ▪ Severe back or chest pain and a ripping, tearing sensation at onset of dissection ▪ Chest tightness moving toward abdomen	▪ Decreased level of consciousness ▪ Distended neck veins ▪ Decreased motor function ▪ Shortness of breath ▪ Decreased urine output, if renal involvement ▪ Tachycardia ▪ Pulse deficits — upper extremities, thoracic dissection
Carotid stenosis	▪ Syncope ▪ Dizziness ▪ Fuzzy or grey vision	▪ Motor weakness contralateral to obstruction

Assessing for Common Peripheral Vascular Disorders — *Continued*

Type	Subjective Findings	Objective Findings
	▪ Amnesia ▪ Decreased sensation contralateral to obstruction ▪ Decreased vision in one or both fields	▪ Decreased cognitive function ▪ Decreased to absent temporal pulses ▪ *Caution*: Never check both carotid pulses simultaneously

SUPPORTING TEST FINDINGS

Laboratory Tests

1. Blood urea nitrogen (BUN) and serum creatinine
   Abnormality: Increased; possible renal insufficiency due to low arterial flow or as a side effect to diagnostic tests; may be noted both preoperatively and postoperatively
2. Prothrombin time, partial thromboplastin time
   Abnormality: May be increased if patient on anticoagulant therapy preoperatively
3. Hemoglobin and hematocrit
   Abnormality: Decreased with hemorrhage
   Indicates blood and oxygen-carrying capacity deficit
4. Arterial blood gases (ABGs)
   Abnormality: Decreased pH reflecting acidosis, due to severe hemorrhage
5. Blood glucose
   Abnormality: Increased postsurgically due to trauma or underlying diabetic condition

Diagnostic Tests

1. Angiography: Aortography/arteriography
   Abnormality: Obstruction, narrowing or alternate pathways of aorta, carotids, or femoral arteries

2. Chest X-ray
   Abnormality: Mediastinal widening and pleural effusion indicative of aortic dissection or aneurysm
       Widening of thoracic aorta in thoracic aneurysm
       Calcification within abdominal aortic aneurysm
3. Computed tomography/magnetic resonance imaging
   Abnormality: Widened anterioposterior diameter of aneurysm
       Leakage at site of aneurysm
       Aortic dissection
4. Carotid Doppler ultrasound
   Abnormality: Thrombotic vessel from ulcerative plaque
5. Digital subtraction angiography
   Abnormality: Carotid stenosis
       Anatomic abnormalities of external carotid arteries, aortic arch, subclavian and vertebral arteries
6. Oculoplethysmography
   Abnormality: Occlusion of artery; decreased blood flow to the ophthalmic artery, a branch of the internal carotid
7. Electroencephalography
   Abnormality: Abnormal electrical activity of brain, which might be etiology of behavioral changes
8. Transesophageal echocardiography
   Abnormality: Intimal calcification in aortic dissection
       Pericardial effusion
       Left ventricular wall motion abnormalities
9. Electrocardiography
   Abnormality: Myocardial infarction (MI)
       Left ventricular hypertrophy related to chronic hypertension

Planning/Intervention

COLLABORATIVE MANAGEMENT

Postoperative Procedures

1. Monitor and support tissue perfusion.
   a. Administer ordered intravenous (IV) fluid resuscitation.
   b. Assist with insertion of central lines and monitor vital

signs and hemodynamic parameters every hour, or as needed, until stable.

c. Place patient on cardiac monitor and report arrhythmias.

d. Monitor intake and output every hour. Report urine output >30 mL/h, significant changes in output, and change in color of the urine.

e. Obtain specimens and report abnormal laboratory studies, particularly decreased hemoglobin and hematocrit, low arterial blood pH, increased BUN and serum creatinine, elevated cardiac enzymes, prolonged clotting times, and decreased platelet count.

f. Administer ordered supplemental oxygen as indicated.

g. Assess neurologic signs every hour, as indicated.

h. Check pulses distal to operative site every hour, or as needed.
   1) Carotid endarterectomy: temporal pulse
   2) Femoral-popliteal bypass: pedal pulses
   3) Abdominal aortic aneurysm: femoral, popliteal, pedal pulses

i. Maintain head of bed flat, unless otherwise instructed. Do not flex legs at hips or knees.

Drug Therapy

1. Opioid analgesics
   Example: morphine sulfate (Duromorph)
   Action: Decreases acute severe episodes of preoperative and postoperative pain
   Caution: Inhibits baroreceptors and may decrease blood pressure and pulse
      Do not use in hypovolemia; may also constrict pupillary reaction, affecting neurologic signs

2. Inotropic agents
   Example: dopamine hydrochloride (Intropin)
   Action: Increases myocardial contraction and blood pressure, as well as renal blood flow
   Caution: Needs close observation to maintain a normotensive state and keep graft patent (open)

3. Antihypertensives
   Examples: labetalol (Normodyne)
      sodium nitroprusside (Nipride)

Action: Lowers blood pressure by decreasing peripheral vascular resistance

Caution: Closely monitor vital signs and hemodynamics to prevent shock

4. Anticoagulants

Example: heparin sodium (heparin)

Action: Inhibits normal clotting mechanism; does not dissolve already existing clots, but prevents their growth; lowers platelet count when administered in high doses

Caution: Monitor clotting times, platelet count to prevent postoperative bleeding

Observe for signs of hematoma/hemorrhage; avoid concomitant use of aspirin-containing substances

NURSING MANAGEMENT

Monitoring and Managing Clinical Problems

1. Tissue Perfusion, altered: peripheral
   a. Monitor tissue perfusion.
      1) Assist with insertion of an arterial line and continuously monitor blood pressure for hypotension/hypertension.
      2) Monitor neurologic vital signs for decreased cerebral perfusion.
      3) Observe anatomy distal to the operative site for possible signs of ischemia.
         a) Carotid endarterectomy—Decreased level of consciousness and possibly restlessness and confusion
         b) Peripheral vascular surgery—Cool skin temperature, pale to blanched color skin, and a change in sensation from normal to tingling, burning
      4) Palpate the peripheral pulses distal to the surgical site every hour, and as needed.
      5) Monitor intake and output hourly. Note fluid overload and high output.
      6) Auscultate abdomen for return of bowel sounds.
      7) Auscultate pulse flow at graft site and distal to graft with Doppler.
      8) Observe for signs of hematoma around operative site.

9) Apply pulse oximeter and continuously monitor oxygen saturation.

b. Promote tissue perfusion.

1) Maintain supplemental oxygen, as needed. (Patient may be mechanically ventilated if the vascular repair was for an aortic aneurysm or aortic dissection).

2) Investigate any drop in blood pressure immediately by:
   a) Noting color and amount of drainage on dressings and from tubes
   b) Checking for edema around surgical site and in dependent areas
   c) Auscultating heart and lungs for abnormal and adventitious sounds

3) Avoid flexion of the extremities.

4) Wrap the feet in a warm blanket.

5) Mark the location of the pulses with indelible ink.

6) Administer IV fluids, as ordered, to provide adequate vascular volume, and prevent shunt collapse.

7) Apply antiembolism stockings, as ordered.

8) Avoid administering medications in the operative extremity.

9) Turn every 2 hours; administer skin care. Note any signs of redness or pressure areas.

10) Administer appropriate vasodilators or vasopressors as needed.

11) Avoid nursing actions that increase blood pressure and place added strain on graft site.

12) For carotid endarterectomy, place ice pack on neck at site of surgery to prevent undue swelling.

13) Report any signs that might indicate decreased blood flow to the brain.
   a) Decreased level of consciousness
   b) Headache on same side as surgery
   c) Pupillary changes to dilated sluggish or unequal in size
   d) Change in motor strength, activity
   e) Visual problems
   f) Decreased respiratory drive
   g) Difficulty communicating verbally

2. Pain — Incisional site pain
   a. Monitor pain status.
      1) Note patient's complaints of pain.
      2) Observe patient for restlessness, agitation, if patient unable to talk.
      3) Monitor patient response to pain treatment.
   b. Provide pain relief.
      1) Administer ordered pain medication.
      2) If pain unrelieved by medication or if acutely severe, investigate for further cause.
3. Injury: high risk for
   a. Monitor potential for injury.
      1) Observe patient for ability to turn self.
      2) Auscultate lungs for crackles or decreased breath sounds.
      3) Observe patient's gag reflex.
      4) Monitor vital and neurologic vital signs hourly.
      5) Monitor patient's response to increased activity postoperatively by noting changes in pulmonary artery pressure (PAP), arterial blood pressure, oxygen saturation, and cardiac rate and rhythm.
      6) Monitor dressing drainage amount and color.
      7) Monitor for and report signs of hematoma formation.
      8) Monitor abdominal girth after abdominal aneurysm repair.
   b. Monitor for and promote safety postoperatively.
      1) Place patient on cardiac monitor and report any arrhythmias.
      2) Observe operative site for signs of hematoma formation; change dressing as ordered, observing site and drainage.
      3) Maintain nasogastric tube and check position every 8 hours.
      4) Check drainage via nasogastric tube for possible bleeding or occult blood.
      5) Once nasogastric tube is removed, closely monitor ability to swallow oral fluids after carotid endarterectomy.
      6) Auscultate airway for patency and identify partial obstruction (most important in the carotid endarterectomy).

      7) Allow patient to dangle legs off bedside prior to standing or moving to chair.

      8) Observe patient's level of consciousness, behavior, and color closely while increasing activity.

4. Injury: high risk for — Monitor for complications.

  a. Fluid Volume Deficit (Acute Loss) — Postoperative bleeding

    1) Monitor vital signs for hypotension, tachycardia.

    2) Monitor for increase in abdominal girth and pain.

    3) Observe for hematoma at operative site.

    4) Monitor for peripheral pulse deterioration.

    5) Note and report bloody nasogastric drainage.

  b. Tissue Perfusion, altered: gastrointestinal — Bowel ischemia

    1) Auscultate for bowel sounds and measure for increased abdominal girth to determine presence of prolonged postoperative ileus.

    2) Assess patient for abdominal pain.

    3) Monitor for and report diarrhea.

    4) Monitor for increased temperature, white blood cell count.

  c. Tissue Perfusion, altered: cerebral — Brain or spinal ischemia, graft reocclusion or thrombosis

    1) Assess for cranial nerve damage post carotid endarterectomy.

      a) Difficulty swallowing, speaking, with hypoglossal and vagus nerve damage

      b) Asymmetry of smile with facial nerve damage

      c) Difficulty with movement and strength of arm and shoulder with accessory nerve damage

      d) Upper airway obstruction with hypoglossal nerve damage

    2) Observe for deterioration in cerebral function after carotid endarterectomy.

      a) Decreased level of consciousness

      b) Inequality in pupillary size and reactivity

      c) Inequality in strength and movement of extremities

      d) Abnormal change in respiratory pattern

      e) Decreasing blood pressure with widening pulse pressure

  d. Tissue Perfusion, altered: renal

1) Monitor vital signs, cardiac monitor for change in hemodynamics before, during, and after dialysis.
2) Observe for serial BUN, serum creatinine, and serum electrolyte abnormalities before, during, and after dialysis.
3) Monitor for behavioral changes due to serum electrolyte, BUN, and serum creatinine abnormalities.
4) Observe for signs of fluid overload, such as:
   a) Increased pulse, blood pressure, respiratory rate
   b) Distended neck veins
   c) Peripheral edema
   d) Increased central venous pressure and PAP
5) Maintain dialysis, as ordered, to decrease fluid and electrolyte overload.
6) Maintain strict intake and output, restricting fluid intake as indicated.

Monitoring, Managing, and Preventing Life-Threatening Emergencies

1. MI
   a. Closely observe the postoperative aortic dissection repair with valve replacement for a deterioration hemodynamically:
      1) Decreased blood pressure with increased heart rate
      2) Increased respiratory rate with abnormal lung sounds
      3) Increased PAP
      4) Decreased cardiac output
   b. Monitor serum cardiac enzymes postoperatively for increase.
   c. Ask the patient to describe location, amount, and characteristics of pain.
   d. Observe cardiac monitor and report any arrhythmias, abrupt changes in pattern.
   e. Auscultate for S_3 or S_4 heart sounds and crackles in lungs indicating possible myocardial weakness.
2. Hypertensive crisis
   a. Continuously monitor blood pressure before, during, and after instituting antihypertensive drug therapy.

b. Monitor hourly neurologic vital signs with fine motor function and report abnormalities.

c. Monitor hourly urine outputs and report significant changes.

d. Assess peripheral pulses hourly and report significant changes.

e. Observe cardiac monitor for change in rate or presence of arrhythmias.

f. Assess and medicate patient for chest pain, as indicated.

g. Auscultate lungs for presence of abnormal and adventitious lung sounds.

h. Auscultate heart for extra sounds or bruits.

3. Acute renal failure from acute tubular necrosis related to continued hypotension, infection, and use of nephrotoxic agents

a. Administer ordered IV fluids.

b. Regulate fluid intake to achieve fluid and electrolyte balance.

c. Administer buffering agents to maintain acid-base balance.

d. Monitor for changes in level of consciousness and intervene quickly as indicated to preserve neurologic function.

e. Manage nutrition.

1) Restrict protein intake to maintain anabolism while limiting load on kidneys. Amount will vary depending on patient's weight and activity level and whether or not the patient is on dialysis.

2) Restrict dietary potassium intake.

3) Restrict fluids.

4) Provide adequate calories to prevent catabolism.

5) Administer ordered supplemental vitamins.

6) Administer ordered blood transfusions to maintain adequate level of red blood cells for optimum tissue oxygenation.

7) Initiate renal replacement therapy (RRT), as indicated.

a) BUN >100 mg/dL

b) Serum creatinine >9 mg/dL or lower for patients with reduced muscle mass

c) Signs of pulmonary edema, pericarditis, uncontrollable acidosis, hyperkalemia, and central nervous system dysfunction related to uremia

8) Prepare patient for ordered RRT: hemodialysis, continuous ultrafiltration, continuous RRT, or peritoneal dialysis.

4. Hypovolemic shock caused by graft rupture

   a. Monitor hemodynamic parameters continuously.
   b. Titrate fluids and inotropic agents to maintain a systolic blood pressure of at least 80 mm Hg.
   c. Administer ordered supplemental oxygen.
   d. Obtain blood specimens and monitor ABGs and hemoglobin and hematocrit results and report significant changes.
   e. Palpate pulses and monitor capillary refill to assess peripheral perfusion.
   f. Monitor hourly urine output to assess renal function.
   g. Auscultate abdomen for decreased bowel sounds and note presence of any gastric bleeding.
   h. Monitor for decreased alertness and attention span, drowsiness, or excessive sleeping indicating a deterioration in the level of consciousness.

5. Cardiopulmonary arrest

   a. Call for help.
   b. Begin cardiopulmonary resuscitation.
   c. Follow with advanced cardiac life support.

Systemic Inflammatory Response Syndrome and Multiple Organ Dysfunction Syndrome (Multiple System Organ Failure)

Systemic inflammatory response syndrome (SIRS), which has a mortality rate of 40–60%, is an overall inflammatory response to a variety of severe injuries and illnesses affecting virtually all body systems and results in two or more of the following:

1. Temperature >38°C (100°F) or less than 36°C (96.8°F)
2. Heart rate >90 bpm
3. Respiratory rate >20 breaths per minute with a P_{aCO_2} of less than 32 mm Hg
4. White blood cell count >12,000 mm³ or <4,000 mm³ or 10% immature neutrophils (bands)

Multiple organ dysfunction syndrome (MODS), a progression of SIRS, occurs when there is alteration in functioning of two or more organs requiring intervention to prevent organ failure. Currently, there is no known prevention or cure for MODS, so supportive care is the primary treatment. It has a mortality rate of 90–100%. Greater than three organ systems dysfunctioning results in a nearly 100% mortality. There are two forms of MODS:

1. One organ sustains the primary insult and dysfunction progresses to other organ systems.
2. Dysfunction is present in multiple organs from the beginning event.

MODS is evidenced by all the criteria for SIRS plus:

1. An imbalance of oxygen supply and demand
2. Failure of the capillaries to extract the delivered oxygen
3. Evidence of organ dysfunction that requires therapy

Multiple system organ failure (MSOF) is a term often used to apply to the above two syndromes. SIRS/MODS is a progressive syndrome that is difficult to stop and often results in patient death. The syndrome has been seen more frequently as technologic advances have salvaged more critically ill and injured patients.

Etiology/Pathophysiology

1. Risk factors for developing SIRS include:
   a. Septic on admission
   b. Critically ill on admission
   c. Very young or very old (greater than 85 years)
   d. Impaired immunity
   e. Dysfunction of one organ system on admission
   f. Multiple trauma
2. Metabolic responses seen in SIRS/MODS:
   a. Generalized intracellular and extracellular edema
   b. Increased energy expenditure resulting in glycolysis (breakdown of fats for energy)
   c. Autocannibalism (a significant total body protein catabolism causing rapid reduction of muscle mass) that is relatively unresponsive to exogenous amino acids
3. Phases of SIRS
   a. Hyperdynamic phase, or compensated stage, when the patient is able to compensate for the responses
   b. Hypodynamic phase, or decompensated stage, when compensation is no longer possible
4. Pathophysiology
   a. Once SIRS occurs, humoral immune mediators are released resulting in:
      1) Cardiac dysfunction caused by pancreatic release of myocardial depressant factor
      2) Pulmonary dysfunction caused by leaky pulmonary capillary membranes, microemboli, and vasoconstriction and leading to ventilatory failure and adult respiratory distress syndrome
      3) Central nervous system dysfunction caused by cerebral hypoperfusion
      4) Renal dysfunction caused by renal vasoconstriction and hypoperfusion and leading to acute tubular necrosis
      5) Hematologic dysfunction caused by overstimulation of the coagulation cascade and leading to disseminated intravascular coagulopathy
      6) Gastrointestinal dysfunction caused by vasoconstriction and hypoperfusion and leading to gut failure and release of gram-negative bacteria into the system, and eventually, gram-negative sepsis

Assessment/Analysis

ASSESSMENT FINDINGS

Subjective Findings

1. History of an injury or illness that puts the patient at risk for SIRS/MODS
2. Anxiety
3. History of rapid patient deterioration

Objective Findings

1. Hyperdynamic phase of SIRS
   a. Increased respiratory rate from hypoxemia
   b. Decreased urine output from decreased renal perfusion
   c. Change in level of consciousness from decreased cerebral perfusion
   d. Strong, bounding pulse
   e. Flushed, warm skin
   f. Decreased blood pressure
   g. Wide pulse pressure
   h. Increased heart rate
   i. Crackles in lungs from leaking pulmonary capillary membranes
2. Hypodynamic phase of SIRS
   a. Pale, cool, clammy skin
   b. Decreased respiratory rate
   c. Coma
   d. Anuria
   e. Increased or decreased temperature
   f. Weak thready pulse
   g. Increased heart rate
   h. Decreased blood pressure
   i. Crackles, rhonchi, and wheezes
3. MODS
   a. Change in the level of consciousness (confusion, agitation, lethargy)
   b. Decrease in the Glascow Coma Scale score to <6 (See Appendix N)
   c. Hypothermia or hyperthermia
   d. Low or high respiratory rate

e. Signs of hypoxia—restlessness, confusion, air hunger
f. Severe dyspnea
g. Rigid, boardlike abdomen with abdominal pain possibly indicating organ perforation
h. Diarrhea
i. Evidence of overt bleeding—bruising, prolonged bleeding from puncture sites and wounds
j. Evidence of occult bleeding—coffee-ground emesis, tarry stools, signs and symptoms of shock, rapid change in the level of consciousness
k. Oliguria
l. Sediment present in urine
m. Jaundice
n. Gastrointestinal bleeding from mucosal erosion
o. Ventricular tachycardia or fibrillation
p. Bradycardia
q. Hypotension with mean arterial pressure <50 mm Hg
r. Anasarca (generalized body edema) caused by fluid moving out of the vasculature and into the tissues (third spacing)
s. Crackles and wheezes in lungs and increasing peripheral edema caused by cardiovascular failure
t. Absent bowel sounds indicting paralytic ileus

SUPPORTING TEST FINDINGS

Laboratory Tests

1. Arterial blood gases
   Abnormality: Respiratory alkalosis, hypoxemia, and metabolic acidosis in the hyperdynamic phase
   Severe hypoxemia with metabolic and respiratory acidosis in the hypodynamic phase
   Hypoxemia, hypercapnia, and deterioration from baseline values with MODS
2. Mixed venous oxygen saturation
   Abnormality: May have normal or increased values in the hyperdynamic phase
   Decreased values in the hypodynamic phase and MODS
3. White blood cell (WBC) count
   Abnormality: WBC count is increased with increase in

immature neutrophils (shift to the left) in the hyperdynamic phase

WBC decreases in the hypodynamic phase and
MODS

4. Coagulation studies increased prothrombin time and
partial thromboplastin time, and fibrin split products;
decreased fibrinogen and platelet count

Abnormality: In the hyperdynamic phase:

All of the above plus positive findings for disseminated intravascular coagulation in the hypodynamic
phase and MODS

5. Blood glucose

Abnormality: Increased in the hyperdynamic phase

Decreased in the hypodynamic phase and MODS

6. Serum lactate

Abnormality: Increased indicating lactic acidosis in the
hypodynamic phase and MODS

7. Serum electrolytes

Abnormality: Increased anion gap in the hypodynamic
phase and MODS

8. Renal function tests

Abnormality: Increased blood urea nitrogen and serum
creatinine and abnormal urine values in the hypodynamic phase and MODS

9. Liver function tests

Abnormality: Increased liver enzymes (to twice normal),
serum amylase, serum lipase, and serum bilirubin in
the hypodynamic phase and MODS

10. Serum cardiac enzymes

Abnormality: Increased in hypodynamic phase and
MODS

Diagnostic Tests

1. Chest X-ray

Abnormality: Bilateral pulmonary infiltrates

2. Hemodynamic monitoring

Abnormality: Increased cardiac output (CO), decreased
systemic vascular resistance, decreased pulmonary artery pressure (PAP), decreased pulmonary artery
wedge pressure (PCWP), decreased central venous
pressure (CVP) in hyperdynamic phase

Decreased CO; increased systemic vascular resis-

tance; increased or decreased PAP, PCWP, and CVP in hypodynamic phase and MODS
3. Endoscopy
   Abnormality: Gastric mucosal erosion

Planning/Intervention

MEDICAL MANAGEMENT

Procedures

1. Prevent organ injury.
   a. Provide ventilatory support through intubation and mechanical ventilation.
   b. Control body temperature to adjust for hyperthermia or hypothermia.
   c. Administer buffering agents to reverse acidosis.
2. Provide supportive care.
   a. Control the infection.
      1) Obtain a specimen of all secretions for culture testing.
      2) Prepare the patient for surgical intervention to remove sources of infection.
   b. Arrest and reverse the progress of the syndrome.
      1) Prevent translocation of bacteria from the gut with enteral feeding of glutamine, an immunonutrient that maintains gut integrity and stimulates the immune system.
      2) Prepare for continuous arteriovenous hemodiafiltration, which has been used successfully in trauma patients.
   c. Provide metabolic support.
      1) Measure oxygen consumption with increased flow rates until lactic acid level returns to normal.
      2) Provide adequate nutrition. Enteral route is preferred over parenteral. Use a formula that is high in protein and has medium-chain triglycerides for lipids.

Drug Therapy

1. Volume expanders

Examples: Ringer's solution, Ringer's lactate, normal saline solution, albumin, dextran, hetastarch, plasma, packed red blood cells

Action: Prevent hypotension and oliguria by replacing intravascular volume; crystalloids, colloids, blood or blood products may be used

Caution: May cause fluid overload

2. Inotropic agents

   Examples: norepinephrine (Levophed)
   dopamine (Intropin)
   dobutamine (Dobutrex)

   Action: Improves cardiac contractility; increases CO and organ perfusion

   Caution: Can cause oliguria, increased myocardial oxygen demand, ventricular arrhythmias, and vasoconstriction

3. Vasodilators

   Examples: nitroglycerin (Tridil)
   nitroprusside (Nipride)
   chlorpromazine (Thorazine)
   phentolamine (Regitine)

   Action: Reverse vasoconstriction and improve tissue perfusion

   Caution: Can cause hypotension
   Nipride can cause cyanate toxicity

4. Antibiotics

   Examples: ticarcillin (Timentin)
   ceftazidime (Fortaz)
   gentamycin (Garamycin)

   Action: Bacteriocidal
   Broad-spectrum antibiotics that kill aerobic and anaerobic gram-negative and gram-positive bacteria
   Before the source is identified, at least a two-drug combination should be given
   When the source is identified, therapy may be tailored to the cause

   Caution: Can cause allergic reaction, nephrotoxicity, and ototoxicity

5. Diuretics

   Examples: furosemide (Lasix)
   bumetanide (Bumex)

   Action: Increase urine output by increasing sodium and

chloride excretion in the loop of Henle; used to treat oliguria

Caution: Can cause hypokalemia and dehydration

6. Corticosteroids

Example: hydrocortisone (Hydrocortone)

Action: Stabilize capillary walls thus decreasing fluid shifts out of the vasculature

Caution: Can cause hypokalemia, hypernatremia, nausea, and petechiae

NURSING MANAGEMENT

Monitoring and Management of Clinical Problems

1. Tissue Perfusion, altered: peripheral, high risk for — Monitor patients at risk for SIRS and recognize onset during the early phases.
   a. Assess for risk factors.
   b. Be alert for early warning signals, such as:
      1) Increased or decreased temperature
      2) Increasing heart rate
      3) Tachypnea
      4) Increased or decreased WBCs
      5) Subtle changes in sensorium
   c. Report findings consistent with the development of SIRS.

2. Protection: altered, high risk for — Monitor for progression of SIRS.
   a. Monitor for subtle changes in assessment findings that may indicate deterioration from the hyperdynamic phase to the hypodynamic phase.
   b. Measure hemodynamic parameters frequently and report changes.
   c. Assess the patient frequently, paying particular attention to serial findings to identify deterioration in previously uninvolved organ systems.
   d. Analyze changes in laboratory values to determine deterioration of multiple organs.
   e. Monitor patient responses to medications and treatments, and report significant findings.

3. Infection: high risk for — Monitor for infection and promote an aseptic environment to prevent concomitant (nosocomial) infections.

a. Use aseptic technique when providing care.
b. Monitor invasive tube sites for signs and symptoms of infection.
c. Wash hands frequently.
d. Monitor serial WBCs for signs of infection.
e. Culture suspicious secretions from the patient.
f. Immediately report signs and symptoms of infection.
g. Monitor the patient's temperature every 4 hours and more frequently if fever develops.
h. Administer medications ordered to prevent or fight infection and monitor patient's response to them.

4. Nutrition: altered, less than body requirements — Promote adequate nutrition.
   a. Administer enteral (preferred route) or parenteral nutrition, as ordered.
   b. Enteral nutrition
      1) Keep head of bed elevated, if possible, to prevent aspiration.
      2) Check residuals every 4 hours to assess absorption. Report high residuals.
      3) Flush enteral feeding tube every 4 hours.
      4) Change feeding apparatus every day to prevent bacterial contamination.
   c. Parenteral nutrition
      1) Deliver through a central line.
      2) Change the bag and tubing every day to prevent bacterial contamination.
      3) Monitor blood glucose readings every 6 hours and cover elevations with sliding-scale regular insulin.
   d. Monitor serum albumins and transferrins to assess the adequacy of the nutrition therapy.

5. Recognize complications.
   a. Tissue Integrity: impaired — Skin breakdown
      1) Use pressure-relieving devices (e.g., pads, mattresses, specialty beds) to prevent breakdown.
      2) Turn the patient every 2 hours, if possible.
      3) Assess the skin every 4 hours to identify and intervene in the early stages of breakdown.
      4) Consult the enterostomal therapy nurse for definitive treatment of skin breakdown.
   b. Fluid Volume Deficit — Third spacing of fluid

1) Assess the patient every 4 hours for edema, ascites, or anasarca.
2) Weigh the patient daily and report significant increases.
3) Accurately measure intake and output and report significant disparities.
4) Monitor lung sounds every 4 hours and report changes.
5) Administer diuretics, as ordered, to increase urine output.

Monitoring, Managing, and Preventing Life-Threatening Emergencies

1. SIRS/MODS (MSOF)
   a. These are life-threatening emergencies.
   b. Because of the high percentages of death associated with these syndromes, preparation of the family for the patient's impending death is necessary.
2. Cardiopulmonary arrest
   a. Call for help.
   b. Begin cardiopulmonary resuscitation.
   c. Follow with advanced cardiac life support.

3 NEUROLOGIC DISORDERS

Increased Intracranial Pressure

Increased intracranial pressure (IICP), or intracranial hypertension, is a sustained pressure greater than 15 mm Hg exerted within the skull; a sustained intracranial pressure (ICP) greater than 20 mm Hg is known as malignant intracranial hypertension.

Etiology/Pathophysiology

1. Etiology
   a. Trauma
      1) Head injury
      2) Post craniotomy
   b. Post cardiac arrest
   c. Cerebral hematomas, tumors
2. Major determinants of ICP
   a. Brain tissue: (occupies 80% intracranial space) volume increases due to tumors or cerebral edema. Cerebral edema is caused by an increase in the water content of the brain tissue.
   b. Blood: (occupies 10%) Cerebral blood volume (CBV) is primarily controlled by the venous system. Under a limited regulatory mechanism, when a rapidly growing hematoma or tumor causes ICP increases, the CBV is displaced to compensate. This compensatory mechanism is finite; and after a certain point, even a very slight increase in lesion size can cause a major change in ICP.
      1) Cerebral blood flow (CBF) is directly related to the blood pressure in the brain tissue (cerebral perfusion pressure [CPP]), and the cerebrovascular resistance. CPP should be maintained at no lower than 50–60 mm Hg to support brain function.
      2) CBF is maintained at a constant level by a compensatory mechanism known as *autoregulation*.
         a) Autoregulation operates within a mean arterial pressure of 60–150 mm Hg. Above 150 mm Hg, the blood–brain barrier is disrupted, and cerebral edema results.
         b) Autoregulation affects the brain in two ways:
            1] Maintaining arterial pressures by vasoconstricting or vasodilating arterioles in response to systemic pressure
            2] Vasodilating in response to:
               a] Buildup of hydrogen ions and CO_2 in the blood
               b] Drop in oxygen concentration
      3) Hyperemia exists when the CBF exceeds the metabolic demand of the tissue.

    c. Cerebrospinal fluid: (occupies 10%) volume increases due to abnormalities in overproduction, circulation, drainage, or reabsorption

3. Other factors influencing ICP
    a. Arterial and venous pressures
        1) Elevated systemic blood pressure produces increased CBF and intracranial blood volume, leading to IICP, if autoregulation is impaired.
        2) Decreased systemic blood pressure causes decreased CBF and intracranial blood volume, leading to lowered oxygen content in the brain. Hypoxia causes vasodilation of cerebral arteries and brain ischemia with subsequent edema.
    b. Posture: The following slows or obstructs venous return from the cranium.
        1) Neck flexion
        2) Hip flexion, which increases intra-abdominal pressures.
        3) Incorrect positioning resulting in slumping, which increases intrathoracic pressures.
    c. Blood gases
        1) Acidosis, or abnormally low oxygen levels in the blood, cause vasodilation of cerebral arteries and subsequent brain tissue ischemia and swelling.
        2) Respiratory alkalosis, or abnormally low carbon dioxide levels in the blood caused by overzealous hyperventilation, lead to vasoconstriction of the cerebral arteries and subsequent ischemic damage.
    d. Temperature
        1) A temperature elevation of $1°C$ causes a $7-10\%$ increase in cerebral metabolic demand. If metabolic needs are not met, ischemia is inevitable.

Assessment/Analysis

ASSESSMENT FINDINGS

Subjective

1. Headache
2. Visual changes

   a. Decreased acuity
   b. Diplopia

Objective

1. Level of consciousness deteriorates with increasing ICP
   a. Affect: animated to flat
   b. Attention span and memory deteriorate from normal, to limited, to absent.
   c. Orientation loss to time, place, and person
   d. Wakefulness deteriorates from alert to drowsy, confused, restless, lethargic, stuporous, comatose.
2. Vomiting often projectile and not associated with nausea
3. Sensory and motor losses deteriorate with IICP.
   a. In the early stages, there may be no loss noted or there may be hemiparesis on the contralateral side of the lesion.
   b. In later stages, hemiplegia, decorticate or decerebrate posturing, or bilateral flaccidity of extremities may be present.
4. Pupillary changes
   a. In metabolic coma, pupils still respond to light.
   b. Increased ICP pupillary changes
      1) Early during the course of supratentorial lesions, pupils are in midposition (3.5 mm), or when the pupil and iris are observed together, half of the diameter is pupil and half is iris. The pupil then dilates on the side of the brain lesion.
      2) During late IICP in supratentorial lesions, the pupil on the same side as the brain lesion is fixed and dilated.
      3) With brainstem herniation, pupils become bilaterally fixed and dilated.
5. Elevation in body temperature occurs in late stages
6. Seizure activity
7. Blood pressure variations
   a. Widened pulse pressure and hypertension may accompany a rising ICP. If accompanied by bradycardia, this signals a late sign in increased ICP (Cushing's triad).
   b. Hypotension may accompany hemorrhage and shock, as well as the terminal stage of neurologic injury.

8. Respiratory pattern may change as the respiratory centers of the brain are affected by the rise in ICP.
   a. Cheyne-Stokes respiration: crescendo-decrescendo breathing followed by apnea
   b. Central neurogenic hyperventilation: sustained hyperventilation causing an increased PaO_2 and decreased $PaCO_2$
   c. Apneustic respiration: respirations with brief pauses at the end of inspiration
   d. Cluster respiration: periods of irregular breaths alternating with apnea
   e. Ataxic respiration (commonly known as agonal): grossly irregular and random inspiration and expiration

SUPPORTING TEST FINDINGS

Laboratory Tests

1. Serum electrolytes
   Abnormality: Increased serum sodium
   Decreased serum potassium and chloride
   Electrolytes may be altered due to diuretic therapy
2. Serum osmolality
   Abnormality: Increased due to hyperosmolar agents used to pull fluid off brain and the effect corticosteroids have on promoting diuresis
3. Urine specific gravity
   Abnormality: Decreased following diuretic therapy and with diabetes insipidus associated with increased ICP
   Increased with syndrome of inappropriate secretion of antidiuretic hormone (SIADH)

Diagnostic Tests

1. ICP monitoring
   Abnormality: Plateau waves (A waves) signal a neurologic emergency. These occur in patients with ICP >15–20 mm Hg and an amplitude ranging between 50–100 mm Hg. They indicate low oxygen supply to brain cells, causing significant damage.

Types and Advantages of ICP Monitoring*

Intraventricular Catheter	Subarachnoid Screw	Epidural/Subdural Catheter or Sensor
▪ Most accurate for ICP	▪ Direct ICP measurement	▪ Less invasive and easier to insert
▪ Direct access to cerebrospinal fluid for drainage or sample	▪ Direct access for volume-pressure response	▪ Less chance of altered monitoring due to occlusion of sensor
▪ Direct access to measure volume-pressure response		▪ Greater mobility for transporting
▪ Direct access to instill drugs		▪ May remain in place longer if dura is not penetrated

*ICP = intracranial pressure.

2. Computed tomography scan
   Abnormality: Hematomas, arteriovenous malformations, cerebral infarctions, brain abscesses, contusions, tumors, hydrocephalus
3. Positron emission transaxial tomography
   Abnormality: Absence of brain cellular metabolism and blood flow due to brain trauma, and vascular and electrical abnormalities
4. Magnetic resonance imaging
   Abnormality: Cerebral edema, hemorrhage, hematomas, infarction, and vessel or bone lesions

5. Brain scan
   Abnormality: Ischemia, cerebral infarction, hematomas, hemorrhages, and tumors
6. Electroencephalography
   Abnormality: Foci of abnormal electrical activity
7. Cerebral angiogram
   Abnormality: Cerebrovascular abnormalities and arterio-venous malformations
8. Electrocardiography
   Abnormality: Arrhythmias

Planning/Intervention

COLLABORATIVE MANAGEMENT

Procedures

1. Ensure adequate oxygenation.
   a. Obtain specimens and monitor results of arterial blood gas (ABG) values.
   b. Apply pulse oximeter and monitor oxygen saturation in response to activity.
   c. Have emergency resuscitation equipment nearby and be prepared for possible intubation.
   d. Anticipate ventilator assistance for respiratory stability.
   e. Preoxygenate carefully before performing limited suctioning.
2. Promote cerebral venous drainage.
   a. Elevate head of bed 20–30 degrees, or as indicated.
   b. Anticipate physician insertion of ICP monitoring with intermittent drainage via ventricular catheter.
3. Maintain normothermia.
   a. Apply hypothermia blanket.
   b. Provide privacy with minimal clothing.
4. Restrict fluid intake to prevent fluid overload.
   a. Maintain strict intake and output.
   b. Administer piggyback medications in minimal concentrations.
5. Protect patient from further injury.
   a. Assess corneal reflex to prevent corneal abrasions.
   b. Assess gag and swallow reflexes to protect airway.

    c. Insert gastric tube to prevent aspiration of stomach contents.

    d. Perform gastric aspirate analysis to monitor hyperacidity and possible gastrointestinal bleeding as side effects of stress and steroids.

    e. Institute and monitor gastric tube feedings to prevent malnutrition.

    f. Institute and maintain cardiac monitor to assess cardiac irritability and fluctuations in rate.

6. Monitor and promote fluid and electrolyte stability.

    a. Assist with insertion of central catheter and monitor hemodynamic pressures.

    b. Adjust intake to maintain a slightly dehydrated state.

      1) Monitor urine output, and report signs and symptoms of SIADH or diabetes insipidus.

      2) Infuse only 0.45% or 0.9% normal saline solution intravenously (IV), as ordered.

      3) Limit fluid intake to 1,200–1,500 mL/d.

    c. Monitor results of serial laboratory studies.

      1) Serum osmolality for increase or decrease

      2) Electrolyte imbalances

      3) Blood urea nitrogen or serum creatinine increase

Drug Therapy

1. Diuretics

   Example: Loop diuretic—furosemide (Lasix)

   Action: Reduces ICP by decreasing sodium to the brain, decreasing total body water content, and slowing cerebral spinal fluid production

   Caution: May contribute to electrolyte imbalance causing cardiovascular alterations

   Example: Osmotic diuretic—mannitol (Osmitrol)

   Action: Reduces ICP by increasing serum osmolality causing fluid to be pulled from brain tissue with an intact blood–brain barrier to balance the osmotic gradient; also acts as a free radical scavenger

   Caution: Not effective when blood–brain barrier is not intact; over time, drug moves into injured tissue and can be instrumental in increasing cerebral edema; drug can increase CBF

2. Antipyretics

   Example: acetaminophen (Tylenol)

Action: Reduces ICP by reducing temperature; ICP is increased by hypermetabolism; metabolic rate increases 7–10% each time body temperature increases 1°C (about 2°F)

3. Corticosteroids

Examples: dexamethasone (Decadron)
hydrocortisone (Solu-Cortef)
methylprednisolone (Solu-Medrol)

Action: May be helpful in decreasing ICP by affecting autoregulation and restoring CBF

Caution: Controversial with brain trauma

Must be tapered gradually due to possible adrenal insufficiency

Can contribute to major gastrointestinal irritation and stress ulceration

4. Anticonvulsants

Examples: diazepam (Valium)
phenobarbital (Luminal)
phenytoin (Dilantin)

Action: Reduces seizure activity, which can increase cerebral metabolism and ICP

Caution: Administer slowly into a large vein; observe cardiac and respiratory function closely

Check IV site to prevent extravasation

5. Neuromuscular blocking agents

Example: pancuronium bromide (Pavulon)

Action: Reduces ICP by causing skeletal muscle paralysis and allowing mechanical ventilator to totally control respirations and maintain optimal oxygenation status

Caution: Does not cause sedation

Can increase patient anxiety and ICP

Does not replace the need for pain control and sedation

Patient must be on mechanical ventilator

Interferes with accurate motor function assessment

6. Sedatives — analgesics

Examples: morphine sulfate (Duromorph)
pentobarbital (Nembutal)

Action: Helps decrease anxiety and relieves pain; often used in conjunction with neuromuscular blocking agents

Caution: May alter neurologic assessment findings

May cause hypotension, cardiac depression

Patient must be fully supported with ventilation, ICP and hemodynamic monitoring, gastric and urinary catheters

Barbiturate coma is controversial therapy; must be certain all barbiturates have been eliminated from the body before criteria for brain death can be established

7. Antihypertensives

Examples: nitroprusside sodium (Nipride)
labetalol (Normodyne)

Action: Causes vasodilation, decreases peripheral vascular resistance, and depresses cardiac contractility to lower blood pressure which, when increased, increases cerebral edema found in injured brain tissue

Caution: Vasodilation also can increase CBF and ICP; monitor for adverse effects as seen on ICP monitor

8. Vasoconstrictor

Example: phenylephrine (Neo-Synephrine)

Action: Elevates both systolic and diastolic blood pressures by arterial constriction to prevent ischemia during a hypotensive crisis

Caution: Careful monitoring is necessary to prevent hypertensive crisis and disruption of the blood–brain barrier; titrate as soon as possible

NURSING MANAGEMENT

Monitoring and Managing Clinical Problems

1. Gas Exchange: impaired — hypoxia and hypercapnia. Hypoxemia causes vasodilation and increased CBV, resulting in increased ICP.
   a. Monitor for hypoxia and hypercapnia.
      1) Monitor for adequate airway with appropriate head positioning or mechanical airway.
      2) Assess breath sounds frequently for abnormal and adventitious sounds.
      3) Obtain blood specimens and monitor ABGs for increased $PaCO_2$ and decreased PaO_2, pH; report significant changes.
      4) Apply pulse oximeter and monitor oxygen saturation in response to nursing care activities.

     5) Assess for deteriorating level of consciousness; correlate findings with ABGs.
  b. Promote adequate cerebral gas exchange.
     1) Maintain patient at normotensive state.
     2) Limit suctioning and do not suction within 30 minutes before obtaining specimen for ABGs.
     3) Preoxygenate with 100% O_2 before suctioning. Do not vigorously hyperventilate; alkalosis can cause vasoconstriction and subsequent elevations in ICP.
     4) Passively turn patient while monitoring oxygen saturation.

2. Tissue Perfusion, altered: cerebral
  a. Facilitate cerebral venous drainage.
     1) Elevate head of bed 20–30 degrees or as ordered.
     2) Maintain head in alignment with trunk without pillow.
     3) Avoid having the patient flex at the hip.
     4) Do not place the patient in the prone position.
     5) Prevent increased intrathoracic or intra-abdominal pressures.
       a) Limit suctioning.
       b) Prevent coughing.
       c) Limit hiccoughing.
       d) Insert nasogastric tube.
       e) Prevent Valsalva maneuver, preventing the patient straining for stool and passively turning the patient or using a kinetic bed.

3. Tissue Perfusion, altered: cerebral, high risk for — hypertension causes cerebral edema in a damage blood–brain barrier and hypotension causes decreased CBV, CBF, and increases ischemia to brain tissue.
  a. Administer vasopressors to maintain systolic blood pressure within 70–140 mm Hg systolic range.
  b. Correct hypertension to within 70–140 mm Hg systolic range. Do not lower blood pressure excessively if there is an IICP. The increased blood pressure is a compensatory mechanism to aid in blood flow to the brain. Lowering the systolic pressure could compromise this CBF.

4. Hyperthermia — increases brain metabolism, CBF, and CO_2 production.
  a. Use minimal bedcovering to cover patient.

   b. Administer cool-water sponging.

   c. Apply hypothermia blanket, as indicated.

   d. Administer ordered acetaminophen, as indicated.

   e. Prevent shivering, which would increase cerebral metabolism and hypoxemia.

   f. Do not increase fluids to lower temperature.

5. Injury: high risk for—seizures increase cerebral metabolic rate by producing large amounts of CO_2, burning glucose, and using oxygen.

   a. Protect body position and extremities during seizures without restraining or interfering with activity.

   b. Observe ICP monitor for abnormal increases, if available.

   c. Assess neurologic vital signs after seizure.

   d. Keep padded siderails in upright position and bed in lowest position.

   e. Have emergency resuscitation equipment in close proximity.

   f. Take skin or tympanic temperatures; avoid taking temperature orally.

   g. Administer ordered anticonvulsants, as indicated.

6. Nutrition: altered, less than body requirements—hypermetabolism increases CO_2 production and uses excessive amounts of calories and oxygen.

   a. Monitor daily weights.

   b. Monitor for hyperthermia, abnormal oxygen consumption.

   c. Administer adequate calories and proteins via enteral feedings, as ordered.

   d. Control muscle activity, seizures via use of sedation and neuromuscular blocking agents.

Monitoring, Managing, and Preventing Life-Threatening Emergencies

1. Herniation syndrome—a downward protrusion of the brain from the cranium through the tentorium due to increased pressure within the cranium

   a. Monitor for change in behavior and deterioration in level of consciousness.

     1) Difficulty concentrating and restlessness in early stage

     2) Coma in late stage

    b. Note any respiratory pattern change.
      1) Ranges from no change to possibly Cheyne-Stokes respirations in early stage
      2) Shallow, grossly irregular to respiratory arrest in late stage
    c. Assess pupillary size and reaction.
      1) Unilaterally sluggish to nonreactive dilated pupils in early stage
      2) Bilaterally fixed and dilated pupils in late stage
    d. Assess motor response.
      1) Contralateral hemiparesis to hemiplegia in early stage
      2) Ipsilateral rigidity, decorticate or decerebrate posturing, or flaccidity with occasional decerebrate movement in mid to late stage
    e. Assist physician with oculocephalic and oculovestibular tests.
      1) An abnormal response for an oculocephalic test would be for the eyes to look straight ahead regardless of head movement. This indicates pontine-midbrain damage.
      2) An abnormal response for an oculovestibular test would be no eye movement regardless of ice-water instillation into the ear.
2. Status epilepticus/serial seizures—a series of tonic-clonic motor movements with or without restoration periods between each episode. The major clinical concern in the patient already experiencing IICP is increased cerebral metabolism.
    a. Administer anticonvulsants and monitor for additional seizures or respiratory compromise after medicating.
    b. Observe for respiratory depression and/or laryngospasm during seizure.
    c. Administer phenytoin or phenobarbital to prevent recurrence.
3. Malignant intracranial hypertension—a sustained ICP >20 mm Hg resulting in neuronal damage and ischemia
    a. Administer ordered vasopressors, as indicated.
    b. Monitor vital signs and neurologic vital signs continuously.
    c. Have emergency resuscitation equipment nearby.

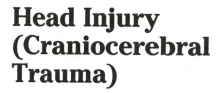

Head Injury (Craniocerebral Trauma)

Head injury (craniocerebral trauma) is defined as injury to the skull, brain, or both.

Defining Head Injury Terms

Closed head injury	A blunt injury in which there is no penetration of the skull and therefore no contact with the outside environment
Open head injury	A head injury causing direct exposure of the cranial contents to the environment
Coup injury	Brain tissue injury located directly at the site of impact on the skull
Contrecoup injury	Brain tissue injury located at the pole opposite the site of impact on the skull, which can be caused by the brain's movement inside the cranium
Focal injury	Injury to a limited area of the brain directly from the initial insult

Continued

Defining Head Injury Terms — *Continued*

Diffuse injury	Injury involving the entire brain
Primary injury	Injury that occurs with direct impact
Secondary injury	Injury that results from the initial impact and often results in a cascade of pathophysiologic events that lead to a poor prognosis or death

Etiology/Pathophysiology

1. Mechanism of injury
   a. Primary injury
      1) Skull fractures
         a) Linear fracture: a low-velocity injury causing a crack in the skull
         b) Comminuted fracture: a direct-impact injury causing fragmentation of bone at the fracture
         c) Depressed fracture: an inward depression of skull fragments, which may have debris mixed within wound
         d) Basilar skull fracture: a fracture located at the base of the cranium, where the bones are very fragile and integrated closely with the dura. It carries a high risk for cerebrospinal fluid leakage and infection via a dural tear in the ear or nose.
      2) Brain injuries
         a) Acceleration-deceleration injury is caused by the brain tissues bouncing within the cranium.
         b) Rotational injury is caused by the shearing or tension created by the friction of brain surface and inner cranium upon impact.
         c) Missile or impalement injuries include both focal and diffuse brain injury.
   b. Secondary head injuries
      1) Cerebral edema: swelling of brain tissue due to excess water content. This swelling may be localized or throughout the entire brain, depriving different areas of oxygen and glucose. This malnourishment of cells prevents adequate performance of the sodium pump, which further increases fluid accumulation. Cerebral edema contributes to increasing intracranial pressure (ICP).
      2) Increased ICP: increased pressure within the cranial vault, which can cause the following:
         a) Decreased cerebral perfusion pressure and ischemia
            1] Cerebral perfusion pressure is the blood pressure present throughout the brain mat-

ter. It is determined by the mean arterial pressure minus the ICP and is normally between 70–100 mm Hg.

2] Minimum cerebral perfusion pressure needed to deliver nutrients to the brain is usually 60 mm Hg.

3] If the ICP increases, the cerebral perfusion pressure decreases with eventual ischemia to brain tissue.

b) Decreased cerebral blood flow (CBF)

1] Cerebral edema leads to increased brain mass, which impinges on cerebral vessels, slowing the blood flow and nutrients to the brain.

2] This increase in carbon dioxide waste and decrease in oxygen activates the regulatory mechanisms to correct acidosis. Vasodilation occurs, resulting in increased blood flow and volume.

3] This added volume only compounds the increased ICP, with eventual failure of the autoregulatory system, and destruction of the blood–brain barrier.

4] CBF passively responds to systemic arterial blood pressure rather than responding to ICP. Perfusion pressure lowers and blood flow slowly fades with the compression of cerebral vessels from the increased pressure.

2. Location of injury

a. Focal injuries are those injuries occurring in a localized area. (See Table, "Focal Brain Injuries".)

b. Diffuse injuries incorporate a large portion of brain tissue.

1) Concussion: reversible disruption of axons on the nerve pathway involved in wakefulness

2) Diffuse axonal injury: widespread damage to the brain axons due to a high impact acceleration-deceleration force

3) Hypoxic brain injury: a widespread damage to the brain caused by lack of oxygen to the cells

Assessment/Analysis

ASSESSMENT FINDINGS

Subjective

1. Headache
2. Tingling, paresthesia
3. Loss of feeling in extremity, paralysis

Objective

1. Changes in the level of consciousness: Level of consciousness varies, but generally it deteriorates as the secondary injury evolves with cerebral edema and increased ICP. The Glasgow Coma Scale is used with the head-injured patient. It is divided into three areas of eye opening, best verbal response, and best motor response, and assesses for arousal as well as mentation.

Describing Level of Consciousness*

Fully conscious	Awake, alert, and oriented to person, place, and time; comprehends and is able to express the written and spoken word
Confusion	Has difficulty with memory and following commands; may have hallucinations, be agitated, or disoriented to time, person, or place
Lethargy	Oriented to time, person, and place but very slow in mental, motor, and speech functions
Obtundation	Follows simple commands when stimulated and can answer with simple phrases
Stupor	Unresponsive except when vigorously stimulated; answers with inappropriate sounds or may open eyes; appropriate in avoiding painful stimuli

Continued

Describing Level of Consciousness — *Continued*

Coma	Does not appear to respond to stimuli; eyes closed; levels of coma differentiated by purposeful, nonpurposeful, or unresponsive motor movement

*To ensure continuity of assessment, all personnel should be using the same term to describe the patient's condition.

2. Cranial nerve dysfunction (see Table Assessing Cranial Nerves.)
   a. Common nerve injuries with head injury:
      1) Optic (CN II)
      2) Abducens (CN VI)
      3) Facial (CN VII)
      4) Acoustic (CN VIII)
   b. Noting abnormalities during cranial nerve assessment helps locate the area of brain dysfunction. Generally, the cranial nerves can be placed in three groups, corresponding to specific areas of the brainstem.
      1) Alteration in group I indicates damage to midbrain
         a) Olfactory (CN I)
         b) Optic (CN II)
         c) Oculomotor (CN III)
         4) Trochlear (CN IV)
      2) Alteration in group II indicates damage to the pons
         a) Trigeminal (CN V)
         b) Abducens (CN VI)
         c) Facial (CN VII)
         d) Acoustic (CN VIII)
      3) Alteration in Group III indicates damage to the medulla
         a) Glossopharyngeal (CN IX)
         b) Vagus (CN X)
         c) Spinal accessory (CN XI)
         d) Hypoglossal (CN XII)

Assessing Cranial Nerves

Number	Cranial Nerve	Testing	Function	Testing Method
I	Olfactory	Sensory	Smell	Deferred in critical care
II	Optic	Sensory	Vision	Ask the patient to read the menu or newspaper, or ask "How many fingers do I have up?"
III	Oculomotor	Motor	Movement of eyes, upper eyelids	III, IV, and VI tested together; check all quadrants of extraocular field by having the patient follow an object with the eyes; check pupillary response:
IV	Trochlear	Motor	Movement of eyes	Consensual response— light in one eye constricts the pupil in the other eye
VI	Abducens	Motor	Movement of eyes	Direct response—light in one eye constricts the pupil in that eye
V	Trigeminal	Motor	Chewing movement of jaw	Ask the patient to "bite down"; check strength in cheeks

Continued

243

Assessing Cranial Nerves—*Continued*

Number	Cranial Nerve	Testing	Function	Testing Method
VII	Facial	Motor	Facial expression	Ask patient to smile; observe for unilateral or bilateral function
VIII	Acoustic	Sensory	Hearing	Whisper numbers; have patient repeat them
IX	Glossopharyngeal	Motor	Swallow, gag reflex	Have patient swallow water or check gag reflex by stimulating the pharynx with a cotton swab
X	Vagus	Motor	Swallow, gag, and cough reflex	
XI	Spinal accessory	Motor	Movement of head and shoulders	Ask patient to shrug shoulders; push against shoulder; check strength
XII	Hypoglossal	Motor	Movement of tongue	Ask patient to push tongue against his cheek; check cheek strength

3. Pupil size and reactivity
   a. Pinpoint—indicates pontine hemorrhage or opiate overdose
   b. Small, but larger than pinpoint—could indicate normal reaction in bright room, pontine hemorrhage, bilateral diencephalic lesions, metabolic coma, or be drug related
   c. Midposition and nonreactive—pupil and iris are equal in surface area—indicates midbrain damage
   d. Large—unilateral, sluggish to fixed
   e. Dilated—bilateral, fixed—indicative of severe anoxia or death; a dilated pupil that reacts sluggishly or not at all to light indicates ocular nerve compression, usually from edema or a lesion on the same side as the dilation
4. Pupil shape
   a. Ovoid, or slightly oval—indicates increased ICP with ominous sign toward herniation
   b. Keyhole or irregular shaped—generally indicates previous surgery or trauma to the pupil
5. Excessive sweating on the face, and sometimes the neck and chest, may be seen in diffuse axonal injury.
6. Nausea and vomiting
7. Onset of seizure activity
8. Leakage of cerebral spinal fluid (CSF) and blood from ear or nose
   a. Commonly seen with basilar skull fractures
   b. CSF tests positive for dextrose.
   c. CSF produces yellow halo around bloody drainage on sheet or gauze.
9. Presence of Battle's sign: bruising over mastoid process of temporal bone seen 24 hours after basilar skull fracture injury
10. Presence of periorbital bruising or "raccoon eyes" noted with basilar skull fractures.
11. Bradycardia, which occurs with increased ICP as blood pressure increases and is a late and ominous sign of increased ICP and possible herniation
12. Widened pulse pressure as a result of increased ICP, an ominous sign of increased ICP and herniation
13. Abnormal respiratory pattern dependent on location and extent of injury and increased ICP; becomes more significant with pons and medulla involvement

14. Hyperthermia may be seen on admission or appear within the first few days after head injury; may decrease, only to re-elevate sporadically; may be due to hypothalamic dysfunction or infection
15. Changes in motor function usually occur contra-laterally, or on the opposite side, of where the lesion is located.
    a. Abnormalities noted in the conscious patient
        1) Inability to grasp with hands, or inequality of handgrasps
        2) Inability to extend and hold arms above body at equal distance
        3) Weakened resistance in hands and arms, when tested
        4) Inability to flex or extend upper leg, knee, and ankle on either or both sides
        5) Weakened resistance when pressing either/both feet against the examiner's hands
        6) Abnormal gait, if able to walk
        7) Involuntary movements
    b. Abnormalities noted in the unconscious patient
        1) Increased resistance to extension of extremity
        2) Flaccid or loose extremity movement with passive motion
        3) Constant inflexible muscle condition with or without noxious stimuli, indicating cerebral damage
            a) Abnormal flexion or decortication: a flexion of the upper extremities with extension of ankles, indicative of hemispheric dysfunction
            b) Abnormal adduction or decerebration: hyperextension of arms and legs, which can develop to arching of the back and hyperextension of the neck and head; indicates movement of brain tissue in a head-to-toe motion, as in herniation
            c) Generally, as herniation progresses, abnormal movement goes from decortication to decerebration to flaccidity.
            d) Both decerebration and decortication may occur simultaneously on different sides of the

body, or with movements vacillating between the two types. This perplexing movement is due to the obscurity of injured tissue within the deep cerebral hemisphere and the upper portion of the brainstem.

16. Positive Babinski's reflex indicates damage to the corticospinal tract

SUPPORTING TEST FINDINGS

Laboratory Tests

1. No laboratory test specifically diagnoses head injury.

Diagnostic Tests

1. Computed tomography scan
   Abnormality: Hematoma
   Intracranial shift, herniation
2. Magnetic resonance imaging
   Abnormality: Small hemorrhages associated with diffuse axonal injury
   Posterior fossa lesions
   Brainstem lesions
   Nonhemorrhagic contusions and shearing injuries
3. Positron emission tomography
   Abnormality: Areas of decreased metabolism secondary to injury
4. Transcranial Doppler ultrasound
   Abnormality: Abnormal blood flow velocity in the head-injured patient with intracranial hypertension
   Vasospasm in subarachnoid hemorrhage
5. Auditory evoked potentials
   Abnormality: Prolonged conduction or absence of waveforms, indicating brainstem dysfunction or brain death secondary to head trauma
6. Skull X-ray
   Abnormality: Skull fractures
7. Radionuclide scintigraphy
   Abnormality: Subdural hematomas, tumors
   Vascular lesions
   Cerebral or bone lesions that disrupt the blood–brain barrier

Planning/Intervention

COLLABORATIVE MANAGEMENT

Procedures

1. Monitor and promote neurologic function.
   a. Monitor vital signs hourly or as needed until stable.
   b. Perform neurologic assessment using Glasgow Coma Scale.
   c. Be prepared to assist with instituting ICP monitoring if Glasgow Coma Scale is less than or equal to eight.
   d. Assist physician in oculovestibular reflex (caloric stimulation) testing.
   e. Assess oculocephalic reflex (doll's eye phenomenon).
2. Reduce or prevent increased ICP.
   a. Elevate head of bed 20–30 degrees once X-ray of cervical spine confirms no injury.
   b. Keep neck in neutral position between flexion and extension to aid in venous drainage.
   c. Assist with insertion of endotracheal tube and patent airway to prevent ventilatory insufficiency.
   d. Obtain specimens and monitor arterial blood gases (ABGs) to prevent vasodilation of cerebral vasculature due to hypercarbia and hypoxia.
   e. Maintain hypothermia blanket with rectal probe to inhibit hypermetabolism and subsequent ischemia with cerebral edema.
   f. Maintain seizure precautions to prevent increased cerebral metabolism and subsequent elevations in ICP.
   g. Restrict intravenous (IV) fluids to 1,200–1,500 mL/24 h.
   h. Prepare patient for intracranial surgery, as ordered.
3. Support body functions and prevent complications.
   a. Maintain indwelling urinary catheter patency to prevent bladder distention.
   b. Insert nasogastric tube after all anterior fossa, basilar skull or midface fractures have been ruled out. If basilar or midface fracture present, insert nasogastric tube after endotracheal intubation complete, to prevent aspiration. Monitor nasogastric tube contents for coffee-ground or blood return.

c. Administer total parenteral nutrition to prevent hypercatabolic state when paralytic ileus is present.
d. Administer enteral feedings when intestinal motility present.
e. Assist with insertion of arterial line to aid in the collection of ABGs.
f. Assist with the insertion of a pulmonary artery catheter for hemodynamic monitoring.

Drug Therapy

1. Corticosteroids
   Examples: methylprednisolone (Solu-Medrol)
       dexamethasone (Decadron)
   Action: Stabilize cell membranes and prevent lysosomal rupture, as well as reduce edema and CSF production
   Caution: Although there have been positive results for reducing edema around tumors, studies are inconclusive on the success of methylprednisolone and head injury
2. Diuretics
   Examples: furosemide (Lasix)
       mannitol (Osmitrol)
   Action: Reduce total body water by removing water and electrolytes, thereby reducing cerebral edema, a common complication of head injury
       Mannitol, an osmotic diuretic, increases serum osmolality to create an osmotic gradient that pulls the fluid from the brain's internal environment into the systemic circulation; this requires an undamaged, or intact, blood–brain barrier
       Furosemide works at the loop of Henle, where it inhibits the reabsorption of chloride and sodium
   Caution: Can cause electrolyte imbalance, cardiac arrhythmias secondary to diuresis
       Mannitol may produce a rebound effect approximately 12 hours after administration, with an increase in ICP
3. Anticonvulsants
   Examples: diazepam (Valium)
       phenytoin (Dilantin)
       phenobarbital (Luminal)
   Action: Inhibit seizure activity, a complication of head injury, by different actions:

Diazepam produces calm and smooth muscle relaxation

Phenytoin alters ion transport and may also decrease synaptic transmission

Phenobarbital produces a sedative effect by interfering with the impulse transmission of the cerebral cortex

Caution: Phenobarbital can cause respiratory distress, circulatory collapse, coma when given in large doses; have emergency equipment ready

Phenytoin can cause cardiovascular collapse; administer slowly IV, with emergency equipment nearby

4. Neuromuscular blocking agents

Example: pancuronium (Pavulon)

Action: Induces skeletal muscle relaxation by blocking neuromuscular transmission, aiding in the ventilatory management of the head-injured patient

Caution: Causes almost immediate respiratory depression, lasting 20–60 minutes; patient is totally ventilator-dependent during this time; patient's level of consciousness cannot be determined while motor movement is compromised by drug

5. Hormone

Example: vasopressin (Pitressin)

Action: Increases tubular reabsorption of water and sodium to counteract the complication of diabetes insipidus in the head-injured patient

Caution: Stimulates smooth muscle contraction around vessels, causing vasoconstriction of splanchnic, coronary, gastrointestinal, and other smooth muscles; observe for angina, myocardial infarction depending on dose

Investigational Drugs

Tromethamine (THAM), superoxide dismutase (SOD), and polyethylene glycol conjugated superoxide dismutase (PEG-SOD) are being used experimentally to reduce the sequelae of head injury. THAM reduces cerebral acidosis, intracranial pressure, and vasoconstriction caused by prophylactic hyperventilation in the acute head injury phase.

Continued

Investigational Drugs — *Continued*

SOD and PEG-SOD scavenge for superoxide anions that assist in neuronal death following ischemia from brain injury.

NURSING MANAGEMENT

Monitoring and Managing Clinical Problems

1. Tissue Perfusion, altered: cerebral, high risk for
   a. Monitor/assess cerebral tissue integrity.
      1) Note and report scalp lacerations, open head wounds, and drainage from same.
      2) Note and report amount and color of any drainage from ears, nose, or mouth that might be CSF.
      3) Monitor ABG analysis for hypoxia and hypercarbia.
      4) Assess unassisted respiratory rate, rhythm, and lung sounds.
      5) Assess ventilated patient's reaction to change in ventilator settings, especially when placed on positive end-expiratory pressures, which increase intrathoracic pressures and eventually ICP.
      6) Monitor ICP and calculate cerebral perfusion pressures (mean arterial pressure − ICP).
      7) Monitor blood pressure and report deteriorating trend of increased pulse pressure and hypertension or hypotension.
      8) Monitor temperature and report elevations.
   b. Promote cerebral tissue integrity.
      1) Clean and cover all head wounds as ordered, using sterile technique.
      2) Check drainage from the nose, mouth, or ear for presence of dextrose or positive Halo test, which would indicate CSF.
      3) Refrain from cleaning orifices immediately following injury to prevent introducing bacteria through a possible dural tear.
      4) Suction only as necessary.
      5) Oxygenate before and immediately after suctioning. Do not hyperventilate; this will cause a re-

bound cerebral vasoconstriction with subsequent cerebral ischemia.

6) Space nursing activities most stressful to patient, performing them as smoothly as possible, when necessary.

7) Observe ICP monitor, if available, to ascertain patient's greatest elevations in ICP in response to nursing care.

8) Elevate head of bed and keep head in neutral position after cervical-spine X-ray is cleared of any abnormalities.

9) Maintain nasogastric suction of stomach contents to lower intra-abdominal pressure and diaphragm.

c. Assess for increased intracranial pressure

1) Assess and report any deterioration in level of consciousness.

2) Assess cranial nerve function and report any abnormalities.

3) Assess sensory-motor function and report any abnormalities.

4) Observe and report alterations in ICP with turning, suctioning, bathing, mouth care, and stimulation from visitors.

2. Fluid Volume Excess or Defecit: high risk for

a. Monitor fluid and electrolyte balance.

1) Assess intake and output for trending over several hours, days.

2) Assist with insertion of arterial line and monitor hemodynamic parameters.

3) Monitor blood pressure and heart rate, and report significant changes.

4) Obtain specimens and monitor blood urea nitrogen, and serum creatinine, osmolality, and electrolytes. Report abnormalities.

5) Monitor cardiac arrhythmias associated with the use of diuretics.

6) Assess for clinical signs of dehydration or overhydration.

7) Monitor urine specific gravity.

8) Monitor daily weights. Note and report significant changes.

b. Promote fluid and electrolyte balance.

1) Regulate fluid intake according to output, keeping patient slightly dehydrated, as ordered.
2) Administer ordered diuretics, urea, and glucose and assess patient response to treatment.

c. Assess for any complications in fluid and electrolyte balance.

1) Syndrome of inappropriate secretion of antidiuretic hormone
   a) Monitor intake and output for fluid retention (<500 mL in 24 hours).
   b) Observe daily weights for increase.
   c) Monitor for low serum osmolality and urine osmolality equal to or greater than serum osmolality.
   d) Monitor for concentrated urine specific gravity (>1.030).
   e) Note any signs of hyponatremia, including lethargy, confusion, muscle weakness, cramping, headache, seizures, and loss of consciousness.
   f) Assess for signs of fluid overload, including distended neck veins, increased respiratory rate, and crackles on lung auscultation.

2) Diabetes insipidus
   a) Monitor hourly output for >200 mL/h for 2 consecutive hours, with no diuretic therapy.
   b) Observe daily weights for decrease.
   c) Monitor for high serum osmolality and low urine osmolality every 1–2 hours.
   d) Monitor for dilute urine and specific gravity <1.005.
   e) Note any signs of dehydration, including lethargy, listlessness, sunken eyeballs, and poor skin turgor.
   f) Replace fluids, as indicated.
   g) Administer ordered vasopressin.

3) Neurogenic pulmonary edema
   a) Monitor lung sounds for acute increase in respiratory rate, crackles, and wheezing.
   b) Assess lung secretions for increase in amount and change in amount, color, and texture.
   c) Monitor vital signs for elevated blood pressure and rapid thready pulse.

3. Nutrition: altered, less than body requirements — hyperdynamic cerebral metabolism
   a. Monitor and assess for catabolism.
      1) Weigh daily at same time, with same amount of covering.
      2) Compare caloric intake with estimated metabolic rate.
      3) Assess intake and output for significant changes or trends.
      4) Assess cerebral perfusion pressure if ICP monitoring is available.
      5) Observe for shivering and elevated temperature.
      6) Monitor for and report seizure activity.
      7) Monitor effect of patient activity on SvO_2.
   b. Promote cerebral metabolism.
      1) Keep patient normothermic by using hypothermia blanket and checking temperature each hour, or as needed.
      2) Administer anticonvulsants for seizures, as ordered.
      3) Administer total parenteral nutrition solutions, as ordered, if ileus present.
      4) Begin enteric feedings as soon as ileus is resolved.
      5) Provide for oxygenation with proper ventilation.

Monitoring, Managing, and Preventing Life-Threatening Emergencies

1. Herniation syndrome
   a. Supratentorial herniation
      1) Subfalcine (cingulate) herniation: a unilateral swelling with brain tissue shifted laterally under the midline dural fold, falx cerebri
      2) Central (transtentorial) herniation: the head-to-toe pushing of contents, displacing the upper brainstem and midbrain through the tentorial notch
      3) Uncal herniation: a swelling of the temporal lobe or lateral middle fossa, displacing the medial portion of the temporal lobe down into the tentorial notch
   b. Infratentorial herniation

1) Upward transtentorial herniation with midbrain compression
2) Downward transtentorial herniation through foramen magnum

c. Nursing management
   1) Monitor for difficulty concentrating and restlessness, early signs of deteriorating level of consciousness. Coma is a late sign.
   2) Note any respiratory pattern change. Cheyne-Stokes respirations are an early sign of herniation; grossly irregular respirations to respiratory arrest occur in late stage.
   3) Assess pupillary size and reaction. Early on herniation pupils are unilaterally sluggish to nonreactive. Bilaterally fixed and dilated pupils are a late sign.
   4) Assess motor response. Contralateral hemiparesis and hemiplegia are early signs. Ipsilateral rigidity, decorticate posturing, decerebrate posturing, and flaccidity with occasional decerebrate movements are mid to late signs.
   5) Assist physician with oculocephalic (doll's eye phenomenon) and oculovestibular (ice-water caloric) tests.
      a) An abnormal response for an oculocephalic test would be for the eyes to look straight ahead regardless of head movement. This indicates pontine-midbrain damage.
      b) An abnormal response for an oculovestibular test would be no eye movement regardless of ice-water instillation into the ear.

Focal Brain Injuries*

Type	Pathophysiology	Signs and Symptoms	Prognosis	Nursing Actions
■ Cerebral contusion—actual bruising of the brain due to an acceleration-deceleration injury	■ Damage may be asymmetric ■ May be a coup-contrecoup injury ■ Bruising and edema from capillary hemorrhage ■ Frontal and temporal area most often affected	■ Confusion and restlessness ■ Loss of consciousness lasting from a few minutes to weeks ■ Alert with hemiparesis suggests frontal contusion ■ Agitation and disorientation suggests temporal contusion ■ Aphasia suggests frontal-temporal contusions ■ Deep coma and	■ May have secondary injury from increased ICP	■ Observe for change in level of consciousness, pupils, respiratory pattern, and motor responses ■ Ensure safety by reorienting patient

		decerebrate posturing suggests brainstem contusion		
■ Cerebral laceration—an actual tear in the brain tissue caused by a shearing force	■ Tearing of brain tissue with a break in the meningeal layers ■ Usually at an area of uneven cranial surface ■ May be present with skull fracture or cerebral contusion	■ No specific symptoms ■ Clinical presentation reflects contusion or fracture	■ Dependent on extent of damage and secondary injury	■ Observe for deterioration in level of consciousness and abnormal pupils, respiratory pattern, and motor response indicating bleeding ■ Monitor open head injury for infection
■ Epidural hematoma—	■ Often results from temporal	■ Momentary unconsciousness	■ Dependent on proper	■ Monitor level of consciousness,

Continued

257

Focal Brain Injuries* — Continued

Type	Pathophysiology	Signs and Symptoms	Prognosis	Nursing Actions
bleeding between the skull and dura mater	bone fracture and middle meningeal arterial bleeding ■ Produces symptoms when quantity of blood experts pressure on the brain	after injury followed by a period of awakeness and lucid thinking lasting up to several hours ■ Followed by a rapid deterioration in level of consciousness ■ Pupils dilate ipsilateral to lesion and motor responses are abnormal when hematoma expands	assessment and treatment ■ If hematoma is surgically evacuated and bleeding stops, prognosis is good	pupillary changes, motor responses, and vital signs ■ Report significant changes

Acute subdural hematoma— Bleeding between the dura mater and arachnoid layers, associated with brain contusion and laceration	■ Often results from venous or small cerebral artery bleeding in the frontal or temporal areas	■ Headache ■ Rapid deterioration from confusion, agitation, and difficulty thinking to coma ■ Ipsilateral pupil dilation ■ Hemiparesis with increasing ICP	■ Prognosis good with immediate craniotomy, which prevents secondary injury and permanent damage	■ Monitor level of consciousness, respiratory rate and pattern, motor function, pupil response, and vital signs
Subacute subdural hematoma— Bleeding between the dura mater and arachnoid layers, associated with less severe brain	■ Results from less severe venous or small cerebral artery bleeding often in the frontal or temporal areas	■ Similar to acute subdural hematoma but symptoms occur from 2 days up to 2 weeks after injury	■ May require craniotomy if midline shift seen on computed tomography scan	■ Monitor changes in ICP, response to drug therapy, and results of laboratory tests

Continued

259

Focal Brain Injuries* — *Continued*

Type	Pathophysiology	Signs and Symptoms	Prognosis	Nursing Actions
contusion and intracerebral bleeding				
■ Chronic subdural hematoma—Blood clot between the dura mater and arachnoid layers	■ Blood encased in membrane and cell lysis causes osmotic gradient, pulling of fluid into and enlargement of space	■ Symptoms develop from 2 weeks to several months after injury ■ Gradual onset of symptoms may be attributed to senility or cerebral atrophy ■ Gradual onset of headache ■ Behavioral changes ■ Ipsilateral pupil dilation with	■ May require craniotomy for gelatinous hematoma	■ Monitor vital signs and neurologic vital signs for evidence of rebleeding after surgery

		sluggish light response		
■ Intracerebral hematoma— Bleeding into the brain mass, associated with contusion or laceration	■ Generalized usually over the frontal and temporal lobes and deep in the hemispheres	■ Ipsilateral pupil dilation ■ Decreasing level of consciousness ■ Contralateral hemiparesis ■ Abnormal respirations, and pupillary and motor response with transtentorial herniation	■ Poor prognosis ■ Usually permanent neurologic deficits	■ Supportive postoperative care ■ Prepare family for poor prognosis
■ Subarachnoid hemorrhage— Bleeding into the subarachnoid space between the pia and	■ Usually results from direct disruption of major vessels caused by trauma or from a	■ Excruciating headache ■ Sudden loss of consciousness ■ Nausea and vomiting	■ Immediate surgical removal of hematoma may reduce or prevent increasing ICP,	■ Monitor for signs and cerebral edema and increasing ICP and intervene immediately

Continued

Focal Brain Injuries—Continued

Type	Pathophysiology	Signs and Symptoms	Prognosis	Nursing Actions
arachnoid	ruptured cerebral aneurysm	■ Dizziness and vertigo ■ Sweating, chills, fever ■ Photophobia and diplopia ■ Nuchal rigidity ■ Seizures ■ Positive Kernig's and Brudzinski's signs	brain ischemia, and permanent damage	
■ Brainstem injury—Damage to brainstem tissue, usually as a result of secondary injury	■ Generally occurs with diffuse axonal injury from trauma, increasing ICP, and subsequent herniation	■ Immediate onset of coma from moment of injury ■ Level of consciousness and respiratory pattern indicates level of damage	■ With continued brainstem compression, vital organ functions will cease ■ Surgery will not restore function	■ Monitor and treat increasing ICP ■ Support respirations

*ICP = intracranial pressure.

Acute Spinal Cord Injury

Acute spinal cord injury is a traumatic injury to the spinal cord that interrupts the nerve impulses between the peripheral and central nervous systems, impairing both sensory and motor function.

Etiology/Pathophysiology

1. Occurs most often in male patients under age 30 years
2. Most common causes
   a. Motor vehicle accident
   b. Falls
   c. Diving accident
   d. Gunshot wound
3. Mechanism of injury
   a. Hyperextension
      1) Falling forward, hitting chin, and snapping head backward
      2) Fracture in posterior spinal column
      3) Injury to anterior ligaments
      4) Greatest stress point at C4 and C5
   b. Hyperflexion
      1) Anterior dislocation or fracture
      2) Tearing of posterior ligaments
      3) Sudden deceleration, such as with diving or head-on collision
      4) Greatest stress point C-5, C-6, T-11, T-12, and L-1
   c. Vertical compression (or axial loading)
      1) Vertical force placed on spinal column
      2) Occurs when landing on feet or buttocks during a fall or jumping and diving
   d. Rotational
      1) Extreme lateral rotation
      2) Ruptures posterior ligament and may cause neurologic deficit
   e. Penetration
      1) Sharp object enters the spinal cord.
      2) Shattered vertebral column produces bone fragments.
      3) Cut across a portion or all of the spinal cord caused by complete or incomplete transection

Types of Spinal Cord Injury

Type	Etiology/ Pathophysiology	Prognosis/ Functional Levels
Concussion	Severe shaking of the spinal cord. Brief disturbance of cord function. No identified pathophysiology	Lasts up to 48 hours with no residual neurologic dysfunction
Contusion	Vertebral fractures or dislocations compresses cord from direct trauma. Microscopic hemorrhages and edema cause ischemia and bruising of the cord tissue	Surgery may be needed. Prognosis depends on the length of time injury remains untreated, degrees of cord ischemia, and presence of collateral circulation
Laceration	Actual tearing of cord tissue that may accompany compression following fracture, contusion, and edema	Damage is permanent. Functional level depends on section of cord damaged
Transection	Complete or incomplete severing of the cord	Damage is permanent below the level of cord injury

4. Pathophysiology
   a. Usually spinal cord is not completely severed at the time of injury. Primary injury initiates a domino effect caused by chemical and vascular changes.
   b. Within minutes of injury, tiny hemorrhagic lesions and inflammation occur in the central cord. Within 4 hours of injury, the affected tissue is denied oxygen, producing swelling and ischemia.
   c. Spinal shock occurs with injury above T-4–T-6, interrupting the sympathetic pathways of the autonomic nervous system.
      1) Without sympathetic influence, the parasympathetic system dominates, slowing heart rate and dilating peripheral vessels and resulting in decreased cardiac output (CO) and blood pressure.
      2) Vasodilation and subsequent cooling, as well as inability to shiver and produce more heat, cause low body temperature.
      3) Usually resolves in about 4–6 weeks but may last longer in severe injury. Return of perianal reflexes signals resolution of spinal shock.
      4) With upper motor neuron injury, deep tendon reflexes will return but they may be hyperactive and spastic. Babinski's reflex will be positive.
      5) With lower motor neuron injury, deep tendon reflexes and Babinski's reflex will be absent and flaccidity will be present.
      6) Incomplete spinal cord syndromes have the potential for partial recovery. Spinal shock symptoms vary with incomplete lesions and depend on the section of cord involved.

Incomplete Spinal Cord Transections

Type	Vertebral Injury	Section of Cord Affected	Function Lost
Anterior cord syndrome	Flexion and compression injury	Anterior portion. (Posterior section controlling pathways for light touch, proprioception, and vibration are spared)	Motor, pain, temperature, and sensation below the level of the lesion
Brown-Séquard's syndrome	Penetration injury	Right or left side of cord penetrated	Ipsilateral motor, touch, position, and vibration
Central cord syndrome	Hyperextension injury	Central portion affected by edema and compression between disks	Greater loss of motor and sensory in upper extremities

Assessment/Analysis

ASSESSMENT FINDINGS

Subjective

1. Loss of mobility and sensation below level of injury
2. Pain immediately above the level of the injury due to heightened sensitivity
3. Mild tingling and hyperesthesia after spinal shock in incomplete transection

Objective

1. Respiratory function varies with level of injury and edema. The higher the injury, the greater the respiratory insufficiency. Respiratory arrest occurs with injury above C-4.
2. Weak or absent cough or gag reflex and shallow respirations indicate respiratory insufficiency.
3. Abnormal thoracic expansion and contraction during respiratory cycle.
4. Abnormal heart rate associated with complications: bradycardia with neurogenic shock, tachycardia with hypovolemic shock.
5. Hypotension occurs with cervical lesions and during neurogenic shock due to the temporary loss of sympathetic input. Hypertension occurs after the acute stage. Life-threatening hypertensive crisis may result from noxious stimuli, creating an exaggerated sympathetic response (autonomic hyperreflexia).
6. Hypothermia resulting from inability to vasoconstrict and maintain core body temperature (loss of sympathetic tone).
7. Bladder distention or overflow caused by atonic bladder muscle.
8. Altered reflexes and motor and sensory function
   a. Total flaccid paralysis and loss of reflexes below level of injury within 60 minutes of injury (spinal shock). Can last for several weeks.
   b. Ascending deterioration in motor function for 72 hours after injury, indicating progression of spinal cord edema and subsequent ischemia and necrosis.

c. Return of reflexes signals resolution of spinal shock.
   1) Anal reflexor response if lesion is incomplete. Test for this by inserting a finger through the anus. If the patient is able to contract perianal muscle or can feel the presence of the finger, the lesion is incomplete.
   2) Positive bulbocavernosus reflex in male patients indicates an upper motor neuron lesion; its absence indicates a lower motor neuron lesion. Test for this reflex by inserting a finger in the rectum and by gently pulling on the end of the urinary catheter or pinching the distal end of the penis. Rectal sphincter contraction denotes a positive response.
   3) Changes from flaccid paralysis to spastic paralysis in a patient with upper motor neuron injury. Patients with lower motor neuron injury will continue to have flaccid paralysis.
9. Absent bowel sounds in acute stage or spinal shock, indicating paralytic ileus.
10. Lung sounds will be moist or diminished.

SUPPORTING TEST FINDINGS

Laboratory Tests

1. No laboratory tests diagnose spinal cord injury.

Diagnostic Tests

1. Cervical-spinal X-rays
   Abnormality: Disconfiguration and malalignment of the vertebral bodies
2. Computed tomography scan
   Abnormality: Injury to spinal cord
      Possibly head, intrathoracic, and intra-abdominal injuries
3. Myelography
   Abnormality: Dural defects or avulsed nerve roots
4. Pulmonary function studies
   Abnormality: Decreased vital capacity and tidal volume with respiratory insufficiency resulting from paralysis of intercostal muscles

Planning/Intervention

COLLABORATIVE MANAGEMENT

Procedures

1. Maintain adequate oxygenation to spinal cord and vital organs.
   a. Administer ordered supplemental oxygen via face mask, endotracheal intubation, or tracheostomy.
   b. Initiate mechanical ventilation with either intermittent mandatory ventilation, synchronized intermittent mandatory ventilation, pressure support ventilation, or positive end-expiratory pressure, as indicated.
   c. Obtain specimens and monitor arterial blood gases (ABGs) to determine onset of respiratory insufficiency.
   d. Place patient on cardiac and blood pressure monitors, and continuously monitor cardiac rhythm and arterial blood pressure.
   e. Assist with insertion of central venous line and monitor fluid status for overload.
   f. Assist with insertion of pulmonary artery line and monitor pulmonary artery pressure (PAP) and pulmonary capillary wedge pressure (PCWP) to maintain fluid balance and CO.
   g. Administer ordered crystalloid and colloid solutions for fluid resuscitation and volume expansion.
   h. Administer ordered vasopressor therapy to increase compromised CO.
2. Reduce injury to the spinal cord.
   a. Maintain patient in correct body alignment, initially using traction, skull tongs, or halo brace, as ordered.
   b. Do not turn the patient until a physician reviewing the X-rays has determined it is safe to do so.
   c. Place patient on a kinetic bed. Or, if one is not available, log-roll the patient, with the help of three staff members, with one stabilizing the head in a neutral position.

d. Maintain strict intake and output to keep patient slightly dehydrated to prevent spinal cord edema.
e. Monitor body temperature routinely to detect hypothermia present in spinal shock. Institute measures to maintain normal temperature and prevent hyperthermia.
f. Administer ordered steroids to help decrease cord edema.
g. Prepare patient for surgery to stabilize the spinal column, as indicated.

Functional Levels of Injury*

■ C-1–C-3	■ Quadriplegia	■ Ventilator dependent ■ Full care dependent
■ C-4	■ Quadriplegia	■ Respiratory compromised ■ Limited self-care
■ C-5	■ Quadriplegia	■ Respiratory independent but tidal volume 300 mL ■ Intercostal muscles not functional ■ Improved hand-mouth coordination, but dependent for major care
■ C-7–C-8	■ Incomplete quadriplegia	■ Potential for independent living. Transfers and activities of daily living independent
■ T-1–T-10	■ Paraplegia	■ Lung expansion increases ■ Independent in daily care ■ Manages own bowel and bladder ■ Walks with braces

*To plan care, be aware of the type of injury associated with the level of injury.

Drug Therapy

1. Inotropic agents

   Example: dopamine (Intropin)

   Action: Combats hypotension and decreased CO from peripheral vascular dilation and pooling of blood, clinical symptoms of shock

   Caution: Increases myocardial oxygen demand

2. Corticosteroids

   Example: methylprednisolone (Depo-Medrol)

   Action: Decreases spinal cord edema if administered within the first 8 hours after injury; high-dose treatment is investigational

   Caution: May exacerbate gastric irritation and bleeding and increase susceptibility to infection

3. Autonomic nervous system agents

   Example: atropine

   Action: Aids in increasing heart rate during massive parasympathetic outpouring of neurogenic shock

   Caution: Unpredictable cardiac response; increases myocardial workload; use cautiously in patients with cardiovascular compromise

4. Anticoagulant

   Example: sodium heparin (Heparin)

   Action: Prevents clotting of blood pooled in the periphery, particularly the legs, during vasodilation stage of spinal shock

   Caution: Increases risk of gastric hemorrhage

   Monitor gastric pH and coagulation time

5. Histamine$_2$-receptor antagonist

   Examples: ranitidine (Zantac)
   cimetidine (Tagamet)

   Action: Slows gastric acid secretion by inhibiting histamine at the histamine$_2$-receptor sites in the gastric parietal cells

   Caution: Cimetidine may cause false-positive findings on Hemoccult gastric test within the first 15 minutes after taking the drug orally

   May cause pulse and blood pressure changes and paralytic ileus

6. Antacids

   Examples: magnesium hydroxide/aluminum hydroxide (Maalox, Mylanta)

Action: Neutralizes gastric acid

Investigational Drugs*

Drug	*Rationale*
Opioid antagonist naloxone (Narcan)	Thought to inhibit release of endogenous opioids that decrease microcirculation and contribute to secondary injury
Calcium channel blocker nimodipine (Nimotop)	Thought to improve neurologic deficit by increasing spinal cord blood flow when used in conjunction with Adrenalin

*Two drugs are being researched for their potential use in treating spinal cord injury.

NURSING MANAGEMENT

Monitoring and Managing Clinical Problems

1. Breathing Pattern: ineffective
   a. Monitor for adequate ventilation.
      1) Monitor respiratory rate and rhythm. A stable respiratory status can quickly become unstable as edema ascends.
      2) Monitor level of consciousness for deterioration resulting from buildup of CO_2.
      3) Note use of accessory muscles for breathing. Note chest and diaphragmatic expansion for abnormalities.
      4) Assess adequacy of cough, gag, and swallow reflex.
      5) Monitor pulmonary vital capacity and tidal volume and note any significant reductions.
      6) Auscultate lungs hourly for crackles or decreased sounds.
      7) Obtain specimens and monitor ABGs for decreased pH and Pao_2 and increased $Paco_2$.
   b. Promote adequate respirations.

1) Maintain neutral cervical ailgnment with no pillow until diagnostic tests have determined the extent and location of injury.

2) Auscultate lungs hourly, or as indicated, for abnormal or adventitious sounds.

3) Have emergency resuscitation equipment nearby and be prepared to assist with emergency intubation and institute mechanical ventilation.

4) Provide humidified oxygen to keep secretions moist.

5) Preoxygenate and instill 0.9% normal saline solution before suctioning.

6) Auscultate bowel sounds hourly and note absent bowel sounds indicating paralytic ileus. If this occurs, insert a nasogastric tube to prevent vomiting and possible aspiration.

2. Tissue Perfusion, altered: peripheral
   a. Monitor cardiovascular status.
   1) Apply a cardiac monitor and monitor for cardiac arrhythmias secondary to spinal shock, pulmonary edema, or autonomic dysreflexia.
   2) Monitor blood pressure and pulse, and report significant changes. In the acute stage, hypotension accompanies spinal shock; hypertension could signal autonomic dysreflexia.
   3) Assess skin for cyanosis.
   4) Monitor for increased PAP and PCWP indicating fluid overload.
   b. Promote cardiovascular stability.
   1) Administer ordered crystalloid solutions to maintain fluid balance without overhydration.
   2) Administer ordered colloid solutions to expand plasma volume.
   3) Administer vasopressors to maintain a systolic blood pressure ≥100 mm Hg
   4) Elevate lower extremities to combat blood pooling in dilated peripheral veins, as indicated.
   5) Administer atropine for acute symptomatic bradycardia and note response on cardiac monitor.

3. Physical Mobility: impaired
   a. Monitor for complications of immobility.
   1) Assess skin for areas of redness or breakdown.

    2) Assess for redness and edema in lower extremities, which might signal deep vein thrombosis.

    3) Monitor extremities for alignment, wasting, and contractures.

    4) Monitor stools for consistency, color, and amount.

    5) Monitor urine output for amount, color, odor, and clarity.

  b. Prevent complications.

    1) Massage bony prominences.

    2) Turn by log-rolling patient, when permitted, or place patient on kinetic bed.

    3) Administer total parenteral nutrition if patient has paralytic ileus.

    4) Administer enteral feedings once ileus has resolved.

      a) Insert feeding tube and check position in stomach before administering feeding.

      b) Stay with the patient for initial and bolus enteral feeding, observing for aspiration.

    5) Perform range-of-motion exercises to promote full joint mobility.

    6) Institute bowel retraining program as soon as possible to promote adequate evacuation.

    7) Monitor hourly urine output and maintain catheter patency.

    8) Discontinue indwelling urinary catheter as soon as possible to decrease the chance of infection.

    9) Administer antibiotics prophylactically or to treat infection.

4. Injury: high risk for

  a. Monitor for occult injury.

    1) Assess cardiac monitor and arterial blood pressure continuously for signs of internal bleeding.

    2) Monitor for deterioration in the level of consciousness and cranial nerve function to assess neurologic status.

    3) Monitor respiratory excursion for unilateral movements; observe for mediastinal shift.

    4) Assess heart sounds for muffling and extra heart sounds.

  b. Promote stability of vital organ function.

    1) Report significant changes in vital signs and neurologic status.

2) Prepare patient for ordered diagnostic tests.
3) Auscultate lungs for abnormal and adventitious sounds.
4) Measure abdominal girth initially and every 8 hours.
5) Do not clean ears or nares without physician's approval. Check any drainage for presence of glucose or a yellow halo surrounding bloody drainage on gauze.
6) Cleanse any wounds with bactericidal soap and apply antibiotic ointment, as indicated.
7) Insert nasogastric tube and report significant change in color or amount of drainage.
8) Apply antiembolic stocking or sequential compression devices to legs. Remove for 20 minutes every 8 hours. Report any redness or edema.
9) Check urine output for amount, color, odor, and clarity.

Monitoring, Managing, and Preventing Life-Threatening Emergencies

1. Cardiopulmonary arrest
   a. Call for help.
   b. Begin cardiopulmonary resuscitation.
   c. Follow with advanced cardiac life support.
2. Autonomic hyperreflexia (autonomic dysreflexia)
   a. Seen after the acute stage of spinal injury and characterized by a hypersympathetic response to noxious stimuli.
   b. Commonly seen in patients with injury above T-8.
   c. Prevent onset.
      1) Monitor urine output hourly for an abrupt decrease.
      2) Observe indwelling urinary catheter position to ensure adequate drainage.
      3) Assess dependent areas for redness or pressure marks and massage bony prominences every 2 hours.
      4) Use anesthetic ointment during bowel assessment.
      5) Remove antiembolic stockings and observe toenail integrity. Note and report redness or edema of cuticles.
   d. Monitor for signs of complication.

      1) Monitor for rapid rise in blood pressure and bradycardia.
      2) Note increased anxiety.
      3) Investigate complaints of headache.
      4) Assess for sweating and flushing of skin above the level of the injury and pallor and pilomotor spasm below the level of injury.

  e. Manage clinical presentation.
      1) Raise head of bed to create postural hypotension.
      2) Administer ordered antihypertensives, as indicated.
      3) Monitor blood pressure every 5 minutes or continuously if arterial line is present.

  f. Remove source of irritation.
      1) Insert indwelling urinary catheter, if indicated.
      2) Ensure catheter patency.
      3) Check for fecal impaction by using anesthetic ointment to lubricate the anus. Remove any impaction.
      4) Check for pressure areas and treat any breakdown.
      5) Obtain specimens and monitor laboratory results for decreased hemoglobin and hematocrit levels, indicating internal bleeding.
      6) Remove any wind drafts that may stimulate the skin.

3. Hemorrhage
  a. Monitor for tachycardia; tachypnea; hypotension in recumbent position; cool, pale, clammy skin of blood loss; capillary refill greater than 3 seconds; changes in the level of consciousness; increasing abdominal girth; rigid abdomen; guaiac-positive stools or nasogastric drainage indicating internal bleeding.
  b. Manage hemorrhage.
      1) Administer ordered colloid solutions.
      2) Prepare patient for emergency surgery.
      3) Insert large-bore intravenous catheters in both arms and assist with central line for fluid administration and hemodynamic monitoring.

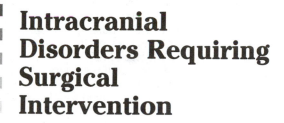

Intracranial Disorders Requiring Surgical Intervention

Intracranial disorders include intracranial abscesses, aneurysms, arteriovenous malformations, hydrocephalus, hematomas, and tumors. Any of these disorders may be treated surgically with a postoperative period in critical care.

1. Brain abscess—a collection of purulent material within brain tissue, causing focal signs with elevated intracranial pressure (ICP) and cerebrospinal fluid (CSF) pressure
2. Cerebral aneurysm—a weakening of the cerebral artery wall, causing a dilation of the vessel wall
3. Arteriovenous malformation (AVM)—one of four cerebral vascular malformations caused by a problem during embryonic development and consisting of a tangled collection of abnormally thin-walled, dilated blood vessels that are missing the capillary connection of arterial to venous system. The tangle of abnormally dilated vessels has increased flow and cerebral pressure and is highly susceptible to rupture.

4. Hydrocephalus — an excess of CSF within the brain, caused by either an obstruction of flow, an abnormal amount of CSF produced, or not enough being circulated or reabsorbed

5. Hematoma — a blood clot found within the layers (meninges) of the brain or within the grey matter itself. Usually caused by trauma, the hematoma is either fed from an arterial or venous source, or may expand due to osmotic pull of fluid as the blood cells lyse.

6. Tumor — an abnormal cellular growth, usually spherical in shape, which infiltrates brain tissue and causes cerebral edema and increased ICP

7. Several types of intracranial surgery are performed to treat these disorders.
   a. Burr hole — a circular opening in the skull to evacuate hematomas, or to initiate further invasive brain surgery
   b. Craniotomy — a surgical window in the skull made by sawing between multiple burr holes
      1) Supratentorial craniotomy — access to areas above the tentorium, i.e., frontal, parietal, temporal, and occipital lobes of cerebrum
      2) Infratentorial craniotomy — access to areas below the tentorium, i.e., cerebellum, medulla, midbrain, and pons
   c. Craniectomy — surgical removal of a portion of the skull without replacement
   d. Cranioplasty — replacement of missing cranium with a plastic insert to restore skull contour and integrity

Etiology/Pathophysiology

1. Brain abscess
   a. Infections originating in other parts of the body and carried to the brain via the blood (approximately 50%)
   b. Infection spreading from the middle ear, mastoid, or sinuses or caused by trauma to the head (surgery or compound skull fractures)
   c. The abscess evolves from a soft swollen grouping of polymorphonuclear leukocytes to a more liquified form with a wall of varying thickness. There may be offshoots of the abscess. These offshoots as well as the abscess itself grow, acting like a space-occupying lesion, and increase ICP.
2. Cerebral aneurysm
   a. Associated with cerebral vascular disease that is influenced by hemodynamic stress. There may be a predisposition to vessel wall fragility within families.
   b. Aneurysms usually occur in the bifurcations and branches of large basilar arteries, in the circle of Willis area. Upon rupturing, blood will spread and form a hematoma before the bleeding aneurysm is sealed off by platelets and fibrin.
   c. This hematoma may be within the brain tissue (intracerebral hematoma), the ventricles (intraventricular hematoma), subdural space (subdural hematoma), or subarachnoid space (subarachnoid hematoma).
   d. The clot impinges on precious space, occludes the venous flow of CSF, and irritates the brain tissue, which causes inflammation and subsequent edema. All contribute to increasing ICP and lowering cerebral perfusion pressure.
3. AVMs
   a. The AVM may occupy a small area, or extend over an entire hemisphere. It may be cone shaped and extend from the surface of the brain to the inner ventricles, with nonfunctioning brain tissue serving for support of the AVM. Most AVMs are located in the supratentorial area of the cerebral hemisphere.
   b. Because of their overperfused venous system, there is a greater tendency to rupture. There is also a tendency

to steal blood away from adjacent normal brain tissue, causing ischemia. This, together with the displacement of normal tissue with nonfunctioning tissue, adds to progressive neurologic deficits.

c. Rupture usually leads to hematoma formation in either the subarachnoid space, the intracerebral tissue (or brain tissue), or the ventricles of the brain.

4. Hydrocephalus

a. Sometimes there is a lack of CSF flow between the ventricles and the subarachnoid space. This is commonly caused by a tumor within or adjacent to the ventricular system blocking the flow.

b. There also may be a decrease in reabsorption of CSF due to the arachnoid villi being clogged by debris produced from bleeding or infection.

5. Hematomas

a. Focal injuries caused by trauma and bleeding within the brain tissue itself or on the brain surface layers

b. Their blood supply may be arterial or venous in origin. This bleeding is caused by either direct trauma to the vessel or is due to the shearing energy of the blow, which tears the arteries or veins, causing rupture.

c. The brain's function becomes compromised as secondary increased pressures occur when blood displaces brain tissue.

6. Tumors

a. Most primary brain tumors have an idiopathic origin, but are congenital or hereditary.

b. A tumor generally grows shaped like a ball until the lesion comes in contact with a more rigid structure, requiring a change in contour. Some spread throughout the brain tissue without forming a definite mass. Growth occurs as cells multiply and by-products accumulate within the lesion.

c. Tissues adjacent to the tumor begin to swell, altering the cell wall permeability and subsequent electrical potential. These electrically hyperactive cells can spawn seizures. Edema continues in a spiraling manner, with eventual increased ICP.

Assessment/Analysis

ASSESSMENT FINDINGS

Subjective Findings

1. The major complaint preoperatively is headache, but findings depend on the size and location of the lesion and the amount of pressure exerted on adjacent tissues.
   a. Headache due to increased ICP is usually worse in the morning because of rapid eye movement during sleep and a buildup in carbon dioxide levels in the blood, causing vasodilation of the cerebral arteries.
   b. The pain may be located throughout the entire cranium, or localized frontally or suboccipitally.
   c. Headache due to AVMs is recurrent, migraine-like, and refractory to all pain medication.
   d. Headache due to a brain abscess is localized to the abscess.
2. Postoperative findings include the following:
   a. Headache associated with meningeal irritability or scalp incision
   b. Tingling, paresthesia
   c. Loss of feeling in extremity, paralysis

Objective Findings

1. Level of consciousness deteriorates when lesions increase in size, causing increased ICP. (See Table Describing Level of Consciousness, p 241.)
2. Abnormalities during cranial nerve assessment help locate the area of brain dysfunction. Generally, the cranial nerves can be placed in three groups, corresponding to specific areas of the brainstem.
   a. Alteration in group I indicates damage to the midbrain
      1) Olfactory (CN I)
      2) Optic (CN II)
      3) Oculomotor (CN III)
      4) Trochlear (CN IV)
   b. Alteration in group II indicates damage to the pons

    1) Trigeminal (CN V)
    2) Abducens (CN VI)
    3) Facial (CN VII)
    4) Acoustic (CN VIII)

  c. Alteration in group III indicates damage to the medulla
    1) Glossopharyngeal (CN IX)
    2) Vagus (CN X)
    3) Spinal accessory (CN XI)
    4) Hypoglossal (CN XII)

3. Pupil changes in size, shape, and reactivity that are indicative of focal lesions
  a. Pinpoint—indicates pontine hemorrhage or opiate overdose
  b. Small, but larger than pinpoint—could indicate normal reaction in bright room, pontine hemorrhage, bilateral diencephalic lesions, metabolic coma, or be drug-related.
  c. Midposition and nonreactive—pupil and iris are equal in surface area—indicates midbrain damage
  d. Large—unilateral, sluggish to fixed—indicates a facial lesion on same side of brain
  e. Dilated—bilateral, fixed—indicates severe anoxia, or death. A dilated pupil that reacts sluggishly or not at all to light indicates ocular nerve compression, usually from edema or a lesion on the same side as the dilation.

4. Change in pupillary shape
  a. Ovoid, or slightly oval—indicates increased ICP with ominous sign toward herniation
  b. Keyhole or irregular shaped pupils—generally indicate previous surgery or trauma to the pupil

5. Abnormal reflexes
  a. Presence of positive Babinski's reflex indicates damage to the corticospinal tract and is seen with dorsiflexion of the great toe, with or without fanning of the other toes.
  b. Lower extremity reflexes are increased in hydrocephalus.

6. Nausea and vomiting
  a. Characteristic of brain tumors in the posterior fossa,

vomiting is unrelated to meals and occurs early in morning with headaches.
  b. Characteristic immediately before and at the time of cerebral aneurysm rupture
7. Seizure activity
  a. Characteristic of arteriovenous malformations, focal seizures occur in the majority of patients.
  b. Patients with aneurysms have seizures related to cerebral edema and increasing ICP.
  c. Patients with brain abscesses have focal or generalized seizures.
8. Bradycardia — a late and ominous sign of increased ICP and possible herniation
9. Widened pulse pressure as a result of increased ICP — an ominous sign that may indicate herniation
10. Abnormal respiratory pattern dependent on location and extent of injury and increased ICP. Becomes more significant with pons and medulla involvement.
11. Hyperthermia may be seen on admission or appear within the first few days after head injury. May decrease, only to re-elevate sporadically. It may be due to hypothalamic dysfunction or infection.
12. Changes in motor function usually occur contralaterally, or on the opposite side from where the lesion is located.
  a. Abnormalities noted in the conscious patient include the following:
    1) Inability to or inequality of handgrasps
    2) Inability to extend and hold arms above body at equal distance
    3) Weakened resistance in hands and arms when tested
    4) Inability to flex and extend upper leg, knee, and ankle on either or both sides
    5) Weakened resistance when pressing either/both feet against the examiner's hands
    6) Abnormal gait, if able to walk
    7) Involuntary movements
  b. Abnormalities noted in the unconscious patient
    1) Increased resistance to extension of extremity
    2) Flaccid or loose extremity movement with passive motion

3) Constant inflexible muscle condition with or without noxious stimuli indicates cerebral damage.
   a) Abnormal flexion or decortication, a flexion of the upper extremities with extension of ankles, indicative of hemispheric dysfunction
   b) Abnormal adduction or decerebration, hyperextension of arms and legs, which can develop to arching of the back and hyperextension of the neck and head. Indicates movement of brain tissue in a head-to-toe motion, as in herniation.
   c) Generally, as herniation progresses, abnormal movement goes from decortication to decerebration to flaccidity.
   d) Both decerebration and decortication may occur simultaneously on different sides of the body, or with movements vacillating between the two types. This perplexing movement is due to the obscurity of injured tissue within the deep cerebral hemisphere and the upper portion of the brainstem.

SUPPORTING TEST FINDINGS

Laboratory Tests

1. Hemoglobin and hematocrit
   Abnormality: Decreased to normal
2. Serum potassium
   Abnormality: Decreased with diuretic and steroid therapy
3. Serum sodium
   Abnormality: Increased in diabetes insipidus, a complication of intracranial surgery
      Decreased in syndrome of inappropriate secretion of antidiuretic hormone (SIADH)
4. Serum osmolarity
   Abnormality: Increased in diabetes insipidus
      Decreased in SIADH
5. Urine specific gravity
   Abnormality: Dilute/decreased in diabetes insipidus and induced diuresis
      Concentrated/increased in SIADH

Diagnostic Tests

1. ICP Monitoring
   Abnormality: Increased postoperatively due to intracranial bleeding, cerebral edema present before or as the result of surgery or meningitis
2. Computed tomography scan
   Abnormality: Intracranial hemorrhage from surgical trauma
   Pneumocephalus
   Hydrocephalus
3. Magnetic resonance imaging
   Abnormality: Hydrocephalus
   Ischemic/infarcted areas
   Hemorrhage
   Lesions of brainstem, basal skull
4. Lumbar puncture
   Abnormality: Increased pressure due to hydrocephalus
   Decreased pressure due to CSF leak

Planning/Intervention

COLLABORATIVE MANAGEMENT

Procedures

1. Monitor and provide for adequate cerebral perfusion to the surgically traumatized brain.
   a. Maintain integrity of ventriculostomy for ICP monitoring and optional continuous or intermittent drainage of CSF, as ordered. Monitor continuously for increased pressures, which ultimately compromise cerebral perfusion.
   b. Maintain patency of arterial line and monitor arterial line pressures for hypotension or hypertension, and report significant changes.
   c. Maintain patency of central lines and monitor pulmonary artery pressures continuously for elevations that might indicate neurogenic pulmonary edema, and subsequent hypoxia.
   d. Keep head of bed elevated 20–30 degrees in a neutral position, or as ordered, to provide for adequate venous drainage.

    e. Observe cardiac monitor continuously to detect the presence of arrhythmias that reduce cerebral blood flow.

    f. Maintain a $Paco_2$ between 27–30 mm Hg for adequate cerebral blood flow.

2. Provide adequate oxygenation to the respiratory compromised patient.

    a. Maintain patency of airway.

    b. Maintain mechanical ventilation and report patient noncompliance/bucking ventilator.

    c. Suction every 2 hours, or as needed, to provide adequate pulmonary toilet.

    d. Preoxygenate patient before suctioning.

    e. Obtain specimens and monitor arterial blood gases (ABGs), and report significant changes.

    f. Apply pulse oximeter and monitor oxygen saturation to ensure adequate oxygenation.

3. Provide adequate fluid and nutrition to prevent ill effects of high metabolic rate.

    a. Administer intravenous therapy, as ordered, keeping patient slightly dehydrated. Avoid using 5% dextrose in water.

    b. Monitor hourly outputs and report >200 mL/h for 2 consecutive hours, without diuretic therapy.

    c. Monitor serial laboratory studies for osmolality, specific gravity, and electrolytes. Report any decreases secondary to diuretic therapy, as well as antidiuretic hormone abnormalities.

    d. Calculate daily caloric intake.

    e. Monitor daily weight and compare to baseline.

    f. Institute and maintain enteral feedings as postoperative status stabilizes.

    g. Maintain adequate fluid status for appropriate cerebral blood flow by monitoring hemodynamics.

4. Anticipate and prevent further injury.

    a. Administer ordered antibiotic therapy and monitor for signs and symptoms of infection.

    b. Maintain use of hypothermia blanket for elevated temperature without producing shivering; monitor temperature with tympanic thermometer. Administer antipyretics to maintain normothermia.

    c. Administer ordered anticonvulsants to abolish seizures, which increase cerebral metabolism and subsequently raise ICP.

d. Maintain sterile dressing changes, as ordered, reporting abnormal amounts or color of drainage.

e. Monitor continuously (especially in the patient with posterior fossa craniotomy) for nausea and vomiting, administering antiemetics, as ordered.

f. Administer antacids or histamine$_2$-receptor antagonists to prevent gastric irritation and ulcer formation.

Drug Therapy

1. Steroids
   Examples: methylprednisolone (Solu-Medrol)
   dexamethasone (Decadron)
   Action: Stabilize cell membranes and prevent lysosomal rupture, as well as reduce edema and CSF production
   Caution: Although there have been positive results for reducing edema around tumors, studies are inconclusive on the success of methylprednisolone and head injury.

2. Antibiotics
   Example: cephalothin (Keflin)
   Action: Kills the bacterium by slowing the final stage of growth; works well against gram-positive and gram-negative organisms.
   Caution: Can cause anaphylaxis.
   Monitor closely during administration. Most cephalosporins can cause false-positive urine glucose with Benedict's test or Clinitest. Does not affect Dextrostix or TesTape. Probable false-positive results with serum and urine creatinine, urine protein, and ketosteroids.

NURSING MANAGEMENT

Monitoring and Managing Clinical Problems

1. Breathing Pattern: ineffective
   a. Monitor/assess for patent airway.
      1) Monitor respiratory rate, rhythm, and depth.
      2) Assess for adventitious breath sounds, such as crackles or wheezes.
      3) Assess for ineffective airway by identifying snoring, absence of sounds in all lobes.

      4) Monitor ABGs for decreased PaO_2 and increased $Paco_2$.

      5) Assess lung secretions for color, clarity, and amount.

      6) Monitor for increased inspiratory pressures on ventilator, indicating increased intrathoracic pressure and subsequent increased ICP.

      7) Monitor continuously for cyanosis.

  b. Protect airway and respiratory function.

      1) Turn patient side to side, or as ordered.

      2) Elevate head of bed 30 degrees or as ordered.

      3) Suction after preoxygenating patient. Monitor change in ICP.

      4) If nasogastric tube in place, observe for patency on a continual basis. If no nasogastric tube in place, observe closely for nausea and incontinence of oral secretions.

      5) Institute tube feedings slowly, as ordered. Observe for any adverse reactions. Keep patient turned on side during ingestion of feedings.

      6) Check swallow reflex before giving patient initial postoperative fluids by mouth. Observe soft palate for elevation when touched with tongue depressor.

      7) Resume nasogastric tube suction and NPO status, as ordered, if patient is nauseated or vomiting. Be especially careful with the postoperative infratentorial craniotomy patient. The vomiting center is located in the posterior fossa and will be affected by localized edema.

2. Tissue Perfusion, altered: cerebral

  a. Assess and monitor cerebral tissue perfusion.

      1) Observe for return of preoperative neurologic signs; note any differences between patient's right and left side of body.

      2) Monitor for changes in neurologic signs.

      3) Observe ICP monitor readings during suctioning; report any adverse reactions.

      4) Monitor blood pressure and pulse every 15–30 minutes immediately after surgery, then alter interval as condition warrants.

  b. Promote adequate tissue perfusion.

      1) Notify physician of any changes in neurologic signs, indicating lateralizing or increased ICP.

2) Prevent Valsalva maneuver. Administer stool softener to prevent straining with bowel movement. Provide for routine bowel program.
3) Explain all procedures to patient before initiating them. Observe ICP monitor readings for elevations in ICP to nursing care. Avoid clustering nursing care, which increases ICP.
4) Avoid extreme flexion of hips and knees, which might increase intra-abdominal pressure or restrict venous return from lower extremities.
5) Keep head in the same plane as body; avoid neck flexion from big pillows.
6) Follow specific guidelines for individual patient on elevating head of bed, as ordered.

3. Infection: high risk for
   a. Assess and monitor for infection.
      1) Monitor cranial dressing for blood or CSF drainage.
      2) Monitor incision for drainage, redness, or edema.
      3) Monitor temperature very 2 hours, or as needed.
      4) Assess all invasive line insertion sites for signs of redness or irritation.
      5) Assess all drainage from ventriculostomy, and indwelling urinary catheter for clarity, odor, and amount.
      6) Assess for meningeal irritation, as indicated by:
         a) Nuchal rigidity (neck stiffness)
         b) Photophobia (sensitivity to light)
         c) Headache
         d) Hyperpyrexia (elevated temperature)
         e) Positive Kernig's sign: while flexing hip at 90 degrees, attempt to straighten knee joint to 180 degrees. Positive sign is pain at hamstring on straightening knee.
         f) Positive Brudzinski's sign: flexion of hip and knees with flexion of neck.
   b. Prevent infection.
      1) Wash hands between procedures.
      2) Use sterile technique with dressing changes and when draining ventriculostomy.
      3) Collect ordered specimens for culture and sensitivity testing.
      4) Administer ordered antibiotics.

4. Fluid Volume Excess or Deficit: high risk for
   a. Assess and monitor for fluid and electrolyte imbalance.
      1) Monitor and report urinary output >200 mL in 2 hours, unless output results from diuretic therapy.
      2) Monitor serum electrolytes for abnormalities that might result in arrhythmias.
      3) Monitor serum osmolality and urine specific gravity for abnormalities, indicating postsurgical complications of diabetes insipidus or SIADH.
   b. Promote fluid and electrolyte balance.
      1) Administer ordered replacement fluids.
      2) Insert urinary drainage catheter and measure output every hour.
      3) Notify physician for output >200 mL in 2 hours unless output results from diuretic therapy.
      4) Notify physician if urine specific gravity >1.030 or <1.010.
5. Injury: high risk for — seizures
   a. Assess and monitor for potential injury from seizures.
      1) Monitor for restlessness, change in behavior.
      2) Monitor for seizure activity.
   b. Prevent injury from seizures.
      1) Position patient very carefully, as ordered.
      2) Take temperatures rectally; observe cardiac monitor and ICP monitor.
      3) Keep siderails up, with emergency airway, suction equipment at close proximity.
      4) Administer ordered anticonvulsants.

Monitoring, Managing, and Preventing Life-Threatening Emergencies

1. Increased ICP refractory to all therapies — herniation syndrome
   a. Types of herniation
      1) Supratentorial herniation
         a) Subfalcine (cingulate) herniation — unilateral swelling and brain tissue shifted laterally under the midline dural fold, falx cerebri
         b) Central (transtentorial) herniation — the head-to-toe pushing of contents, displacing the

upper brainstem and midbrain through the tentorial notch

   c) Uncal herniation — swelling of the temporal lobe or lateral middle fossa, displacing the medial portion of the temporal lobe down into the tentorial notch

  2) Infratentorial herniation

   a) Upward transtentorial herniation with midbrain compression

   b) Downward transtentorial herniation through foramen magnum

b. Nursing Management

  1) Monitor for difficulty concentrating and restlessness, an early sign, and onset of coma, a late sign.

  2) Note any respiratory pattern such as Cheyne-Stokes, an early sign, and shallow, grossly irregular breathing to respiratory arrest, a late sign.

  3) Assess pupillary size and reaction such as unilaterally sluggish to nonreactive and dilated pupils, an early sign, and bilaterally fixed and dilated pupils, a late sign.

  4) Assess motor response such as contralateral hemiparesis to hemiplegia, which are early signs, and ipsilateral rigidity, decorticate posturing, decerebrate posturing, or flaccidity with occasional decerebrate movement, which are mid to late signs.

  5) Assist physician with oculocephalic and oculovestibular tests.

   a) An abnormal response for an oculocephalic test would be for the eyes to look straight ahead regardless of head movement. This indicates pontine-midbrain damage.

   b) An abnormal response for an oculovestibular test would be no eye movement regardless of ice-water instillation into the ear.

2. Neurogenic pulmonary edema secondary to sudden increase of ICP

a. Monitor for signs/symptoms of pulmonary edema.

  1) Dyspnea

  2) Restlessness and anxiety

  3) Tachycardia

  4) Lung sounds moist, with crackles

5) Skin cyanotic, cool, and clammy
6) Secretions frothy, pink, large amounts
7) ABGs with a decreased pH, PaO_2, and increased $PaCO_2$; refractory to increased levels of administered oxygen

b. Prevent neurogenic pulmonary edema.

1) Control ICP by:

a) Restricting fluid intake
b) Monitoring intake and output hourly
c) Elevating the head of the bed, as ordered
d) Avoiding the grouping of nursing actions that increase ICP
e) Continuously monitoring ICP for abnormally high pressures that trigger the pulmonary edema
f) Administering ordered diuretics
g) Providing an adequate airway and oxygenation to prevent hypoxia and hypercarbia
h) Maintaining a normotensive state that will provide adequate blood flow to cerebral tissues

Serial Seizures/ Status Epilepticus

A seizure is an unpredictable event involving abnormal activity of the brain cells that oftentimes disturbs consciousness and motor or sensory function. Seizures may occur alone or as a clinical manifestation of approximately 50 different diseases. Commonly seen in critical care, generalized tonic-clonic (or grand mal) seizures, which are convulsive, are the most dangerous.

Serial seizures are separate seizures with restoration periods between each seizure. Treatment for serial seizures is the same as for status epilepticus.

Status epilepticus is a chain reaction of tonic and clonic motor movement lasting approximately 2 minutes with a postictal period of lethargy, stupor, or coma and the immediate onset of another seizure.

Of all idiopathic seizure disorders, 90% are diagnosed in patients by 20 years of age. Seizures occurring after this age are usually the result of trauma or disease.

Etiology/Pathophysiology

1. Causes of seizures
   a. Noncompliance or inadequate dosages of anticonvulsants in patients with diagnosed epilepsy
   b. Brain tumors
   c. Head trauma with subsequent hematoma(s) or metabolic abnormality caused by increased intracranial pressure (ICP)
   e. Liver disease
   f. Renal disease and subsequent electrolyte imbalance
   g. Cerebrovascular disease with decreased cerebral oxygenation
   h. Metabolic imbalances
      1) Decreased blood glucose levels
      2) Decreased cellular oxygen in the brain
      3) Hypercarbia
      4) Electrolyte imbalances
      5) Acid-base imbalance
   i. Withdrawal or overdose of certain drugs
      1) Phencyclidine (also known as PCP or "angel dust") abuse
      2) Cocaine or "crack" abuse
      3) Lidocaine overdose
      4) Abrupt withdrawal of any seizure medication
      5) Alcohol withdrawal
2. Phases of generalized tonic-clonic seizure activity
   a. Preictal or aura phase — a time of uneasiness, visual or auditory sensation felt by the patient, which may occur several hours or days before the actual seizure
   b. Tonic phase — the period of decreased consciousness, excessive muscle contraction, and apnea
   c. Clonic phase — the period of more violent jerking movement accompanied by forceful rapid and deep respirations
   d. Postictal phase — the period of recovery in which muscles are flaccid and consciousness as well as normal pupillary size return. Because of metabolic exhaustion, the patient may complain of headache and fatigue.
3. Pathophysiology

a. Seizures are created by abnormally hyperactive neurons, which form an epileptogenic focus, rapidly and repeatedly depolarizing the cells involved for as many as 1,000 times per second.

b. This hyperactivity of the cells may remain localized, as in partial seizures; or it may spread throughout the entire cerebral cortex, causing generalized seizures.

c. Oxygen and nutritive stores are used up at an incredible rate. The body attempts to compensate with an increase in cerebral blood flow.

d. With serial seizures or status epilepticus, low blood glucose levels and oxygen content occur; anaerobic metabolism takes over. With anaerobic metabolism, cellular lactate levels increase, further complicating the already vicious cycle.

Assessment/Analysis

ASSESSMENT FINDINGS

Subjective

1. Preictal or aura phase
   a. Sense of uneasiness
   b. Nausea
   c. Confusion
   d. Visual or auditory disturbances
2. Postictal phase
   a. Headache
   b. Fatigue
   c. May have memory loss

Objective

1. Tonic phase
   a. Excessive muscle contraction causes the following:
      1) Initial crying out as air is forced out of lungs via the vocal cords
      2) Jaws clamp shut, with possible damage to tongue
   b. Loss of consciousness
   c. Apnea for approximately 15 seconds – 1 minute causes the following:

      1) Cyanosis
      2) Pupils dilated and unreactive to light
      3) Decreased heart rate
  d. Bowel or bladder incontinence may occur.
2. Clonic phase
  a. Powerful rhythmic muscle contractions with facial grimacing
  b. Profuse sweating and salivation
  c. Respirations loud and irregular
  d. Eyes roll back
  e. Increased heart rate
  f. Phase may last up to 5 minutes, with movement slowing until all activity stops.
3. Postictal phase
  a. Muscles are flaccid.
  b. Patient awakens from seizure, confused and lethargic, then returns to sleeping again for several hours.
  c. Pupillary reaction is normal upon awakening from seizure.

SUPPORTING TEST FINDINGS

Laboratory Tests

1. Complete blood count
  Abnormality: Decreased white blood cells with use of anticonvulsants, heavy metals, and barbiturates
    Increased red blood cells with acute poisoning
    Decreased hemoglobin and hematocrit with cirrhosis
    Increased hematocrit with dehydration
2. Urinalysis
  Abnormality: Increased specific gravity with diabetes mellitus
    Increased osmolality with hepatic cirrhosis
    Colorless urine may be due to diabetes mellitus and reddish/dark brown urine may be due to myoglobinuria
3. Serum electrolytes
  Abnormality: Decreased serum sodium may be due to a salt depletion, rather than too much ingested water
    Increased serum phosphorus and serum magnesium may be present

Decreased serum calcium may be present
Either increased or decreased serum potassium
4. Fasting blood glucose
   Abnormality: May be decreased
5. Blood urea nitrogen
   Abnormality: May be increased
6. Serum lactic dehydrogenase (serum glutamic oxaloacetic transaminase), aspartate aminotransferase (serum glutamic pyruvic transaminase), alanine aminotransferase
   Abnormality: May be increased
7. Arterial blood gases (ABGs)
   Abnormality: Metabolic acidosis may be present
8. Serum lactate
   Abnormality: Increased after seizure (especially status epilepticus), but drops to half quickly
9. Serum drug levels
   Abnormality: Presence of phencyclidine, cocaine, or other street drugs in persons using these substances
   Toxic lidocaine levels in patients receiving this drug
   Below therapeutic levels of anticonvulsants

Diagnostic Tests

1. Electroencephalography (EEG)
   Abnormality: presence of delta waves, spikes of sharp waves, asymmetry of wave frequency and amplitude
   Caution: Results are dependent on level of consciousness, medication used in treatment, type of seizure disorder, and timing with seizure activity; some seizure disorder patients have normal EEG between seizures; some patients who are never diagnosed with a seizure disorder have abnormal EEGs.
2. Computed tomography scan
   Abnormality: Cerebral infarctions
   Brain tumors
   Cerebral hematomas
3. Lumbar puncture/cerebrospinal fluid (CSF) analysis
   Abnormality: Bloody CSF indicates possible subarachnoid hemorrhage; meningitis may be present with either clear or cloudy CSF
4. ICP monitoring
   Abnormality: Increased ICP with head trauma

Planning/Intervention

COLLABORATIVE MANAGEMENT

Procedures

1. Implement seizure precautions.
   a. Pad and raise siderails. Place bed in low position.
   b. Obtain suction equipment and keep it available at bedside.
   c. Obtain oxygen equipment and keep it available.
   d. Keep emergency resuscitation equipment available.
   e. Take only skin or tympanic temperatures; avoid oral temperature.
2. Monitor cardiorespiratory stability continuously.
   a. Insert intravenous (IV) line to keep vein open with isotonic solution.
   b. Place patient on cardiac monitor and monitor cardiac rhythm continuously.
   c. **Do not** force airway in mouth or restrain patient's extremities.
   d. Prepare for endotracheal intubation and ventilation with patient having serial seizures or status epilepticus.
   e. Obtain specimens for laboratory analysis to help determine underlying cause.

Drug Therapy

1. Skeletal muscle relaxant
   Examples: diazepam (Valium)
       lorazepam (Ativan)
   Action: Interrupts generalized seizures
   Caution: May cause depression of the nervous, respiratory, and renal systems
       May cause hypertension and tachycardia
       Do not mix with other drugs or add to IV solutions
       Diazepam has a long elimination half-life and may accumulate, leading to persistent sedation
2. Anticonvulsants
   Examples: phenytoin (Dilantin)
       phenobarbital (Luminal)
   Action: Acts on the motor cortex to inhibit the spread of

seizure activity; when used with diazepam, diazepam stops the active seizure and phenytoin prevents further seizures

Phenytoin and phenobarbital are often used together when seizures are refractory to phenobarbital alone

Caution: Phenytoin has a slow onset (15 minutes), as compared to diazepam (1–5 minutes); infuse directly into large vein, having contact with only normal saline to avoid precipitation

When administered incorrectly causes hypotension and major cardiac arrhythmias; monitor blood pressure and cardiac monitor during administration; give slowly and steadily, preferably with an infusion control device

Phenobarbital has an additive effect, making assessment of postictal level of consciousness difficult

Lowers respirations and blood pressure

Additive sedation when given with diazepam can cause severe cardiorespiratory distress

3. Sedatives

Example: pentobarbital (Nembutal)

Action: Produces a barbiturate coma level of consciousness, which controls seizures in patients with status epilepticus who have not responded to diazepam or phenytoin

Caution: Closely observe cerebral function; EEG may be monitored routinely while administering drugs

Essential to intubate and support ventilation while patient is in barbiturate coma

May cause myocardial depression; closely observe cardiac monitor and vital signs; may require vasopressor to offset hypotension

NURSING MANAGEMENT

Monitoring and Managing Clinical Problems

1. Airway Clearance: ineffective
   a. Monitor and assess airway patency.
      1) Assess respiratory pattern and breath sounds after seizure.
      2) Note presence and length of apnea and cyanosis.

 3) Assess ability to handle secretions.
 4) Monitor ABGs with serial seizures or status epilepticus.
 b. Promote effective airway.
 1) After seizure, turn patient to side to facilitate drainage of secretions from mouth and oral pharynx.
 2) Use suction without inserting catheter into mouth; discontinue if patient shows increased restlessness.
 3) Do not pry mouth open or forcefully attempt insertion of airway or any other object during seizure.
 4) Ventilate and oxygenate with resuscitator, when possible.
 5) Have emergency resuscitation equipment nearby.
2. Injury: high risk for
 a. Monitor and assess for possible injury.
 1) Observe body position and extremities during seizures.
 2) Assess ICP readings for increase, if patient on ICP monitoring.
 3) Assess neurologic signs after seizure.
 b. Provide for patient safety.
 1) Discuss safety precautions with patient before seizure, if possible. If patient senses an aura, instruct patient to:
 a) Call for help.
 b) Remove food and dentures, if possible.
 c) Lie flat.
 2) Keep padded siderails in upright position and protect patient's head from injury during ictal phase.
 3) Keep bed in lowest position to floor.
 4) Suction, as needed, without inserting apparatus in mouth.
 5) Have emergency resuscitation equipment nearby.
 6) Take skin/tympanic temperature only; avoid oral temperatures.
 7) Medicate, as ordered, and observe for therapeutic and adverse effects.
3. Tissue Perfusion, altered: cerebral
 a. Monitor and assess for possible ischemia.
 1) Ictal period

      a) Monitor duration, time, number, and description of seizure(s).

      b) Observe and record any cardiac arrhythmias during and after seizure(s).

  2) Postictal period

      a) Assess vital and neurologic signs after seizure and with use of sedatives.

      b) Assess ability to communicate and memory directly after seizure(s).

b. Promote cerebral tissue perfusion.

  1) Medicate for cardiac arrhythmias, as ordered.

  2) Administer ordered oxygen.

  3) Prepare for endotracheal intubation, if necessary.

  4) Administer anticonvulsants necessary to stop or prevent seizure; monitor for therapeutic and adverse effects.

  5) Administer medications to adjust metabolic disorder, as ordered.

Monitoring, Managing, and Preventing Life-Threatening Emergencies

1. Cardiopulmonary arrest
   a. Call for help.
   b. Begin cardiopulmonary resuscitation.
   c. Follow with advanced cardiac life support.

Guillain-Barré Syndrome

Guillain-Barré is an autoimmune response affecting the peripheral nervous system, often rendering the patient paralyzed and unable to breathe without assistance.

Etiology/Pathophysiology

1. Etiology
   a. Unknown but may be precipitated by the following:
      1) Viral illness within past 2–3 weeks
      2) Immunization
2. Pathophysiology
   a. Guillain-Barré is thought to be a demyelination of the cranial and spinal peripheral nerves caused by an autoimmune reaction that destroys the myelin sheath encircling these nerves. This myelin sheath destruction slows and obstructs both motor and sensory nerve impulses, with motor impulses affected the most.
   b. This syndrome commonly starts in the distal portion of the extremitites, advancing from toe to head, creating bilateral muscle weakness and paralysis. If Guillain-Barré does not reverse its ascension, it will paralyze the diaphragm, causing respiratory distress and failure.
   c. Although the motor and sensory pathways are affected, cognitive function is undisturbed. The patient is alert, but may not be able to move, swallow, or speak during the acute phase. Recovery depends on the axonal capability to remyelinate.
3. The cranial nerves most often affected are the VII (facial nerve), IX (glossopharyngeal), X (vagus), XI (spinal accessory), and XII (hypoglossal)
4. Types of Guillain-Barré syndrome
   a. Ascending Guillain-Barré syndrome is the most commonly seen, with sensory and motor deficits progressing from the distal extremities upward to the cranial nerves. This type affects both sides of the body equally; and the patient can become quadriplegic with no reflex, sensory, or motor movement.
   b. Descending Guillain-Barré syndrome progresses opposite ascending, with deficits seen first in the cranial nerves, then in the periphery. Upper extremities more often experience numbness. Respiratory involvement occurs early in the syndrome's process.
   c. Pure motor Guillain-Barré syndrome is much like the

ascending type; however, there are no sensory deficits noted. Pain is usually absent, and it appears like a mild case of ascending type.

d. The rarest form, Miller-Fischer variant, does not exhibit the sensory or respiratory difficulties, but rather has problems with ophthalmoplegia, areflexia, and ataxia.

Assessment/Analysis

ASSESSMENT FINDINGS

Subjective

1. Hypersensitivity, numbness, or tingling often noted in hands and feet only
2. Headaches, stiff neck
3. Photophobia (light sensitivity)
4. Pain beginning as muscle cramping that is located in the back, buttocks, or extremities and is often worse at night
5. Awkward coordination, initially
6. Muscle weakness, progressing to paralysis

Objective

1. Bilateral muscle weakness that usually starts in lower extremities
2. Clumsy gait that may progress to full-blown paralysis within 48 hours to several weeks, peaking at 3 weeks
3. A plateau period of neither improvement nor deterioration is followed by recovery, which may take months to a year or longer.
4. Weak or absent deep tendon reflexes
5. Extreme blood pressure lability
6. Cardiac arrhythmias: slow or fast rates
7. Absent bowel sounds suggesting paralytic ileus
8. Urinary retention
9. Large amounts of dilute urine output suggesting syndrome of inappropriate secretion of antidiuretic hormone
10. Inability to smile, frown, close eyelids, speak, swallow, or chew

SUPPORTING TEST FINDINGS

Laboratory Tests

1. Cerebrospinal fluid analysis
   Abnormality: Increased protein levels with a normal cell count seen in first 10 days of illness
2. Arterial blood gases (ABGs)
   Abnormality: Decreased pH and PaO_2 with respiratory distress
   Increased $PaCO_2$ with respiratory distress
3. Cytomegalovirus titer
   Abnormality: Increased

Diagnostic Tests

1. Electromyelography
   Abnormality: Decreased nerve conduction noted soon after paralysis begins. Normal results are predictive of an early recovery.

Planning/Intervention

COLLABORATIVE MANAGEMENT

Procedures

1. Monitor and promote respiratory integrity.
   a. Monitor lung vital capacity for decreases.
   b. Monitor ABGs for hypoxia and hypercapnia.
   c. Assist with ordered inhalation therapy.
   d. Anticipate endotracheal intubation when vital capacity deteriorates lower than 10 mL/kg.
   e. Maintain mechanical ventilation for low vital capacity.
   f. Anticipate tracheostomy if patient unable to be extubated after 2 weeks.
   g. Apply pulse oximeter and monitor oxygenation saturation response to nursing care.
   h. Observe aspiration precautions.
2. Monitor and promote cardiovascular function.
   a. Monitor vital signs every 2 hours and as needed.
   b. Apply cardiac monitor and observe for arrhythmias and changes in rate.

    c. Anticipate insertion of a temporary pacemaker for severe bradycardia or heart block.

    d. Anticipate insertion of central line and pulmonary artery catheter, as indicated.

3. Monitor and provide for gastrointestinal integrity.

    a. Maintain intravenous (IV), central venous line for total parenteral nutrition and fluids, if ileus present.

    b. Insert nasogastric tube.

       1) To suction if gastric ileus present

       2) For enteral feedings, if no ileus present

4. Prevent complications of immobility.

    a. Provide verbal support to the quadriplegic before initiating kinetic continuous rotation bed.

    b. Apply antiembolism stockings (controversial). Remove every 8 hours for skin care.

    c. Maintain sequential compression boots (controversial).

    d. Assist with physical therapy by performing the following:

       1) Range-of-motion exercises

       2) Rehabilitation exercises

5. Decrease the inflammatory response.

    a. Assist in plasmapheresis therapy regimen, performed at the bedside with a blood cell separator machine.

6. Prevent further complications.

    a. Maintain urinary drainage catheter patency to prevent urinary tract infection or bladder distention.

    b. Monitor and report excessive imbalances in intake and output.

    c. Assist with central IV line insertion; provide proper maintenance, as indicated.

Drug Therapy

1. Anticoagulant

   Example: sodium heparin (Heparin)

   Action: Prophylaxis for deep vein thrombosis or pulmonary embolism

   Caution: Excessive anticoagulation can cause hemorrhage.

      Cumulative anticoagulant effect when used with aspirin or nonsteroidal anti-inflammatory agents

2. Opioid analgesics
   Example: morphine (Duromorph)
   Action: Decreases pain and anxiety in the ventilated patient
   Caution: This medication can cause respiratory depression. **Use in the mechanically ventilated patient only!**
3. Antibiotics
   Example: cefoperazone (Cefobid)
   Action: Decrease bacterial growth and prevent infection while patient is hospitalized and receiving routine invasive procedures
   Caution: Can cause abdominal cramps and diarrhea
4. Corticosteroids
   Example: hydrocortisone (Solu-Cortef)
   Action: Decreases the inflammatory reaction
   Caution: May cause gastric irritation and altered immune response; can also mask symptom of infection
5. Vasopressor
   Example: dopamine (Intropin)
   Action: Elevates blood pressure and improves cardiac output (CO)
   Caution: May cause vasoconstriction, electrocardiogram changes, and arrhythmias

NURSING MANAGEMENT

Monitoring and Managing Clinical Problems

1. Airway Clearance: ineffective
   a. Assess and monitor for respiratory distress.
      1) Observe respiratory rate and pattern, noting trends reflecting respiratory muscle strength.
      2) Assess for adventitious sounds, indicating retained secretions.
      3) While patient is not intubated, monitor all drinking and eating. Raise head of bed slowly before allowing drinking and note any difficulty swallowing.
      4) Monitor chest excursion and vital capacity. Record results and note trend.
      5) Note level of consciousness; report any deterioration or change in behavior.
      6) Obtain specimens and monitor ABGs for decreased pH, PaO_2, and increased $PaCO_2$.

      7) Note color, amount, and consistency of airway secretions.
  b. Promote adequate respiratory function.
      1) Auscultate lung sounds every 2 hours, or as often as necessary, for deterioration in breath sounds as well as depth of inspiration.
      2) Notify doctor of decline in respiratory function as reflected by:
         a) Increased respiratory rate, decreased depth
         b) Change in behavior, level of consciousness
         c) Deterioration of ABGs
      3) Raise head of bed and place patient in semi-Fowler's position, turning every 2 hours.
      4) Maintain ordered supplemental oxygen.
      5) Have emergency resuscitation equipment available for intubation.
      6) Maintain mechanical ventilation in the respiratory-dependent patient.
      7) Maintain ventilator alarm parameters at a level sensitive to abrupt change in patient's respiratory status.
      8) Suction the intubated patient via endotracheal or tracheostomy tube, as needed.
      9) Hyperventilate with 100% oxygen before and after suctioning.
2. Nutrition: altered, less than body requirements
  a. Monitor fluid and nutritional status.
      1) Monitor intake and output hourly.
      2) Note caloric and protein intake.
      3) Monitor serial serum albumin for decreases.
      4) Assess patient's ability to swallow.
      5) Assess bowel sounds every 4–8 hours.
      6) Monitor for signs of dehydration, such as:
         a) Dry mucous membranes and fissures on tongue
         b) Low urine output <30 mL/h
         c) "Tenting" of skin when pinched
         d) Postural hypotension (dizziness and blood pressure drop when going from supine to a sitting position.
      7) Assess for dehydration versus cardiac pump failure.
         a) Decreased blood pressure and tachycardia

(heart rate >100 bpm) possibly indicating de-hydration or pump failure

b) Central venous pressure of <1 mm Hg, suggesting dehydration

c) Pulmonary artery pressure >25 mm Hg, suggesting pump failure

d) Pulmonary capillary wedge pressure <4 mm Hg, suggesting dehydration or >12 mm Hg suggesting pump failure

e) CO <4 L/min, suggesting pump failure

8) Assess gastric pH for possible stress-induced ulcer.

b. Promote nutritional/fluid status.

1) Infuse ordered IV fluids.

2) Institute ordered enteral feedings, while closely monitoring for abdominal cramping, nausea, or vomiting.

3) If patient unable to tolerate enteral feedings, begin total parenteral nutrition.

3. Physical Mobility: impaired

a. Assess and monitor for physical mobility and motor strength.

1) Assess and note cranial nerve function, primarily oculomotor, trigeminal, abducens, facial glosso-pharyngeal, vagus, accessory, and hypoglossal (See Table Assessing Cranial Nerves, p 243).

2) Assess and note movement and strength in arms, legs, feet, and hands.

3) Assess and note deep tendon reflexes using a reflex hammer.

b. Promote mobility and strength.

1) Perform range-of-motion exercises every 8 hours.

a) Be aware of overtiring patient.

b) Stop exercise if pain occurs.

c) Remember that patient may not be able to communicate pain caused by exercise.

d) Individualize the exercise plan.

2) Reposition/turn patient at least every 2 hours.

a) Support extremities while turning.

b) Question patient about pain when turning.

4. Infection: high risk for

a. Assess and monitor for infection.

    1) Assess temperature for elevation.
    2) Assess lungs for decreased or moist breath sounds.
    3) Assess patient's gag and swallow reflex.
    4) Monitor and note urine output for color, clarity, and odor.
    5) Monitor and note secretions suctioned from lungs for color and consistency.
    6) Obtain specimens for ordered culture and sensitivity testing.

  b. Promote infection-free environment.
    1) Use sterile technique for insertion of invasive lines and tubes.
    2) Obtain specimens for ordered culture and sensitivity testing.
    3) Perform nasotracheal suction every 2 hours, as needed.
    4) Report any change in patient status that might signal possible infection.
    5) Monitor for bladder distention from urinary retention due to autonomic effects of Guillain-Barré syndrome.

5. Skin Integrity: impaired, high risk for
  a. Monitor for any skin impairment.
    1) Assess skin for signs of redness or edema at IV sites.
    2) Assess pressure points on hips, coccyx, ankles, heels, shoulders, and ears.
    3) Assess nares around nasogastric tube for signs of skin breakdown.

  b. Promote healthy skin integrity.
    1) Massage back and pressure points every 2–4 hours.
    2) Turn every 2 hours or place patient on kinetic bed.
    3) Apply antiembolism stockings. Remove every 8 hours; apply lotion; note any calf redness and reapply stockings after 20–30 minutes.

6. Incontinence: functional
  a. Monitor for proper bowel elimination.
    1) Auscultate bowel sounds every shift.
    2) Note color, consistency, and size of each bowel movement.
    3) Check for incontinence of bowel during acute stage.

    4) Check for impaction during the recovery stage.
    5) Monitor cardiac rate and rhythm during impaction checks.
  b. Promote proper bowel elimination.
    1) Note last bowel movement on patient chart.
    2) Provide for privacy during bowel checks.
    3) Question patient about previous bowel habits before onset of symptoms. Attempt bowel stimulation at same time of day.
    4) Administer fluids (enteral and IV) to promote hydration of stool.
    5) Administer stool softeners and suppositories, as ordered.

Monitoring, Managing, and Preventing Life-Threatening Emergencies

1. Respiratory arrest due to premature extubation or disconnect from ventilator during diaphragm paralysis
  a. Set alarm parameters at sensitive levels that will trigger early.
  b. Never turn off alarms for suctioning or clearing ventilator tubing of water.
  c. Observe patient on a continuous basis.
  d. Investigate all unusual cardiac arrhythmias with auscultation of lungs.
  e. Have emergency resuscitation equipment nearby.
  f. Call for help.
  g. Begin ventilating patient.
  h. Begin cardiopulmonary resuscitation, if patient in cardiopulmonary arrest.
  i. Follow with advanced cardiac life support.

4 RENAL DISORDERS

Acute Renal Failure

Acute renal failure (ARF) is a rapid deterioration or cessation in kidney function demonstrated by progressive azotemia (increased levels of blood urea nitrogen [BUN]) and serum creatinine and usually by decreased urine output. Anuria (<50 mL/24 h), oliguria (<400 mL/24 h), or polyuria (>1800 mL/24 h) may exist.

Etiology/Pathophysiology

1. Risks for development of ARF
   a. Medical history of diabetes mellitus, hypertension, gout, malignant disease, cardiovascular disease, or calculi
   b. Family history of calculi, gout, or hypertension
   c. Hypotensive episodes; any illness or situation that reduces blood flow to kidneys: sepsis; burns; jaundice; advanced age; recent surgery
   d. Multiple organ failure due to tissue ischemia
   e. Use of drugs with potential for nephrotoxicity (especially aminoglycosides, angiotensin converting enzyme [ACE] inhibitors)
   f. Use of multiple drugs
   g. Major trauma, crush syndrome, severe allergic reactions
   h. Exposure to environmental nephrotoxic agents
2. Causes
   a. Prerenal — ARF caused by decreased blood flow to the kidneys without direct damage to the kidney parenchyma
      1) Inadequate intravascular volume from the following:
         a) Excessive fluid losses due to vomiting and diarrhea
         b) Anaphylaxis
         c) Excessive diuresis
         d) Hemorrhage
         e) Burns
         f) Salt-wasting nephropathy
         g) Pancreatitis
      2) Redistributed volume from the following:
         a) Peripheral vasodilation because of sepsis or vasodilating drugs
         b) Third spacing as seen with peritonitis, burns, postoperative status, or ileus or as seen with low-protein state
      3) Reduced cardiac output (CO) from the following:
         a) Acute myocardial infarction
         b) Cardiogenic shock

    c) Congestive heart failure (CHF)

    d) Cardiomyopathies

    e) Pericardial tamponade

    f) Acute or chronic valvular disease

    g) Dysrhythmias

    h) Acute pulmonary embolus

    i) Abdominal aortic aneurysm

4) Renal artery thrombosis or stenosis

5) Use of drugs such as ACE inhibitors or calcium channel blockers

b. Intrarenal—ARF due to direct damage to the kidney parenchyma; the most common form (75%) is acute tubular necrosis (ATN); 25% is due to glomerulonephritis. Risk for any of these is increased if prerenal azotemia or other preexisting renal disease is present.

1) Prolonged ischemic damage due to any of the prerenal causes that results in an inadequate blood flow to the kidneys; may include such situations as:

    a) Inadequate renal perfusion during cardiac or vascular surgery or during cardiopulmonary bypass

    b) Episodes of hypotension (sepsis, hypovolemia)

    c) Any cardiovascular disease that acutely or chronically limits blood flow to kidneys

2) Nephrotoxic damage due to exposure of the nephrons to toxic substances such as:

    a) Pigments (hemoglobin, myoglobin—with such diseases as rhabdomyolysis)

    b) Protein (as occurs with multiple myeloma)

    c) Inflammatory mediators

    d) Radiographic contrast dye

    e) Drugs (antibiotics, nonsteroidal anti-inflammatory drugs)

    f) Organic solvents (ethylene glycol)

    g) Heavy metals (lead, mercury, arsenic, uranium)

    h) Pesticides, fungicides

3) Glomerulonephritis results from processes that affect small renal vessels, including:

    a) Hemolytic uremic syndrome

    b) Scleroderma
    c) Malignant hypertension
    d) Vasculitis
    e) Infections (streptococcal, varicella, hepatitis)
    f) Systemic lupus erythematosus

c. Postrenal—ARF due to any obstruction to the flow of urine. Obstruction may cause hydronephrosis when the accumulated urine has increased pressures within the kidney(s) and damaged nephrons. Renal dysfunction is reversible if cause is discovered early. Postrenal ARF should be suspected for any sudden anuria or decrease in urine output that has no other obvious cause.

  1) Mechanical obstruction may involve ureters or urethra; possible sources include:
    a) Calculi
    b) Blood clots
    c) Benign or malignant prostatic hypertrophy
    d) Obstruction of indwelling catheter
    e) Urethral strictures
    f) Edema
    g) Tumors within or adjacent to ureters or urethra
    h) Uncorrected congenital malformations

  2) Functional obstruction from the following:
    a) Diabetic neuropathy
    b) Pregnancy
    c) Drugs (ganglionic-blocking agents)
    d) Spinal-cord disease

3. Pathology for development of ARF with prerenal azotemia (progressively increased serum levels of nitrogenous wastes):

a. Initially, reduced flow through the renal arteries; ischemia occurs.

b. Reduced flow causes reduced glomerular filtration rate (GFR).

c. The kidney responds to the low flow by causing increased renin-angiotensin activity.

  1) Vasoconstriction of afferent arteriole further decreases GFR.

  2) Decreased blood flow through the glomerulus results in a decrease in glomerular hydrostatic pressure.

    d. The sympathetic stimulation that occurs with the decreased blood flow causes blood flow in the kidney to shift from the outer to the inner cortex; this causes an additional decrease in GFR.

    e. Flow of filtrate through tubules is slow and allows a larger amount of urea to be reabsorbed; this accounts for the increase in BUN : creatinine ratio from 10 : 1 to as high as 40 : 1.

4. Pathology for intrarenal ARF with ATN
    a. Involves damage to the tubules
       1) Backleak
          a) Tubular membrane loses integrity, and this allows filtrate to be reabsorbed.
          b) Can occur anywhere along the length of the tubule.
       2) Tubular obstructions
          a) Because of cellular debris from sloughing of damaged and dying cells or because of presence of such elements as hemoglobin and myoglobin
          b) Pressure is increased in Bowman's capsule, and this opposes glomerular hydrostatic pressure and further diminishes GFR.
       3) Glomerular abnormalities
       4) Changes in renal hemodynamics — increased vasoconstriction
       5) Cellular edema occurs with the ischemic injury.
       6) Inability of tubules to concentrate urine
    b. If ATN is due to kidney exposure to toxins:
       1) Initial injury is to the tubules.
       2) Pathophysiology is similar to other causes but damage to the tubular basement membrane may be absent or if present is less severe.
       3) Urine production often remains >400 mL/24 h.
       4) Recovery is usually more rapid.

5. Renal parenchyma can be damaged by:
    a. Prerenal or postrenal problems
    b. A combination of causes: if nephrotoxicity causes ATN damage, it is worsened if there is also hypotension, infection, or dehydration.

6. Oliguric ARF follows a pattern from insult to recovery:
    a. Onset is time from insult to time when urine volume

changes, 0–2 days; at the end of this time, systemic effects of ARF are first seen.
   b. Oliguric-anuric phase is time during which urine production is usually <400 mL/24 h for 8–14 days.
   c. Diuretic phase is time during which there is an increase in urine production to <400 mL/24 h, and there is stabilization of laboratory values (no further increases); late in this phase, serum BUN and creatinine levels begin decreasing, although normal levels are not reached; lasts about 10 days
   d. Convalescent phase is the period of 4–6 months during which laboratory values slowly decrease until normal or optimum levels are reached.
7. Nonoliguric ARF
   a. Causes less severe damage; tubules have only epithelium involved
   b. Results in inability to concentrate urine
   c. Has a more rapid recovery
   d. Has three phases: onset, diuretic, and recovery
   e. If treated early, an oliguric ARF may become a nonoliguric ARF, but true existence of a nonoliguric ARF as a result of treatment is controversial.

Assessment/Analysis

ASSESSMENT FINDINGS

Subjective Findings

1. Patient reports increased or decreased frequency, urgency, decrease in amount of urine, dysuria (pain with voiding), hesitancy, dribbling, difficulty in starting to void
2. Flank pain
3. Cloudy or bloody urine
4. Weight loss or gain
5. Edema (especially in ankles and feet)
6. Polydipsia
7. Changes in vision or hearing
8. History of hypertension
9. Drug use of any of nephrotoxic agents or history of drug abuse

10. Exposure to chemicals or heavy metals at work or at home
11. Recent history of the following:
    a. Major surgery, pelvic surgery
    b. Cardiovascular disease
    c. Major trauma
    d. Allergic reaction
    e. Infection, especially upper respiratory infection with beta-hemolytic streptococcus as infecting agent
    f. Prostate problems
    g. Severe dehydration
    h. Malaise, fatigue, weakness
    i. Anorexia, nausea, vomiting
12. Family or significant others report changes in patient's mental status or behavior or personality

Objective Findings

1. Lethargy, muscle weakness, or general inactivity
2. Confusion
3. Dry and pale mucous membranes
4. Skin turgor may be normal, increased, or decreased
5. Edema
6. Rapid, regular, and deep respiratory rate
7. Increased heart rate; irregular rhythm
8. If hemodynamic monitoring is available, decreased central venous pressure (CVP) and pulmonary capillary wedge pressure (PCWP)
9. Elevated blood pressure
10. Crackles, rhonchi, or frank pulmonary edema

SUPPORTING TEST FINDINGS

Laboratory Tests

1. Urine electrolytes
   Abnormality: In urine collected before use of diuretics, urine sodium will be decreased (<20 mEq/L) with prerenal problem and increased (>30 mEq/L) with intrarenal problem (specifically ATN); other urine electrolytes are decreased
2. Urine creatinine
   Abnormality: Decreased; may be as low as 1 mL/min with

oliguric ATN; in nonoliguric ATN, urine creatinine may be 2–15 mL/min

3. Urine osmolality

   Abnormality: In urine specimens collected before using diuretics, urine osmolality will be increased with prerenal problem (> 500 mOsm/L) and decreased or normal with intrarenal problem (specifically ATN — 300–320 mOsm/L or equal to serum osmolality [normally about 285–295 mOsm/L])

4. Urinalysis

   Abnormality: No abnormality with prerenal ARF. In intrarenal ARF, red blood cells (RBCs), casts, and perhaps actual tubular epithelial cells will be present; urine will be positive for blood when tested with reagent strip but not confirmed microscopically, suggesting a pigment nephropathy; increased eosinophils suggests drug-induced damage to tubules

5. Urine pH

   Abnormality: Increased; generally more acidic with prerenal ARF

6. Urine specific gravity

   Abnormality: Moves toward 1.010 for intrarenal ARF, and then does not change, not even when patient's fluid status changes; is increased with prerenal ARF (> 1.020); value varies for postrenal ARF

7. Serum sodium

   Abnormality: Will vary based on fluid balance

8. Serum potassium

   Abnormality: Increased (often to a life-threatening level)

9. Serum chloride

   Abnormality: Increased

10. Carbon dioxide combining power level

    Abnormality: Decreased

11. Serum phosphorus

    Abnormality: Increased

12. Serum calcium

    Abnormality: Decreased

13. Serum magnesium

    Abnormality: Increased

14. Serum creatinine

    Abnormality: Increased; > 1.5 mg/100 mL

15. Ratio of urine creatinine to serum creatinine

Abnormality: For prerenal problems >15:1; for intrarenal problems (specifically ATN) <10:1

16. Serum osmolality
Abnormality: Variable, depending on fluid status

17. Ratio of urine to serum osmolality
Abnormality: Intrarenal ARF: 1:2

18. BUN
Abnormality: Increased (>25 mg/100 mL) but can be increased for a variety of reasons

19. Ratio of BUN to serum creatinine
Abnormality: In prerenal ARF, ratio changes to as high as
40:1 (normal is 10:1)

20. Hemoglobin and hematocrit
Abnormality: Decreased during first week of oliguria

21. Serum uric acid
Abnormality: Increased

22. Arterial blood gases (ABGs)
Abnormality: Decreased pH of 7.40 or lower; decreased
HCO_3

Diagnostic Tests

1. Bladder catheterization
Abnormality: Inability to pass a catheter with urethral obstruction (prostate or tumor)
Immediate flow of large amount of urine, indicative
of neurogenic bladder problem

2. X-Ray — flat plate of the abdomen, also known as a KUB
(for kidneys, ureters, bladder)
Abnormality: Renal calculi (if stones are present, they will
be visible 90% of the time)

3. Renal ultrasound
Abnormality: Slight increase in size of kidneys may be
seen because of parenchymal edema
In postrenal ARF, hydronephrosis may be detected,
or area of obstruction in ureters or in kidneys

4. Retrograde pyelography
Abnormality: Clots, stones, or strictures in postrenal ARF;
used when ultrasound has not allowed identification of
area of obstruction

5. Intravenous pyelogram (Note: Benefit of this test may not
outweigh the risk this has for further damage to renal
parenchyma.)

Abnormality: Stones within the kidney or anywhere along length of ureters to bladder

Altered kidney structures

Can be used to identify residual volume if patient able to void

6. Fluid challenge (Note: A bolus of 200–500 mL is given intravenously [IV], followed by loop or osmotic diuretic IV.)

Abnormality: If urine production/output does not increase to 30–40 mL/h over next hour, helps confirm ATN

7. Radionuclide scan

Abnormality: Vascular occlusion to one or both kidneys or other perfusion abnormalities

Structural changes due to disease or trauma, including integrity of collecting system

8. Renal angiography

Abnormality: Renal artery stenosis, infarcts, or other renal vessel disease, renal cysts, renal tumors, renal abscess, renal changes due to trauma

Planning/Intervention

COLLABORATIVE MANAGEMENT

Procedures

1. For prerenal ARF
   a. Correct low CO (if this is underlying disease process) with ordered medications or assistive devices.
   b. Administer IV fluids to:
      1) Correct hypovolemia to improve blood flow to kidneys
      2) Correct inadequate intravascular volumes by correcting or treating causes such as burns, septic shock, excessive diuretic effect of drug therapy
      3) Support intravascular volume deficit when cause is fluid shift to third space
   c. Mobilize third-spaced fluid by administering ordered medications.
2. For postrenal ARF
   a. Assist with identifying and correcting obstruction.

  1) Prepare patient for surgery, if needed.
  2) Assist with placing ureteral stint(s).
  3) Assist with percutaneous nephrostomy.
  4) Assist with placing suprapubic catheter.
  5) Prepare patient for kidney stone removal.
  b. Assist with placement of indwelling urinary catheter to bypass urethral stricture.
3. For intrarenal ARF
  a. Prevent complications related to continued hypotension, infection, use of nephrotoxic agents by administering ordered IV fluids and medications.
  b. Regulate fluid intake to achieve fluid and electrolyte balance.
  c. Administer ordered buffering agents to achieve acid-base balance.
  d. Closely observe level of consciousness. Report significant changes, and intervene quickly to preserve neurologic function.
  e. Manage nutrition.
    1) Enforce protein restriction to maintain anabolism while limiting the load on kidneys.
      a) Amount will vary depending on patient's weight and activity level and whether or not patient is on dialysis.
      b) Protein needs to be high biologic value.
    2) Restrict dietary potassium.
    3) Restrict fluids.
    4) Provide adequate calories to prevent catabolism.
    5) Administer ordered supplemental vitamins.
    6) Administer ordered blood transfusions to maintain adequate level of RBCs, for optimum tissue oxygenation.
4. Initiate renal replacement therapy (RRT) with any of the following signs/symptoms:
  a. BUN exceeds 100 mg/dL
  b. Serum creatinine exceeds 5–9 mg/dL. Begin at lower serum creatinine levels for patients with reduced muscle mass, such as the elderly
  c. Volume overload and signs of pulmonary edema
  d. Pericarditis
  e. Hyperkalemia that has not responded adequately to other treatment modalities

    f. Uncontrollable acidosis
    g. Central nervous system dysfunction related to uremia (e.g., encephalopathy or seizures)
5. RRT may be accomplished by the following:
    a. Hemodialysis
    b. Continuous ultrafiltration or continuous RRT
    c. Peritoneal dialysis

Comparing Methods of Renal Replacement Therapy

Procedure	Advantages	Disadvantages
■ Hemodialysis	■ Most rapid and efficient method	■ Requires specially trained nurse ■ Requires vascular access and routine site care ■ Risk of infection, graft clotting, hemorrhage, and embolism ■ Contraindicated in hemodynamically unstable patients
■ Continuous ultrafiltration	■ Relies on patient blood pressure, rather than a pump, to drive blood flow ■ Useful for patients who cannot tolerate hemodialysis or peritoneal dialysis, in patients with oliguria	■ Uses arteriovenous access

who require large amounts of fluids, and in multiple system organ failure
- Avoids rapid shifts in osmolality and concentrations of solutes

- Peritoneal dialysis
  - Does not require vascular access
  - Useful when hemodialysis is contraindicated
  - Requires no specially trained staff or special equipment
  - May cause patient less discomfort because fluids and solutes removed at a slower rate

- Slow
- Contraindicated when patient has abdominal adhesions or trauma or sepsis
- May not be used after recent abdominal surgery or with peritonitis

Drug Therapy

1. Fluid challenge — used if question of hypovolemia or to change a nonoliguric ARF to an oliguric ARF
   Example: a variety of IV fluids may be given but normal saline solution is usually the choice; 200–500 mL may be given in 10–20 minutes and repeated once
   Action: Should increase urine output by increasing blood volume reaching glomeruli
   Caution: Fluid overload could occur
2. Loop diuretic
   Example: furosemide (Lasix)
   Action: Thought to have renal vasodilatory effects that improve GFR; effects generally are seen only if ARF is in initial stages; increases renal excretion of water, sodium, chloride, magnesium, hydrogen ion, and calcium
   Caution: When administering IV, avoid giving too fast (<4 mg/min) as this can cause ototoxicity
3. Osmotic diuretic
   Example: mannitol (Osmitrol)
   Action: Increases osmolality of glomerular filtrate, attracting more water into the nephron and improving GFR
   May help reverse an insult if instituted early
   Caution: Do not use when patient is anuric or dehydrated
   Do not use in patient with an active intracranial bleed or a suspected intracranial bleed
4. Cation exchange resin
   Example: sodium polystyrene sulfonate (Kayexalate)
   Action: Binds potassium in the gastrointestinal tract to facilitate removal from the body
   Caution: Can cause constipation; this may be lessened when the powder is mixed in sorbitol as the solution
5. Aluminum hydroxide preparations
   Example: aluminum hydroxide (AlternaGEL)
   aluminum carbonate (Basaljel)
   Action: Given to bind phosphorus and to help manage the calcium/phosphate balance; even when patient is hypocalcemic and hyperphosphatemic
   Caution: Can cause constipation; patient may need to in-

crease bulk in diet or manage with laxatives or stool softeners

6. Antibiotics

   Examples: tetracyclines (Vibramycin)
   aminoglycosides (Gentamycin)
   cephalosporins (Clanfaran)

   Action: Used for treating documented infections; have antimicrobial properties

   Caution: Can contribute to kidney damage
   May be given in reduced dosage and with frequent monitoring of desirable blood levels of the antibiotic

7. Calcium replacement

   Example: calcium gluconate (Kalcinate)

   Action: Has a positive inotropic effect on myocardium and helps counteract the cardiotoxic effects of hyperkalemia

   Caution: Give IV; subcutaneous or intramuscular injections can cause tissue damage; requires controlled administration and electrocardiogram (ECG) monitoring during administration because of risk of dysrhythmias or cardiac arrest

8. Alkalinizing agent

   Example: sodium bicarbonate ($NaHCO_3$)

   Action: Systemic alkalinizer; helps counter the metabolic acidosis that occurs with ARF

   Caution: Acid-base balance values should be available before administering; usually used when HCO_3 is < 10 mEq/L

9. Inotropic agents

   Example: dopamine (Intropin)

   Action: Sympathomimetic effects that may improve CO and renal blood flow

   Caution: The only vasopressor that results in renal vasodilation; occurs only when given in the low-dose range ($0.5-3.0$ μg/kg per minute);
   Drug can cause tissue sloughing if it infiltrates
   Patient must have intravascular fluid deficits corrected before drug is used

10. Hypertonic glucose with insulin

    Example: 500 mL 10% dextrose with 10 U regular insulin added may be infused over 30 minutes

    Action: When glucose is taken into a cell, with the aid of insulin potassium is moved into the cell also; the process provides a decrease in serum K$^+$ that may continue for 2–4 hours

Caution: Serum potassium levels should be followed to identify effects of treatment and recognize any excess effect

NURSING MANAGEMENT

Monitoring and Managing Clinical Problems

1. Fluid Volume Excess or Deficit: high risk for
   a. Monitor for and report trends that may signal increasing fluid load.
      1) Maintain accurate intake and output to identify greater intake than output.
      2) Note pattern of urinary output, if any.
      3) Weigh daily at the same time each day and with the same scale.
      4) Report weight changes; rapid gain may indicate fluid retention; a gain of 1 kg in weight is approximately equivalent to retention of 1 L of fluid.
      5) Monitor hourly blood pressure for increases.
      6) Check for neck vein distention.
      7) Monitor for occurrence of or increase in peripheral edema.
      8) Monitor for occurrence of or increase in extent of ascites or periorbital edema.
      9) Measure hemodynamics, if available: an increased CVP or increased PCWP could signal increased total body fluid.
      10) Note respiratory pattern and effort for shortness of breath.
      11) Auscultate lungs for crackles.
      12) Monitor level of consciousness for deterioration.
   b. Monitor for trends that may signal hypovolemia. May occur in the diuretic phase of ARF, or when some form of renal replacement therapy is used.
      1) Record accurate intake and output.
      2) Note pattern of urinary output, if any.
      3) Monitor for hypotension that may occur with hypovolemia.

    4) Continuously monitor heart rate; increases may be seen with hypovolemia.

    5) Note presence of flattened neck veins.

    6) Note delayed venous filling time.

    7) Note sunken, soft eyeballs.

    8) Monitor hemodynamics, if available; may see decreased CVP or decreased PCWP, which could signal decreased total body fluid.

    9) Monitor respiratory pattern and effort, and initiate ventilatory support as indicated.

   10) Check for lethargy or malaise.

   11) Monitor for poor skin turgor or sticky oral mucous membranes.

  c. Promote fluid balance.

    1) Enforce ordered fluid restriction.

    2) Implement RRT.

    3) Provide adequate fluids (usually IV) when dialysis is started.

    4) Recognize complications.

      a) Hypervolemia

        1] May occur during anuric and oliguric stages of ARF and during diuretic phase of ARF or during dialysis.

        2] Monitor for and promote hemodynamic instability.

          a] Assist with insertion of central line and continuously monitor hemodynamic parameters.

          b] Titrate fluids and inotropic agents to maintain a systolic blood pressure of at least 80 mm Hg.

          c] Position the patient in modified Trendelenburg position (elevation of the legs at 45 degrees), if necessary.

        3] Promote adequate oxygenation.

          a] Administer ordered supplemental oxygen.

          b] Obtain specimens and monitor results of serial ABGs and hemoglobin, and report significant changes.

          c] Monitor capillary refill and monitor skin color to assess peripheral perfusion.

4] Monitor for altered organ and tissue perfusion.

a] Monitor for decreased urine output and elevated renal function tests.

b] Monitor for a falling arterial oxygen concentration, suggesting adult respiratory distress syndrome.

c] Monitor for decreased or absent bowel sounds, suggesting gastroparesis, and bright-red or coffee-ground drainage from nasogastric tube, possibly indicating stress.

d] Check temperature every 4 hours to monitor for hypothermia or hyperthermia.

e] Monitor for decreased alertness and attention span, drowsiness, or excessive sleeping, indicating a downward change in the level of consciousness.

5] Monitor for loss of and replace fluid volume in the vasculature.

a] Provide ordered fluid replacement.

b] Maintain accurate intake and output measurements hourly.

c] Continuously monitor blood pressure.

d] Monitor skin turgor for signs of dehydration.

e] Assess for a new onset of an S_3 heart sound, peripheral edema, and moist crackles in the lungs, indicating fluid volume overload.

f] Closely monitor serum electrolytes and urine studies to assess hydration status.

2. Injury: high risk for

a. Monitor for electrolyte imbalances.

1) Altered serum sodium, potassium, carbon dioxide, calcium, magnesium, phosphorus, and chloride; hyperkalemia is a common problem and its physiologic effects may be intensified when other electrolytes are also out of balance.

2) Continuously monitor cardiac rate and rhythm, and note any changes such as the following:

     a) Peaked T waves (early change)
     b) Prolonged PR interval
     c) Lengthened QRS interval, possibly indicating hyperkalemia; at higher levels ($<7-8$ mEq/L), further changes (absence of P wave, widening of QRS complex) may occur and just precede ventricular fibrillation and cardiac arrest.
   3) Observe for muscle weakness, abdominal cramping, and muscle twitching.
   4) Monitor serial serum calcium levels. Hypocalcemia is usually associated with hyperphosphatemia.
   5) Monitor serial serum potassium levels and treat elevations as ordered.
     a) For hyperkalemia of 6.0 mEq/L or less, may only require conservative treatment.
     b) For hyperkalemia of 6.5 mEq/L or greater, which often includes ECG changes and nausea, active intervention may be required, such as some method of RRT.
   6) Monitor serial serum sodium levels. Hyponatremia may be a sign of fluid overload and a need to initiate dialysis.
  b. Promote electrolyte balance.
   1) Assist patient to follow dietary restrictions for potassium and, if needed, for sodium and phosphorus.
   2) Avoid using medications that contain potassium and phosphorus.
   3) Administer medications to help decrease serum potassium.
   4) Implement dialysis when appropriate.
3. Tissue Perfusion, altered: renal
  a. Monitor blood pressure to ensure optimal renal perfusion and hemodynamic values, if available, to identify changes in CO.
  b. Promote optimum environment for renal repair.
   1) Avoid use of nephrotoxic drugs.
   2) Provide adequate fluids, especially if potentially toxic contrast dye must be used.
   3) When there is urine output with early ARF, use any treatment that promotes increased GFR

and high tubular flow rates to help protect nephrons.

4. Infection: high risk for
   a. Monitor for the following:
      1) Temperature elevation and trends
      2) Increased white blood cell (WBC) count
      3) Change in color, consistency, and amount of pulmonary secretions
      4) Occurrence of exudates from any site
      5) Changes in color or consistency of body excretions
      6) Changes in appearance of sites of invasive lines
   b. Protect the patient from nosocomial infection.
      1) Wash hands between patients.
      2) Restrict patient's exposure to anyone with infection.
      3) Use strict medical asepsis and sterile technique if procedure is invasive.
      4) Assist patient to maintain adequate oral hygiene.
      5) Assist patient to turn, cough, and deep breathe, as appropriate.
      6) Assist patient to receive adequate rest and nutrition.
      7) Avoid using an indwelling urinary catheter.
5. Nutrition: altered, high risk for less than body requirements
   a. Monitor for the following:
      1) Adequacy of patient's dietary intake
      2) Changes in daily weights: losses may be sign of inadequate nutrition
      3) Anorexia and nausea from uremia
   b. Protect patient from the following:
      1) Effects of catabolism
         a) Assist patient in selecting and eating those proteins that are high in biologic value.
         b) Implement total parenteral nutrition when patient is unable to take in enough calories and other nutrients.
         c) Treat nausea and anorexia that often occur with uremia with appropriate medications and nursing interventions (such as more frequent oral care) that help improve appetite.

2) Electrolyte and fluid imbalances by assisting patient to follow dietary restrictions

6. Tissue Perfusion, altered: peripheral
   a. Monitor for the following:
      1) Decreases in hemoglobin and hematocrit levels
      2) Signs/symptoms of anemia: pallor, weakness, fatigue, shortness of breath, and chest pain
   b. Administer medications (androgens, folic acid, and iron preparations) to help prevent severe anemia.
   c. Administer packed RBCs when symptoms of anemia (chest pain, dyspnea), or hematocrit level (may allow to drop to <20%) require replacement.
   d. Assess for evidence of internal or external bleeding that may indicate development of disseminated intravascular coagulopathy.

7. Skin Integrity: impaired, high risk for
   a. Observe dependent areas and pressure points for redness, blanching, and skin tears.
   b. Assess for adequate nutrition.
   c. Assess for changes in fluid balance and development of edematous areas.
   d. Assess for intact mucous membranes.
   e. Turn and reposition patient every 2 hours when patient unable to do so.
   f. Avoid harsh, drying soap and use oil in bath water.
   g. Use skin emollients to minimize dryness.
   h. Use appropriate mattress device or specialty bed for patients at risk.
   i. Avoid tight covers and tight shoes or slippers.
   j. Administer ordered medications for pruritus.

8. Sleep Pattern Disturbance
   a. Monitor the amount of uninterrupted sleep each night.
   b. Assess the patient's sleep history to determine the following:
      1) What helps the patient sleep
      2) Previous sleep patterns
      3) Organize care to allow maximum periods of uninterrupted sleep.
      4) Provide appropriate environment to help promote sleep.

9. Urinary Elimination: altered—high risk for

    a. Identify nephrotoxic drugs ordered for the patient.

    b. Ask whether or not dosages need adjustment when renal failure exists.

    c. Identify drugs that need adjustment in time of administration when hemodialysis is instituted.

10. Urinary Elimination: altered

    a. Monitor for increases in BUN, serum creatinine, and uric acid levels.

    b. Monitor for the development of uremic symptoms, such as:

        1) Fatigue

        2) Nausea and vomiting

        3) Memory impairment

        4) Attention deficit

        5) Pericarditis

        6) Pleuritis

    c. Protect from uremic effects by early implementation of dialysis.

11. Injury: high risk for (hemodialysis)

    a. Access site complications

        1) Monitor for signs and symptoms of infection.

        2) Check pulses and neurovascular status distal to access site.

        3) Care of site

            a) Apply an occlusive dressing.

            b) Observe for any sign of bleeding (may be life-threatening if unnoticed).

        4) If a double lumen catheter is placed for dialysis, remember it is usually only to be used for dialysis. The amount of heparin placed as a flush may be more than usual and should be discarded at the time access is used for dialysis.

        5) Restrict patient's position, as indicated. With femoral placement, the leg must be kept extended to prevent kinking or occluding of the catheters.

        6) For an arteriovenous graft, when newly placed:

            a) Assess for patency by auscultating for a bruit or palpating for a thrill.

            b) Elevate the extremity.

            c) Medicate for pain, as indicated.

            d) Assess for any sign of bleeding.

            e) Do not take blood pressures in the involved arm.

f) Do not draw blood from the access site.
b. Hypotension because of removal of large amounts of fluid volumes or rapid changes in osmolality
  1) Give volume expanders, such as normal saline solution or albumin.
  2) Change dialysis settings (such as the negative pressure) that control the amount of fluid removal.
  3) Assess for patient complaints of nausea, dizziness, chest pain, or back pain.
  4) Assess for occurrence of diaphoresis, restlessness, confusion, and dysrhythmias.
  5) Give inotropic agents, if needed, especially for patients with cardiovascular risk or known CHF.
c. Bleeding because of the heparinization
  1) Assess for any development of bleeding during dialysis.
  2) Adjust heparin dosages, as ordered.
  3) Limit systemic heparinization by instilling heparin infusion into the arterial port and protamine infusion into the venous port.
d. Development of dialysis disequilibrium syndrome
  1) Occurs because of the difference in the rates of urea clearance from blood and cerebrospinal fluid.
  2) May cause cerebral edema.
  3) Monitor for changes in level of consciousness, especially during the last minutes of dialysis and for several hours after completion.
  4) Monitor for early recognition of such symptoms as headache, nausea, vomiting, restlessness, and changes in mental alertness.
  5) Administer ordered preventive medications, such as osmotic diuretics, to modify serum osmolality changes.
  6) If symptoms do occur, discontinue dialysis.
12. Injury: high risk for (peritoneal dialysis)
a. Monitor access sites (entrance and exit sites of a temporary catheter are tunneled into peritoneum) daily.
b. Observe for redness, swelling, and presence of exudate at site.

   c. Record the amount of dialysate infused and amount drained for each cycle.
      1) Higher amounts may be removed with a dialysate that has a higher glucose concentration.
      2) Constipation may slow fluid draining and lead to smaller volumes removed and potential for hypervolemia.
   d. Monitor for any symptoms experienced during therapy; abdominal pain, experienced as the fluid flows in, is not uncommon with initiation of peritoneal dialysis.
   e. Protect the patient from peritonitis by:
      1) Washing hands
      2) Wearing mask, when doing an exchange
      3) Using aseptic technique, when preparing equipment and solutions
      4) Identifying early signs of infection, such as cloudiness of fluid return, fairly sudden onset of abdominal pain (increased pain if already complaining of pain), and elevation of temperature
      5) Culturing the effluent (fluid returned after dwelling in abdomen) if symptoms occur
      6) Culturing access site if drainage or redness
   f. Monitor for hyperglycemia that may occur because of the glucose in the dialysate, especially for patients who are diabetic.
      1) Monitor blood glucose on a routine schedule.
      2) If hyperglycemia is a problem, administer additional insulin coverage and/or change to a dialysate with a lower glucose concentration.
   g. Prevent discomfort during the procedure.
      1) Warm the solution before instilling into abdomen.
      2) Help patient identify a position of comfort.
13. Injury: high risk for [continuous renal replacement therapy (CRRT)]
   a. Potential for fluid imbalance because of the large volumes removed during CRRT.
      1) Note amount of ultrafiltrate (UF) collected hourly.
      2) Check rates on pumps providing replacement fluid to see that they are set correctly. Rates should be based on UF rates and should not exceed the UF rate.

3) If UF amount drops:
  a) Check system for kinks in blood lines and in the line from filter to the bag collecting UF.
  b) Check the position of patient in relation to access site; if it is femoral site, extremity needs to be straight and head of bed at less than a 30-degree elevation.
  c) Check for pressure on the site (Are dressings too tight?).
  d) Reposition the patient from side to back.
  e) Check the level of efferent pump between the hemofilter and the collection bag, and the level of the collection bag; they both should be below the level of the access site.
  f) Check hemofilter for presence of clots; suspect clotting if there is:
    1] An accumulation of small clots in the venous end of the hemofilter
    2] Darkening of blood in the line
    3] Separation of serum in the blood lines
    4] Air present in the UF chamber
4) Anytime clotting is suspected, change the system to prevent movement of clots into the access lines.
5) Anytime UF volume drops and there is a delay or an expected delay in reestablishing the UF rate, decrease or stop the infusion of the replacement fluid.
6) Calculate the desired UF rate based on the amounts of IV fluids needed for a 24-hour period.
  a) IV fluids per hour plus the amount of fluid to be removed per hour = volume desired for hourly UF rate
  b) This includes volumes needed for IV medication administration and for total parenteral nutrition, but may also include an amount added to produce adequate solute removal.
  c) Usually a minimum of 12 L of fluid needs to be exchanged in 24 hours.
b. Monitor neurovascular status distal to arterial/venous access.
1) Check distal pulses every 4 hours.

    2) Check color, warmth, and capillary refill in extremity every 4 hours.

    3) Report any change and anticipate removal of the arterial catheter.

  c. Monitor for electrolyte imbalance.

    1) Monitor serum electrolytes, especially potassium, sodium, calcium, and magnesium.

    2) Be sure that replacement solutions contain the ordered electrolyte concentrations.

    3) Confirm correct infusion rate settings.

Monitoring, Managing, and Preventing Life-Threatening Emergencies

1. Seizures
   a. Can occur if fluid and electrolyte imbalances become severe or if uremia is untreated.
   b. Institute seizure precautions to protect the patient from possible injury.
      1) Pad siderails and keep them raised.
      2) Keep bed in low position.
      3) Have emergency resuscitation equipment for airway management nearby.
      4) Have supplement oxygen available.
      5) Remove all potentially harmful objects from the patient's area.
      6) Restrict smoking.
   c. If seizure occurs:
      1) Protect the airway.
      2) Do not insert anything into the patient's mouth.
      3) Loosen restrictive clothing.
      4) Protect the patient from self-injury during the seizure.
      5) Administer ordered medications.
      6) Dialyze patient, as ordered, to prevent electrolyte abnormalities or uremia that may result in seizures.
2. Encephalopathy
   a. Monitor level of consciousness for any sign of decrease.
      1) Monitor laboratory test values.
         a) Increasing BUN and serum creatinine reflecting increasing uremia

       b) Changes in serum electrolytes
       c) Increasing metabolic acidosis
  b. Institute RRT, as ordered.
  c. Prevent encephalopathy by early recognition and intervention.

3. Metabolic acidosis
  a. Occurs when kidneys are unable to excrete the endogenous acids that are constantly produced.
  b. Becomes life-threatening when untreated.
  c. Monitor for confusion, headache, seizures, and coma, indicating metabolic acidosis.
  d. Monitor ABGs for decreased bicarbonate, decreased pH, and increased anion gap.
  e. Monitor for concomitant hyperkalemia.
  f. Monitor for Kussmaul's respiration.
  g. Treat metabolic acidosis with medications and dialysis, as ordered.

4. Hyperkalemia
  a. Most frequent imbalance; monitoring cardiac rhythm and serum electrolytes allows early recognition and intervention.
  b. Continuously monitor cardiac rate and rhythm, and note any changes, such as:
    1) Peaked T waves
    2) Prolonged PR interval
    3) Lengthened QRS interval as this may indicate hyperkalemia; at higher levels ($>7-8$ mEq/L), further changes (absence of P wave, widening of QRS complex) may occur and just precede ventricular fibrillation and cardiac arrest.
  c. Monitor for nausea, which may occur with a K^+ of 6.5 mEq/L or greater.
  d. Hyperkalemia of 6.0 mEq/L or less may require only conservative treatment.
  e. If hyperkalemia is 6.5 mEq/L or greater, which often includes ECG changes, RRT may be required.
  f. Promote electrolyte balance.
    1) Assist patient to follow dietary restrictions for potassium and, if needed, for sodium and phosphorus.
    2) Avoid using medications that contain potassium.
    3) Administer medications to help decrease serum potassium.

    4) Implement dialysis when appropriate.

5. Sepsis
   a. Infection remains a leading cause of mortality.
   b. Monitor for signs/symptoms of infection, such as:
      1) Elevated temperature; note trends
      2) Increased white blood cell count
      3) Change in color, consistency, and amount of pulmonary secretions
      4) Occurrence of exudates from any site
      5) Changes in color and consistency of excretions
      6) Changes in appearance of sites of invasive lines
   c. Protect the patient from contracting an infection by:
      1) Washing hands frequently
      2) Restricting patient's exposure to anyone with infection
      3) Using strict medical asepsis and sterile technique, if procedure is invasive
      4) Assisting patient to maintain adequate oral hygiene
      5) Assisting patient to turn, cough, and deep breathe, as appropriate
      6) Assisting patient to receive adequate rest and nutrition
      7) Avoiding use of an indwelling urinary catheter
   d. Obtain specimens of suspicious material for culture and sensitivity testing.
   e. Administer medications based on cultures and assessment of effectiveness.

Chronic Renal Failure

Chronic renal failure (CRF) involves significant reduction in the glomerular filtration rate (GFR) that may have existed for years before being recognized; CRF frequently progresses to end-stage renal diseases (ESRD), an irreversible loss of kidney function that requires treatment with renal replacement therapy (dialysis) or kidney transplantation for survival. Azotemia is the abnormal collection of nitrogenous wastes in the blood that results from decreased kidney function. Uremic syndrome is all of the systemic pathophysiologic changes that occur with kidney failure.

Etiology/Pathophysiology

1. Risks
   a. Past history of proteinuria, hematuria, acute nephritis, nephrotic syndrome, recurrent urinary tract infections, childhood or adult occurrence of reflux or urinary obstruction, abuse of antibiotics, analgesics, and other nonprescription drugs
   b. Current history of hypertension, diabetes mellitus, collagen-related diseases, Goodpasture's syndrome, or cardiovascular disease
   c. Family history of polycystic kidney disease, sickle cell disease, renal calculi, gout, malignancy, or hereditary nephritis
2. Causes
   a. Chronic glomerular disease, such as glomerulonephritis, collagen-related diseases, and complications of diabetes mellitus
   b. Chronic vascular disease, particularly hypertension
   c. Congenital anomalies, such as polycystic disease
   d. Interstitial renal disease, such as pyelonephritis, nephrotoxins, and radiation injury
   e. Urinary obstructive disorders, such as calculi and strictures
3. Pathophysiology
   a. Chronic glomerular diseases
      1) Chronic glomerulonephritis
         a) May be due to an infectious process that is chronic or could begin as an acute process that becomes chronic; examples include streptococcal infection, hepatitis B, endocarditis, and other agents that may cause sepsis.
         b) Usually involves an immunologic process with an antigen, endogenous or exogenous, and an antibody creating damage via an antigen-antibody complex or the antibody itself.
         c) Chronic inflammation leads to thickening of the glomerular membrane and loss of filtering ability.
         d) Damage to the glomerulus allows red blood

cells (RBCs) and plasma proteins to pass through.

    e) Loss of protein leads to hypoalbuminemia, and this, along with changes in the kidney's ability to manage sodium and water, leads to edema.

    f) When sufficient glomeruli are affected, symptoms occur and dialysis becomes necessary.

  2) Collagen-related diseases, such as systemic lupus erythematosus

    a) Antigen-antibody complexes are formed that damage tissues in the renal vasculature.

  3) Diabetic nephritis

    a) Causes scarring of the capillary loop or nodular glomerulosclerosis

    b) Progressive microangiopathy affects afferent and efferent arterioles, eventually scarring the glomerulus, tubules, and interstitium.

b. Chronic vascular disease

  1) Hypertension causes degenerative changes in the arterioles in interlobular arteries.

  2) In arteriosclerosis, the larger renal arteries are affected, causing unilateral loss of kidney function resulting from diminished blood supply.

  3) In benign nephrosclerosis, the smaller renal arteries and arterioles are affected with loss of function in those nephrons where renal vasculature is destroyed.

    a) The kidneys become smaller and develop a nodular surface.

    b) There is progressive loss of renal blood flow and renal plasma clearance.

    c) Changes are similar to those seen in an aging individual.

c. Congenital anomalies

  1) Congenital polycystic disease

    a) A slowly progressive disease

    b) Cysts develop throughout the cortex and medulla. Cysts vary in size but cause an overall great increase in the size of the kidneys, sometimes as much as 10 times the normal size.

    c) These cysts occupy or displace renal parenchyma, causing a decrease in renal function.

2) Medullary cystic disease
   a) Similar to polycystic disease
   b) Rapid progression to uremia
d. Interstitial renal disease
   1) Chronic pyelonephritis
      a) A slow, progressive disease that may be associated with acute exacerbations of pyelonephritis.
      b) Infection invades the renal pelvis first, and later, the cortex.
      c) Renal calyx dilation and cortical scarring occur, reducing the number of functioning nephrons.
      d) Urine becomes dilute as the kidney becomes unable to concentrate urine.
   2) Nephrotoxins
      a) Nephrotoxic drugs include nonsteroidal anti-inflammatory drugs; antibiotics, particularly penicillins, cephalosporins, sulfonamides, gentamicin, kanamycin, neomycin, polymyxins, amphotericin B, and streptomycin; anesthetic agents, such as methoxyflurane and halothane; diuretics, such as furosemide and thiazides; probenecid; phenytoin; low-molecular-weight dextrans, rifampin, lithium, gold compounds; and radio-iodinated contrast agents.
      b) Environmental agents that are nephrotoxic include heavy metals such as mercurial compounds, lead, cadmium, bismuth, arsenic, copper, and phosphorus; carbon tetrachloride; ethylene glycol; trichloroethylene; carbon monoxide; and chlorinated hydrocarbons.
      c) Exposure can cause acute tubular necrosis, defects in the tubular transport system, interstitial nephritis, vasculitis, and nephrotic syndrome.
   3) Radiation injury
      a) Causes cell mutation and interrupts cell division.
e. Urinary obstructive disorders
   1) Affect the kidneys bilaterally, unless one kidney is already nonfunctioning or absent.
   2) Cause back pressure that dilates collecting

tubules. Pressure is reflected backward until it reaches the area of glomerulus and interferes with glomerular filtration by:
    a) Pressure changes
    b) Compression of the renal vasculature
  3) Result in additional destruction and loss of kidney function.
4. Disease progression
  a. The speed with which the disease progresses varies.
    1) When nephrons are irreversibly destroyed, remaining nephrons become larger to attempt to compensate for those that have been lost.
    2) There is diminished renal reserve when up to half of the nephrons have been destroyed; however, the disease is often asymptomatic at this stage.
    3) Renal insufficiency develops when more than half of the nephrons are destroyed or are not functioning.
    4) End-stage renal failure occurs when 90% of the nephrons have been lost. Symptoms occur because homeostatic mechanisms are no longer able to keep the body's internal environment stable.
    5) Uremic syndrome occurs when loss of kidney function is severe and no replacement therapy is instituted.

Assessment/Analysis

ASSESSMENT FINDINGS

Subjective

1. History of one or more risk factors
2. Family history of any risk factors
3. Changes in patterns of urine production and symptoms such as frequency, urgency, nocturia, and polyuria
4. Personality changes, emotional lability, discouragement, anxiety, depression, withdrawal, and apathy
5. Headaches
6. Irritability
7. Decrease in or loss of appetite

8. Change in taste and smell
9. Shortness of breath
10. Pleuritic-type chest pain
11. Heart palpitations
12. Easy bruising, bleeding of gums; nosebleeds
13. Pruritus
14. Nausea, vomiting
15. Carbohydrate intolerance
16. Constipation or diarrhea
17. Fatigue
18. Muscle weakness
19. Numbness or tingling of face, tongue, hands, or feet
20. Inability to continue usual daily activities
21. Decreased libido

Objective

1. Skin pallor or with uremic changes, a yellow appearance
2. Dry skin, dry mucous membranes
3. Dysrhythmias
4. Low urine output
5. Color of urine ranging from very dark to nearly clear depending on stage of failure
6. Mental changes ranging from confusion and memory loss to stupor or coma
7. Asterixis
8. Restlessness, insomnia
9. Uremic fetor (urine-like breath odor)
10. Hiccoughs, eructation
11. Poor skin turgor
12. Edema of extremities, face, and dependent areas
13. Hypertension, or loss of control of hypertension, possibly along with orthostatic hypotension
14. Crackles, shortness of breath

SUPPORTING TEST FINDINGS

Laboratory Tests

1. Serum creatinine
   Abnormality: Increased; with diminished renal reserve, may be equal to or twice the normal range (2.4 mg/dL); with progression of failure to that labeled

renal insufficiency, the value may be 5.6–9.6 mg/dL; with end-stage, the value may be 5–10 mg/dL or greater

2. Blood urea nitrogen
   Abnormality: Increased (>25 mg/dL); is progressively higher with each stage of renal failure; varies depending on patient's protein intake and other factors such as level of metabolism, muscle mass; at 100 mg/dL, uremic symptoms are usually present

3. Urine creatinine clearance
   Abnormality: Decreased; at stage of renal insufficiency, may decrease to 10–50 mL/min and with ESRD, <5 mL/min

4. Urine osmolality
   Abnormality: Decreased

5. Urinalysis
   Abnormality: Presence of RBCs, casts, perhaps actual tubular epithelial cells, white blood cells (WBCs), and protein

6. Urine pH
   Abnormality: Increased

7. Urine specific gravity
   Abnormality: Increased or decreased

8. Serum osmolality
   Abnormality: Variable depending on fluid status

9. Ratio of urine to serum osmolality
   Abnormality: Ratio often 1:1, but varies

10. Hemoglobin and hematocrit
    Abnormality: Decreased

11. Serum uric acid level
    Abnormality: Increased

12. Arterial blood gases
    Abnormality: Decreased pH (≤7.4)
    Decreased HCO_3
    If disease has been present for some time, compensation may occur with a resulting decrease in $Paco_2$ and a more normal pH

Diagnostic Tests

1. Flat plate of the abdomen, also known as a KUB for kidneys, ureters, bladder
   Abnormality: Small kidneys due to atrophy

2. Renal ultrasound
   Abnormality: Varies depending on which chronic disease is involved; may see enlarged kidneys with polycystic disease or disease that was obstructive in nature, small kidneys, or one kidney that is normal in size and one that is atrophied
3. Renal biopsy
   Abnormality: Presence of renal disease; helps to identify disease process when other diagnostic methods leave questions; is used to identify potential therapeutic interventions

Planning/Intervention

COLLABORATIVE MANAGEMENT

Procedures

1. Assist with preserving remaining kidney function.
   a. Avoid dehydration.
   b. Monitor for inadequate renal blood flow due to cardiac disease or other events that may cause hypotension.
   c. Prevent infection.
   d. Prevent obstruction to flow of urine.
   e. Avoid use of nephrotoxic drugs and radiographic dyes.
2. Help delay development of uremic syndrome.
   a. Restrict dietary protein, potassium, and sodium based on amount of remaining renal function.
      1) Restrict protein when GFR is close to or below 10 mL/min; usually restrict to 0.5–1 g/kg body weight per day.
      2) Maintain an anabolic state.
   b. Restrict fluids based on volume of urine still being produced.
3. Minimize effects of kidney failure on other body systems, such as the development of anemia.
   a. Ensure adequate fluid intake to maintain fluid and electrolyte balance.
   b. Identify an appropriate time in the disease progression to begin dialysis and/or consider renal transplant.

  1) Assist with preparation for dialysis by preparing patient for the required access device.
  2) Ensure that the patient receives information about renal transplant.
c. Implement ordered interventions to treat other disease processes, such as infection, bleeding problems, dialysis access failure, or cardiovascular problems.
  1) Renal failure effects all body systems.
  2) Some diseases are more likely to occur in patients with CRF.
  3) Preexisting chronic diseases will require continued and perhaps, intensified, management.

Drug Therapy

1. Antihypertensive agents
   Example: clonidine (Catapres)
   Action: Causes vasodilation and slightly decreased heart rate, cardiac contractility, and renin release by stimulating alpha-receptors
   Caution: Use of beta-adrenergic blockers along with this drug can cause tachycardia
      Suddenly discontinuing this drug or decreasing dosage when used chronically also may cause severe hypertension.
2. Diuretics
   Example: furosemide (Lasix)
   Action: Increases the amounts of sodium and water that are excreted by the kidneys and assists in managing the decreased water excretion of CRF
   Caution: Used when patient still is making urine
      Diuretics that are potassium-sparing are not used
3. Aluminum hydroxide preparations
   Example: aluminum hydroxide (AlternaGEL)
      aluminum carbonate (Basaljel)
   Action: Bind phosphorus to help regulate calcium/phosphorus balance when patient is hypocalcemic and hyperphosphatemic
   Caution: May be more effective if patient can follow dose with a full glass of water or fruit juice, but this will vary based on fluid and dietary restrictions
      Can cause constipation, which may require in-

creased bulk in diet or use of laxatives and stool softeners

Take with meals to maximize effects

Phosphate and calcium levels need to be evaluated regularly

4. Stool softeners

Example: docusate calcium (Surfak)

Action: Decreases surface tension of feces and also helps by emulsifying fats and water, to allow penetration of hard, dry feces for softening, which facilitates expulsion

Caution: May allow increased absorption of other medications; stool softeners containing sodium should be avoided

5. Laxatives

Example: psyllium (Metamucil)

Action: Absorbs water in the intestines to help increase the bulk of feces and thus stimulate motility and evacuation

Caution: Requires adequate oral fluid intake; need to plan for this when patient is on fluid restrictions

6. Antiemetics

Example: prochlorperazine (Compazine)

Action: Controls nausea by blocking the dopaminergic receptors in the chemoreceptor trigger zone in the brain

Caution: Can cause sedation and hypotension; also may produce additional central nervous system depression if other depressants are used

7. Antipruritics

Example: diphenhydramine (Benadryl)

Action: Blocks histamine-receptors to decrease pruritus

Caution: Can cause sedation

8. Cardiac glycosides

Example: digoxin (Lanoxin)

Action: When patient has cardiovascular disease, may be used to increase cardiac contractility and improve renal blood flow because cardiac output is improved

Caution: Changes in serum potassium levels with CRF and dialysis therapies may increase digoxin blood levels and risk of digitalis toxicity

9. Androgens

Example: fluoxymesterone (Halotestin)
nandrolone decanoate (Deca-Durabolin)
Action: Stimulates RBC production
Caution: Female patients need to be warned that this medication can cause appearance of male sex characteristics

Use is reserved for those patients who have not responded adequately to diet, vitamin, and iron therapies

10. Vitamins
Example: multivitamin supplements that contain water-soluble vitamins
folic acid (Folate)
Action: Replace those water-soluble vitamins that are lost with dialysis
Folic acid is needed to stimulate production of RBCs and other blood components
Caution: If phosphorus levels have not been normalized, multivitamins containing vitamin D may be contraindicated

11. Calcium replacements
Example: calcium gluconate (Kalcinate)
Action: Calcium replacement used to manage changes in calcium levels related to CRF
Caution: Monitor calcium levels at regular intervals
Hypercalcemia increases risk of digitalis toxicity

12. Iron
Example: ferrous sulfate (Feosol)
Action: Provides supplemental iron to assist in RBC production and treat anemia
Caution: Because of the effects of CRF, there is a greater need to give this with or immediately after meals to minimize gastric distress
Should not take within 1 hour of bedtime

13. Epoietin alfa: recombinant human erythropoietin
Example: erythropoietin recombinant (rHU-EPO)
Action: Stimulates erythrocyte production and helps prevent anemia
Caution: Weekly reticulocyte counts should show increase in 1–2 weeks
May require 2–6 weeks to see effects; patient may require alternative support during this period

14. Cation exchange resin
    Example: sodium polystyrene sulfonate (Kayexelate)
    Action: Binds potassium in the gastrointestinal tract to facilitate potassium removal from the body
    Caution: Can cause constipation; this may be lessened when the powder is mixed in sorbitol as the solution
    Solution stable for 24 hours when refrigerated
15. Blood transfusions
    Example: Packed RBCs
    Action: Replaces RBCs to help manage the anemia
    Caution: Attempt is made to avoid transfusions but may be needed when the hematocrit falls below 20% or if patient has chest pain, dyspnea, or other symptoms of tissue hypoxia
    If the patient might be candidate for renal transplant, "washed" cells are the choice for transfusion

NURSING MANAGEMENT

Monitoring and Managing Clinical Problems

1. Fluid Volume Excess or Deficit
   a. Monitor for trends that may signal increasing or decreasing fluid load.
      1) Changes in pattern of urinary output
      2) Imbalances in intake and output
      3) Changes in daily weight. Weighing needs to be done at the same time each day and with the same scale. A gain of 1 kg in weight is approximately equivalent to retention of 1 L of fluid.
      4) Blood pressure increases (may signal increasing fluid load) or decreases (may signal hypovolemia)
      5) Heart rate increases (may be seen with hypovolemia)
      6) Presence of neck vein distention, indicating fluid overload
      7) Occurrence of or change in peripheral edema
      8) Occurrence of or change in amount of ascites or periorbital edema
      9) Hemodynamic changes, if available: an increased central venous pressure (CVP) or increased pulmonary capillary wedge pressure (PCWP) could

signal increased total body fluid; a decreased CVP or decreased PCWP could signal decreased total body fluid that might occur with diuretic phase of acute renal failure (ARF) or during dialysis.

10) Respiratory pattern and effort reflecting shortness of breath (may be sign of fluid overload and development of pulmonary edema)

11) Auscultate crackles in lung fields (may indicate fluid overload).

12) Deterioration in the level of consciousness (may be a sign of a change in fluid balance)

b. Promote fluid balance.

1) Assist patient to restrict fluids, as appropriate.

2) Implement dialysis, as indicated.

3) Provide adequate fluids (usually by intravenous lines) when dialysis is initiated.

c. Recognize complications.

1) Hypervolemia may occur during anuric and oliguric stages of ARF.

2) Hypovolemia may occur during diuretic phase of ARF or during dialysis.

2. Injury: high risk for

a. Monitor laboratory values of serum electrolytes: serum sodium, potassium, calcium, magnesium, phosphorus, and chloride.

b. Hyperkalemia is a common problem.

1) Its physiologic effects may be intensified when other electrolytes are also out of balance.

2) Monitor cardiac rhythm for changes such as peaked T waves, prolonged PR interval, and lengthened QRS interval as this may indicate hyperkalemia; at higher levels (>7–8 mEq/L), further changes (absence of P wave, widening of QRS complex) may occur and just precede ventricular fibrillation and cardiac arrest.

3) Monitor for symptoms of muscle weakness, abdominal cramping, muscle twitching, and nausea, which may occur with a serum potassium of 6.5 mEq/L or greater.

4) Expect hyperkalemia of 6.0 mEq/L or less to be treated conservatively.

5) Expect hyperkalemia of 6.5 mEq/L or greater,

which often includes electrocardiogram changes, to be treated with dialysis.

c. Monitor for hyponatremia, which may be a sign of fluid overload and a need for dialysis.

d. Monitor for hypocalcemia, which is usually associated with hyperphosphatemia.

e. Promote electrolyte balance.

    1) Assist the patient to follow dietary restrictions for potassium and, if needed, for sodium and phosphorus.

    2) Avoid using medications that contain phosphorus and potassium.

    3) Administer medications to help decrease serum potassium.

    4) Implement ordered dialysis as indicated.

3. Infection: high risk for

  a. Monitor for the following:

    1) Increased temperature; note significant changes

    2) Increased WBC count

    3) Change in color, consistency, or amount of pulmonary secretions

    4) Presence of exudates from any site

    5) Change in color or consistency of body excretion

    6) Changes in appearance at sites of invasive lines

  b. Protect the patient from nosocomial infection by:

    1) Washing hands frequently

    2) Restricting the patient's exposure to anyone with infection

    3) Using strict medical asepsis and sterile technique if procedure is invasive

    4) Assisting the patient with oral hygiene

    5) Assisting the patient to turn, cough, and deep breathe every 2 hours

    6) Ensuring that the patient receives adequate rest and nutrition

    7) Avoiding use of an indwelling urinary catheter

4. Nutrition: altered, less than body requirements

  a. Monitor for:

    1) Adequate dietary intake

    2) Trends in daily weights: losses may be sign of inadequate nutrition

    3) Significance of uremia on patient's appetite and occurrence of nausea

b. Protect from effects of catabolism
   1) Assist patient in selecting and eating those proteins that are high in biologic value.
   2) Implement total parenteral nutrition when patient is unable to take in enough calories and other nutrients.
   3) Institute nursing measures, such as oral care, and administer ordered medications to reduce the nausea and anorexia that often occurs with uremia.
   4) Maintain fluid and electrolyte balance by assisting patient to follow dietary restrictions.
5. Tissue Perfusion, altered — potential for anemia
   a. Monitor for:
      1) Decreased hemoglobin and hematocrit levels
      2) Signs and symptoms of anemia: pallor, weakness, fatigue, shortness of breath, chest pain
   b. Administer ordered medications to help prevent severe anemia.
   c. Administer packed RBCs when symptoms (chest pain, dyspnea), or hematocrit levels (may allow to drop to less than 20%) require.
   d. Recognize potential complications:
      1) Assess for evidence of actual bleeding
      2) Assess for signs/symptoms that may indicate internal bleeding and the development of disseminated intravascular coagulopathy (DIC)
6. Skin Integrity: impaired, high risk for — potential loss of skin integrity
   a. Monitor for:
      1) Redness, blanching, or skin tears on dependent areas and pressure points
      2) Adequate nutrition to prevent skin breakdown
      3) Changes in fluid balance and development of edematous areas
      4) Intact mucous membranes
   b. Turn and reposition patient every 2 hours when patient unable to do so.
   c. Avoid harsh, drying soap and use oil in bath water.
   d. Use skin emollients to minimize dryness.
   e. Use specialty bed or mattress device for patients at risk.
   f. Avoid tight covers, tight shoes or slippers.
   g. Administer ordered medications for pruritus.

7. Sleep Pattern Disturbance—potential sleep deprivation
   a. Monitor for amount of uninterrupted sleep.
   b. Assess patient's sleep history.
      1) What helps the patient sleep
      2) Previous sleep patterns
   c. Organize care to allow for maximum periods of uninterrupted sleep.
   d. Provide an appropriate environment to help promote sleep.
8. Injury: high risk for (Adverse effects from any medication that involves renal system for excretion)
   a. Identify nephrotoxic drugs ordered for the patient.
   b. Ask whether or not dosages need adjustment when renal failure exists.
   c. Identify drugs that need adjustment at time of administration when hemodialysis is instituted.
   d. Digoxin is an example of a drug that requires careful regulation of dose in renal failure. Drug levels are also affected by the serum potassium level.
9. Altered Urinary Elimination—Uremic syndrome
   a. Monitor for increases in blood urea nitrogen, serum creatinine, serum uric acid levels.
   b. Monitor for the development of uremic symptoms
      1) Fatigue
      2) Nausea and vomiting
      3) Memory impairment
      4) Attention deficit
      5) Pericarditis
      6) Pleuritis
   c. Protect from uremic effects by early implementation of dialysis.

Monitoring, Managing, and Preventing Life-Threatening Emergencies

1. Seizures
   a. Can occur if fluid and electrolyte imbalances become severe or if uremia is untreated
   b. Institute seizure precautions to protect the patient from possible injury.
      1) Pad siderails and keep them raised.

      2) Keep bed in low position.
      3) Have emergency resuscitation equipment nearby.
      4) Have supplemental oxygen available.
      5) Remove all potentially harmful objects from the patient's area.
      6) Restrict smoking.
  c. If seizure occurs
      1) Protect the airway.
      2) Do not insert anything into the patient's mouth.
      3) Loosen restrictive clothing.
      4) Protect the patient from self-injury during the seizure.
      5) Administer ordered anticonvulsants.
  d. Institute ordered dialysis to prevent electrolyte abnormalities or uremia that may result in seizures.
2. Encephalopathy
  a. Monitor for decreases in the level of consciousness.
  b. Monitor increasing blood urea nitrogen and serum creatinine reflecting increasing uremia, changes in serum electrolyte balance, increasing metabolic acidosis.
  c. Institute ordered dialysis to remove the nitrogenous wastes that cause it.
  d. Prevent deterioration by early intervention.
4. Metabolic Acidosis
  a. Occurs when kidneys are unable to excrete the endogenous acids that are constantly produced
  b. Becomes life-threatening when untreated
  c. Monitor for neurologic changes indicating metabolic acidosis.
      1) Confusion
      2) Headache
      3) Seizures
      4) Coma
  d. Monitor arterial blood gas values for decreased bicarbonate, decreased pH, and increased anion gap.
  e. Monitor for concomitant hyperkalemia.
  f. Monitor for Kussmaul's breathing.
  g. Treat metabolic acidosis with ordered medications and dialysis.
5. Hyperkalemia
  a. The most frequent imbalance

   b. Continuously monitor cardiac rate and rhythm and note any changes
   1) Peaked T waves (early change)
   2) Prolonged PR interval
   3) Lengthened QRS interval as this may indicate hyperkalemia; at higher levels (greater than 7.0 — 8.0 mEq/L), further changes (absence of P wave, widening of QRS complex) may occur and just precede ventricular fibrillation and cardiac arrest
   c. Monitor for nausea which may occur with a serum potassium of 6.5 mEq/L or greater
   d. For serum potassium of 6.0 mEq/L or below, expect conservative treatment
   e. For serum potassium of 6.5 mEq/L or above, which often includes electrocardiogram changes, expect dialysis
   f. Promote electrolyte balance
   1) Assist patient to follow dietary restrictions for potassium and if needed, for sodium and phosphorus.
   2) Avoid using medications that contain potassium.
   3) Administer medications to help decrease serum potassium.
   4) Implement dialysis when appropriate.
6. Sepsis
   a. Infection remains a leading cause of mortality
   b. Monitor for signs/symptoms of infection
   1) Temperature elevation; note significant changes
   2) Increased WBC count
   3) Change in color, consistency, amount of pulmonary secretions
   4) Occurrence of exudates from any site
   5) Changes in color and consistency of body excretions
   6) Changes in appearance of sites of invasive lines
   c. Protect the patient from nosocomial infection
   1) Wash hands frequently
   2) Restrict patient's exposure to anyone with infection
   3) Use strict medical asepsis and sterile technique if procedure is invasive
   4) Assist patient to maintain adequate oral hygiene
   5) Assist the patient to turn, cough, deep breathe every 2 hours

     6) Ensure that the patient receives adequate rest and nutrition

     7) Avoid using an indwelling urinary catheter

  d. Obtain specimens of suspicious material or sites for culture and sensitivity testing.

  e. Administer antibiotic medications based on cultures and assess effectiveness by monitoring serial WBC levels.

7. Respiratory Failure

  a. Monitor for increasing respiratory distress leading to increasing hypoxemia.

     1) Monitor serial arterial blood gas (ABG) results and report significant changes.

     2) Monitor serial chest X-ray reports.

     3) Auscultate lungs frequently for decreased breath sounds, crackles, and/or rhonchi.

     4) Apply pulse oximeter and continuously measure oxygen saturation.

     5) Administer ordered bronchodilators.

     6) Monitor for air hunger, tachypnea, restlessness, and confusion indicating increasing respiratory distress.

  b. Prepare for immediate intubation if necessary.

  c. Monitor for effective ventilation while on mechanical ventilator.

     1) Reassess lung sounds frequently

     2) Suction as needed to remove sputum and promote a clear airway

     3) Measure compliance frequently and report decreases

     4) Measure peak pressures and report increases

     5) Sedate the patient as needed to control ventilator fighting. Neuromuscular blocking agents may be necessary also.

     6) Monitor serial ABGs for effectiveness of mechanical ventilation. Indications for applying positive end-expiratory pressure (PEEP).

       a) Pao_2 <60 mmHg on an Fio_2 >50%

       b) pH <7.25

       c) $Paco_2$ >45 mmHg

     7) Decrease Fio_2 to <50% as quickly as possible to prevent oxygen toxicity

8) If the patient is on PEEP, remember PEEP holds alveoli open thus increasing functional residual capacity, decreasing shunting, and decreasing hypoxemia. But, PEEP can
   a) Decrease cardiac output
   b) Increase the chance of oxygen toxicity
   c) Cause fluid overload

d. Monitor fluid volume status
   1) Hemodynamically measure cardiac output at frequent intervals
   2) Measure hourly urine output and report output <30% mL/h
   3) Observe for new S_3, increasing pulmonary crackles and rhonchi, edema, weight gain, intake greater than output indicating fluid overload and report positive findings
   4) Observe for weight loss, low cardiac output, intake greater than output, tenting of skin indicating dehydration and report positive findings
   5) Cautiously give intravenous fluids to prevent fluid overload but maintain adequate fluid volume

Comparing Fluid and Electrolyte Disorders

	Extracellular Fluid Volume Deficit	*Intracellular Fluid Volume Deficit*
Definition	Insufficient fluid outside the cell	Insufficient total body water
Cause	Fever with profuse diaphoresis Reduced oral intake Vomiting Diarrhea Fistula or wound drainage Continuous gastrointestinal suction Overdose of cathartics Renal disease Overzealous use of diuretics Diabetes insipidus Hypoproteinemia Hemorrhage Third spacing of fluids	Insufficient water intake Extensive insensible fluid loss Profuse diaphoresis Diabetes insipidus Osmotic diuresis
Assessment findings	Acute weight loss Changes in mental status Seizures	Changes in level of consciousness and mental status Muscle weakness

Continued

Comparing Fluid and Electrolyte Disorders— *Continued*

Extracellular Fluid Volume Deficit	*Intracellular Fluid Volume Deficit*
Muscle cramps	Seizures
Postural hypotension	Altered respiratory rate and rhythm
Dizziness	Urine output <30 mL/h
Vertigo	Skin warm and flushed
Syncope	
Tachycardia	
Pulse weak and thready	
Absence of neck vein distention	
Decreased central venous pressure (CVP)	
Decreased pulmonary artery pressure	
Decreased cardiac output (CO)	
Nausea	
Vomiting	
Anorexia	
Increased thirst	
Urine output <30 mL/h	
Dry skin and mucous membranes	

	Extracellular Fluid Volume Excess	Intracellular Fluid Volume Excess
Laboratory test findings	Increased hemoglobin, hematocrit Increased serum protein	Serum sodium >148 mEg/L Normal to increased hemoglobin and hematocrit Increased serum protein
Treatment	Restore fluid and electrolyte balance using normal saline solution until oliguria is relieved Treat underlying cause	Aggressive fluid replacement, usually with 5% dextrose in water Treat underlying cause
Definition	***Extracellular Fluid Volume Excess*** Excessive amounts of fluid outside the cell	***Intracellular Fluid Volume Excess*** Excessive amounts of total body water
Causes	Increased retention of fluid in intravascular space Serum protein depletion and hyponatremia Cirrhosis Hyperaldosteronism	Renal disease Syndrome of inappropriate secretion of antidiuretic hormone (SIADH) Excessive oral and/or intravenous (IV) intake
Assessment findings	Weight gain >0.5 kg/24 h	Changes in mental status and level of

Continued

Comparing Fluid and Electrolyte Disorders — *Continued*

	Extracellular Fluid Volume Deficit	*Intracellular Fluid Volume Deficit*
	Changes in mental status and level of consciousness Seizures Paralysis Hypertension Tachycardia with bounding pulse Neck vein distention Increased CVP and pulmonary pressures Peripheral edema Shortness of breath Tachypnea Dyspnea Cough Crackles Urine output disproportionately less than fluid intake	consciousness Headache Nausea and vomiting frequently accompanying the headache Weakness Muscle cramps Muscle twitching Seizures
Laboratory test findings	Normal to decreased hemoglobin, hematocrit, serum protein, and blood urea nitrogen (BUN)	Normal hemoglobin and hematocrit Normal to decreased serum protein and BUN

	Hypernatremia	Hyponatremia
Treatment	Serum osmolality about 285 to 295 mOsm/kg Decreased urine sodium Urine osmolality <500 mOsm/kg Urine specific gravity <1.010 Salt and fluid restriction Osmotic diuretics and salt poor albumin to increase fluid excretion Treat underlying cause	Serum osmolality <285 mOsm/kg Decreased urine and serum sodium Urine osmolality <500 mOsm/kg Urine specific gravity <1.010 Strict fluid restriction (fluid replacement limited to urine output) Treat underlying cause
Definition	*Hypernatremia* Excessive amounts of serum sodium	*Hyponatremia* Decreased concentration of serum sodium
Causes	Decreased body intake ■ Inadequate fluid intake ■ Water loss in excess of sodium loss ■ Diarrhea ■ Chronic renal failure ■ Diaphoresis ■ Diabetes insipidus	Sodium dilution ■ Cardiac failure ■ Hepatic insufficiency ■ Nephrotic syndrome (inability to excrete free water) ■ Excessive water ingestion or administration of hypotonic electrolyte-free intravenous solutions

Continued

Comparing Fluid and Electrolyte Disorders — *Continued*

	Hypernatremia	*Hyponatremia*
	Sodium excess ■ High sodium intake without water supplement ■ Hyperaldosteronism ■ Cushing's syndrome ■ Excessive steroid administration	Excessive tap water enemas ■ SIADH Sodium loss ■ Diuretics ■ Salt-poor diet ■ Vomiting ■ Nasogastric suctioning ■ Diarrhea ■ Renal disease ■ Adrenal insufficiency ■ Water replacement only when replacing fluids after diaphoresis and blood loss
Assessment findings	Decreased water intake ■ State of dehydration with thirst ■ Changes in mental status, including restlessness, irritability, agitation, lethargy, confusion, and coma	Sodium dilution ■ Altered cardiac, hepatic, or renal function ■ Changes in mental status and level of consciousness

- Tremors
- Seizures

Sodium excess
- Weight gain <0.5 kg/24 h
- Changes in mental status and level of consciousness
- Seizures
- Paralysis
- Hypertension
- Tachycardia with bounding pulse
- Neck vein distention
- Increased CVP and pulmonary pressures
- Peripheral edema
- Shortness of breath
- Tachypnea
- Dyspnea
- Cough
- Crackles
- Urine output disproportionately less than fluid intake

- Headache
- Nausea and vomiting frequently accompanying the headache
- Weakness
- Muscle cramps
- Muscle twitching
- Seizures

Sodium loss
- Acute weight loss
- Changes in mental status including lethargy, confusion, and coma
- Headache
- Seizures
- Muscle cramps
- Postural hypotension

Continued

369

Comparing Fluid and Electrolyte Disorders — *Continued*

	Hypernatremia	*Hyponatremia*
Laboratory test findings	Decreased water intake ■ Increased hemoglobin and hematocrit ■ Serum osmolality >295 mOsm/kg ■ Serum sodium >148 mEq/L ■ Urinary sodium <20 mEq/L ■ Urine osmolality >500 mEq/L ■ Urine specific gravity >1.015	Serum osmolality <285 mOsm/kg Serum sodium <124 mEq/L Urine sodium <20 mEq/L Urine sodium >30 mEq/L
Treatment	Decreased water intake ■ Fluid replacement therapy, usually an isotonic or hypotonic intravenous solution (5% dextrose solution) ■ Electrolyte replacement therapy Sodium excess ■ Sodium and fluid restriction ■ Hypnotic intravenous fluids ■ Diuretics	Sodium dilution ■ Fluid and sodium replacement therapy using intravenous normal saline (avoid undue haste in correcting the abnormality) Sodium loss ■ Loop diuretics ■ Treat underlying case

	Hyperkalemia Excessive serum potassium	**Hypokalemia** Decreased serum potassium concentration
Definition		
Cause	Acute renal failure, oliguric phase Chronic renal failure, later stage Potassium-sparing diuretics Acidosis Aldosterone deficiency Overly aggressive potassium replacement therapy Medications high in potassium Crush injury, trauma, or burns	Inadequate dietary intake Excessive vomiting Persistent diarrhea Overuse of potassium wasting diuretics Hyperaldosteronism Renal tubular disorder Resistance to antidiuretic hormone (ADH) Use of gentamycin, carbenicillin, or digitalis
Assessment findings	Signs and symptoms highly nonspecific and are often similar to hypokalemia electrocardiogram (ECG) changes ■ Tented, symmetric T waves ■ Shortened repolarization ■ Widened QRS leading to cardiac arrest ■ Reduced R wave amplitude ■ Depressed ST segment	Reduction in overall muscle tone Fatigue Weakness Respiratory muscle weakness Hypotension ECG changes ■ Peaked P wave ■ Prolonged PR interval

Continued

Comparing Fluid and Electrolyte Disorders — *Continued*

	Hyperkalemia	*Hypokalemia*
	■ Prolonged PR interval leading to heart block ■ Flattened to absent P waves	■ Flattened T wave ■ Depressed ST segment ■ Elevated U wave
Laboratory test findings	Serum potassium >5.5 mEq/L	Serum potassium >5.5 mEq/L
		Serum potassium <3.5 mEq/L
Treatment	For serum potassium of 5.5–6.5 mEq/L with adequate renal function ■ Sodium polystyrene sulfonate ■ Loop diuretics For serum potassium >6.5 mEq/L and/or severely impaired renal function ■ Emergency administration of 10% calcium gluconate with continuous cardiac monitoring ■ Administration of 500 ml 10% glucose with 10 units regular insulin, IV over 30 min	For serum potassium 2.5–3.5 mEq/L: ■ Oral potassium therapy ■ Increased dietary potassium ■ Treat underlying cause such as nausea and vomiting, alkalosis For serum potassium <2.5 mEq/L with cardiac dysrhythmias ■ Intravenous potassium chloride at concentrations not exceeding 40 mEq/h ■ If fluids need to be restricted, use intravenous 10–20 mEq of potassium chloride with a volume control

	▪ Sodium bicarbonate 2–3 amps, in 500 mL glucose, IV over 1–2 h or as prescribed ▪ Hemodialysis Avoid rapid correction of hyperkalemia and monitor serum potassium, urine output, and cardiac rhythm	device over 1 h or as prescribed Avoid rapid correction of hypokalemia and monitor serum potassium, urine output, and cardiac rhythm
Definition	*Hyperchloremia* Excessive serum chloride	*Hypochloremia* Decreased concentration of serum chloride
Causes	Gastrointestinal loss of HCO_3 from diarrhea and small-bowel, biliary, or pancreatic drainage Use of carbonic anhydrase inhibitors Renal tubular acidosis	Direct chloride ion loss (HCO_3^- is reabsorbed with chloride depletion) Direct hydrogen ion loss Vomiting, gastric drainage, villous adenoma of the colon Osmotic diuresis Excessive diaphoresis
Assessment findings	Drowsiness Lethargy	Neuromuscular irritability Muscle cramps

Continued

Comparing Fluid and Electrolyte Disorders — Continued

	Hyperchloremia	*Hypochloremia*
	Headache Weakness Tremors Tachypnea Dyspnea Kussmaul's breathing with pH <7.20 Hyperventilation Dysrhythmias	Weakness Hyperactive deep tendon reflexes Tetany Decreased respirations
Laboratory test findings	Serum chloride >106 mEq/L	Serum chloride <96 mEq/L
Treatment	Treat underlying cause of metabolic acidemia Intravenous administration of bicarbonate to increase pH Intravenous fluid therapy with Ringer's lactate	Treat underlying cause of metabolic alkalemia Intravenous fluid replacement with sodium chloride and potassium chloride
	Hypermagnesemia	*Hypomagnesemia*
Definition	Excessive serum magnesium	Decreased serum magnesium concentration

Cause	Renal failure, oliguric phase Excessive use of magnesium-containing compounds Overdose of magnesium replacement therapy Dehydration	Diabetic ketoacidosis Malabsorption syndrome Long-term gastrointestinal suctioning Malnutrition Pancreatitis Renal failure, diuretic phase Hyperaldosteronism Hyperparathyroidism, thyrotoxicosis Toxemia of pregnancy Chronic alcoholism Use of aminoglycosides, cisplatin, digoxin, ethyl alcohol, or mannitol Long-term IV use with Mg replacement
Assessment findings	Coma Lethargy Decreased respiratory rate Bradycardia, which can progress to cardiac arrest Muscle weakness Ascending flaccid paralysis Hypotension ECG changes	Muscle weakness Tremors Laryngeal stridor Muscle spasms Generalized tetany and seizures in severe deficit Confusion to coma Positive Chvostek's and Trousseau's signs

Continued

Comparing Fluid and Electrolyte Disorders—*Continued*

	Hypermagnesemia	*Hypomagnesemia*
	■ Tall, peaked T waves ■ Widening of the QRS complex	Dizziness Anorexia and nausea ECG changes ■ Flat or inverted T wave ■ Possible ST segment depression ■ Prolonged QT interval ■ Prominent U waves ■ Dysrhythmias
Laboratory test findings	Serum magnesium >2.5 mEq/L	Serum magnesium <1.5 mEq/L
Treatment	Hemodialysis or peritoneal dialysis if renal failure is present Calcium gluconate Observe for respiratory distress Monitor continuous ECG, and serum magnesium	Emergency treatment Magnesium sulfate 1–2 g 10–20% solution IV not to exceed 1.5 mL/min Observe patient for signs of magnesium toxicity such as skin flushing, hypotension, weakness, diminished-to-absent deep tendon reflexes, drowsiness, and lethargy

Maintenance magnesium dosage of 10 mEq/24 h

Institute seizure precautions

Monitor ECG since hypomagnesemia will enhance digitalis effect predisposing to digitalis toxicity

	Hyperphosphatemia	**Hypophosphatemia**
Definition	Excessive serum phosphate	Decreased serum phosphate
Cause	Acute and chronic renal failure	Shift of phosphate into cells caused by administration of glucose, insulin, or antacids
	Hyperthyroidism	Refeeding those with protein-carbohydrate malnutrition
	Diphosphonate therapy	Respiratory alkalosis in the presence of the following:
	Phosphate-containing laxatives	■ Gram-negative bacteria
	Overdose of intravenous phosphate	■ Alcohol withdrawal
	Large intake of milk for peptic ulcer management	■ Primary hyperventilation
	Blood transfusions with phosphate leaking from stored blood cells	■ Salicylate overdose
	Necrosis of muscle due to trauma, virus, or heat stroke	■ Heat stroke
	Decreased parathyroid activity with decreased calcium	■ Thyrotoxicosis

Continued

	Hyperphosphatemia	**Hypophosphatemia**
	Hyperthyroidism	Phosphorus wasting in the gastrointestinal or genitourinary tracts
Assessment findings	Symptoms are nonspecific Tingling in the fingertips and around the mouth Numbness Muscle spasms Soft tissue calcification	Lethargy Altered mental status or confusion Muscle weakness, pain, numbness or tingling of fingers Dilated cardiomyopathy Seizures
Laboratory test findings	Total serum phosphorous >4.5 mg/dL; 5–8 mg/dL indicates mild-moderate elevation; and >10 mg/dL, severe elevation Elevated serum potassium and urate, with depressed serum sodium and calcium indicates cell lysis	Serum phosphate <2.5 mg/dL Increased urine calcium, magnesium, bicarbonate and glucose Urine phosphate may be elevated with renal insufficiency; decreased urine phosphate indicates an external etiology
Treatment	Treat underlying cause	Treat underlying cause

	Administer enteric PO_4 binding agents such as aluminum hydroxide calcium, and magnesium Administer volume expanders or carbonic anhydrase inhibitors to increase urine output, if renal function adequate If kidney function compromised, institute dialysis	
Definition	*Respiratory Acidemia* Excessive acidity of body fluids secondary to pulmonary insufficiency and retention of carbon dioxide	*Respiratory Alkalemia* Excessive alkalinity of body fluids resulting from elimination of carbon dioxide more rapidly than the body can produce at the cellular level secondary to alveolar hyperventilation
Cause	Alveolar hypoventilation Drug overdose Respiratory depressants Guillain-Barré syndrome Myasthenia gravis	Alveolar hyperventilation Central nervous system dysfunction of respiratory centers in pons and medulla Pneumonia

Continued

	Respiratory Acidemia	**Respiratory Alkalemia**
	Kyphoscoliosis	Pulmonary embolism
	Massive obesity	Congestive heart failure
	Chronic obstructive pulmonary disease	Interstitial lung disease
	Asthma	Mechanical ventilation
	Adult respiratory distress syndrome	Hypoxia
	Bilateral pneumonia	Gram-negative septicemia
	Congestive heart failure with pulmonary edema	
Assessment findings	Restlessness	Coma
	Irritability	Lightheadedness
	Headache	Giddiness
	Drowsiness	Paresthesias
	Confusion	Weakness
	Coma	Muscle cramps
	Weakness	Seizures
	Tremors	Tetany
	Tachypnea	Hyperactive deep tendon reflexes
	Tachycardia	Seizures
	Hypotension	Deep, rapid breathing

Laboratory test findings	pH <7.35 PaCO₂ >45 mg Hg HCO₃ >26 mEg/L	Tachycardia pH >7.45 PaCO₂ <35 mg Hg HCO₃ <22 mEg/L
Treatment	Vigorous pulmonary toilet and/or mechanical ventilation Supplemental oxygenation as indicated by PaO₂, assessment findings Closely monitor cardiopulmonary and neurologic function and fluid and electrolyte status	Treat underlying disorder Supplemental oxygenation as indicated Patients on mechanical ventilation who manifest neuromuscular irritability may benefit from decreasing the minute ventilation and increasing dead space ventilation
Definition	*Hypercalcemia* Excessive serum calcium	*Hypocalcemia* Decreased serum calcium concentration
Cause	Primary hyperparathyroidism associated with benign adenoma Malignancy (metastatic carcinoma) Prolonged immobilization Alkalemia Excessive administration of vitamin D Hypophosphatemia Hyperthyroid crisis	Idiopathic or iatrogenic (removal of, or damage to, parathyroid glands during neck surgery) hypoparathyroidism Malignancy Alkalemia Alkalosis due to vomiting Alkali ingestion

Continued

Comparing Fluid and Electrolyte Disorders — Continued

	Hypercalcemia	**Hypocalcemia**
	Longstanding thiazide use	Hyperventilation
	Renal tubular acidosis	Chronic renal failure
	Use of sex hormone therapy	Chronic malabsorption
	Aggressive correction of acidemia	Hypomagnesemia or
	Side-effect of many drugs	hyperphosphatemia
		Acute pancreatitis
		Massive transfusions of citrated blood
Assessment findings	Hypertension	Acute episode
	Polydipsia, polyuria, and nocturia	■ Irritability
	Flank and thigh pain	■ Restlessness
	Anorexia, weight loss, nausea	■ Muscle twitching
	Constipation	■ Bronchospasms
	Band keratopathy (i.e., linear deposits	■ Neuromuscular irritability
	of calcium in the cornea)	■ Paresthesia
	Pathological fractures	■ Carpopedal spasms
	ECG changes	■ Seizures
	■ Shortening of the ST segment	■ Tetany, muscle cramps
	■ Shortening of the QT interval	

	■ End of QRS indistinguishable from beginning of the T wave ■ J wave ■ Atrial and ventricular arrhythmias	Chronic ■ Dry, scaly skin ■ Alopecia ■ Mild depression to psychosis ■ Osteoporosis ■ Diarrhea ECG changes ■ Lenghtening of the ST segment ■ Lengthening of the QT interval ■ Atrial and ventricular arrhythmias ■ Cardiac arrest
Laboratory test findings	Serum calcium >10.5 mg/dL Symptoms occur with levels >11–12 mg/24 h per liter	Serum calcium <8.5 mg/100 mL Symptoms occur with levels <7 mg/dL
Treatment	Hydrate with 0.9% sodium chloride solution Administer loop diuretics to promote excretion Administer ordered mithramycin, calcitonin, and steroids Administer ordered IV phosphates with caution	Treat underlying cause Administer IV calcium gluconate for acute hypocalcemia As needed, administer magnesium sulfate Monitor for hypomagnesemia and treat

Continued

Comparing Fluid and Electrolyte Disorders — *Continued*

	Hypercalcemia	*Hypocalcemia*
	Peritoneal dialysis and hemodialysis efficiency Monitor digitalis level for toxicity	
Definition	*Metabolic Acidemia* Excessive acidity of body fluids secondary to an increase in acids other than carbonic acid	*Metabolic Alkalemia* Excessive alkalinity of body fluids resulting from increased loss of acids or increased amounts of bicarbonate
Cause	Increase in unmeasured anions (anions gap greater than 15 mmol/L) such as in: ■ Diabetic ketoacidosis ■ Starvation ketoacidosis ■ Salicylate, ethylene glycol, and methyl alcohol poisoning ■ Lactic acidosis ■ Shock ■ Cardiac arrest ■ Renal failure	Fluid loss from upper gastrointestinal tract such as with vomiting and continuous nasogastric suctioning Rapid correction of chronic hypercapnia Diuretic therapy Corticosteroid therapy Severe hypocalcemia Alkali administration

Without increase in anion gap:

- Diarrhea
- Drainage of pancreatic juice
- Ureterosigmoidostomy
- Obstructed ileal loop
- Ammonium chloride therapy
- Renal tubular acidosis
- Dilutional acidosis
- Hyperalimentation
- Acetazolamide therapy

Assessment findings

Headache
Change in level of consciousness
Drowsiness
Confusion
Coma
Depressed cardiac function
Cardiac dysrhythmias
Decreased peripheral vascular resistance, with hypertension, shock, and tissue hypoxia
Dyspnea
Tachypnea

History of vomiting, diuretic usage, and complaints of weakness may provide clues
Neuromuscular irritability
Muscle cramps
Hyperactive deep tendon reflexes
Tetany
Muscle weakness
Cardiac dysrhythmias

Continued

Comparing Fluid and Electrolyte Disorders—*Continued*

	Metabolic Acidemia	*Metabolic Alkalemia*
Laboratory test findings	Crackles Nausea, vomiting, anorexia pH <7.35; if severe <7.20 PacO$_2$ normal; or decreased with compensation HCO$_3$ <20 mEq/L; if severe <15 mEq/L Anion gap: normal or increased, depending on the underlying cause Normal-to-increased serum potassium	pH <7.45 PacO$_2$ normal or decreased with compensation HCO$_3$ >26–30 mEq/L Decreased serum potassium and chloride
Treatment	Treat underlying disease process For severe metabolic acidemia	Treat underlying disease process Correct volume depletion

administer intravenous sodium bicarbonate to raise pH to >7.20 and bicarbonate levels to >15 mmol/L
Avoid very rapid correction of acidemia
Closely monitor cardiopulmonary status, fluid and electrolyte balance, and neurologic and neuromuscular status

Replace chloride, sodium and potassium
Administer ammonium chloride for compromised cardiac and/or renal function
Administer intravenous acetazolamide to increase renal excretion of bicarbonate
Closely monitor fluid and electrolyte balance

Renal Trauma

Renal trauma includes blunt or nonpenetrating injury (accounts for 70–80% of all renal trauma) or penetrating injury (accounts for 20–30% of all renal trauma). There are five types: renal contusion with or without hematoma, renal cortical lacerations, renal fracture, renal pedicle trauma, and ureteral disruption. Renal trauma commonly occurs with trauma to other organ systems. Of all abdominal trauma, 10–15% has associated renal trauma. It can be associated with injuries to the urinary collecting system (ureters, urinary bladder, and urethra) or the reproductive system. The mortality rate from renal trauma ranges from 6–12%.

Etiology/Pathophysiology

1. Blunt force, caused by rapid deceleration or a direct blow to the flank, sets the kidneys in motion, possibly causing dissection of the pedicles.
2. Motor vehicle accidents account for the majority of renal trauma cases, followed by gunshots, stab wounds, falls, and sports injuries. Seat belts and air bags help to prevent injury.
3. There is a higher incidence of injury in patients with congenital abnormalities or previous renal disorders.
4. Renal contusion with or without hematoma accounts for greater than 90% of all nonpenetrating renal trauma. Bruising to the renal tissue occurs and hematuria is almost always present.
5. Renal cortical lacerations and renal fractures (disruptions in the tissue of the kidney) can produce massive bleeding and extravasation of urine.
6. Renal pedicle trauma, the most life-threatening injury, results in renal vessel injury. Hematuria is most likely to be absent. Hemodynamic instability and other serious injuries are commonly seen. Nephrectomy is frequently required.
7. Ureteral disruption results in extravasation of urine into the retroperitoneal space or abdomen. It is extremely uncommon in nonpenetrating trauma.

Assessment/Analysis

ASSESSMENT FINDINGS

Subjective

1. History of a causative event
   a. Congenital abnormality of the kidneys
   b. History of previous renal disorders
   c. Mechanism of injury consistent with renal injury
2. Complaints of flank, upper abdominal, or back pain that may radiate to the groin or shoulder and may be accompanied by nausea

Objective

1. Presence of major abdominal trauma
2. Changes in the level of consciousness
3. Anxiety, restlessness, or fear
4. Bruising of the thorax and/or abdomen
5. Blood at the urinary meatus (associated with accompanying urethral injury)
6. Turner's sign — bruising over the flank and lower back in the presence of retroperitoneal hematoma
7. Decreasing urine output
8. Hematuria
9. Diaphoresis
10. Tachycardia
11. Kussmaul's respiration
12. Enlarged mass surrounding the kidney
13. Costovertebral-angle pain upon palpation
14. Hypotension or a drop in mean arterial pressure (MAP)

SUPPORTING TEST FINDINGS

Laboratory Tests

1. Urinalysis
   Abnormality: Gross or microscopic hematuria (may not be present in up to 20% of patients)
2. White blood cells (WBCs)
   Abnormality: Increased with infection
3. Hematocrit and hemoglobin
   Abnormality: Decreased with hemorrhage
4. Blood urea nitrogen (BUN)
   Abnormality: Increased with renal trauma or renal failure
5. Serum creatinine
   Abnormality: Increased with renal trauma or renal failure

Diagnostic Tests

1. Intravenous (IV) pyelogram
   Abnormality: Injury evidenced by extravasation of dye from the kidneys or the urinary collecting system
2. Cystogram/urethrogram
   Abnormality: Injury to the urethra or bladder evidenced by extravasation of dye
3. Renal ultrasound

Abnormality: Renal contusion, fracture, laceration, or pedicle trauma to either kidney

4. Flat plate X-ray of the abdomen (kidneys-ureters-bladder [KUB] X-ray)

   Abnormality: Fracture to the overlying bony structures may indicate trauma to the kidneys, ureter, or bladder.

5. Computed tomography scan of the kidney

   Abnormality: Renal contusion, fracture, laceration, or pedicle trauma to either kidney

6. Renal angiography

   Abnormality: Renal contusion, fracture, laceration, or pedicle trauma to either kidney

   Done when other tests are inconclusive

Planning/Intervention

COLLABORATIVE MANAGEMENT

Procedures

1. Treatment depends on degree of injury and ranges from rest and self-repair to heminephrectomy to nephrectomy.

2. Prevent or treat infection.

   a. Monitor temperature every 4 hours.

   b. Observe wounds for purulent drainage. Obtain a specimen of any suspicious drainage for culture and sensitivity testing.

   c. Monitor serial WBCs for increases.

   d. Administer ordered antibiotics.

   e. Cleanse the insertion site of the indwelling urinary catheter every 8 hours; note and report discharge.

   f. Keep the urinary drainage system intact and prevent backflow of urine into the bladder with patient movement.

3. Alleviate pain.

   a. Monitor pain level in the patient by using a 1–10 scale with 10 being the most severe pain.

   b. Administer ordered analgesics, as indicated, for pain.

   c. Assess response to pain medication and report failure to control pain.

4. Maintain hemodynamic stability.

    a. Assist with insertion of hemodynamic monitoring catheters.

    b. Monitor hemodynamic parameters every 4 hours, or as needed, to assess stability.

    c. Administer medications and IV fluid to correct hemodynamic instability.

5. Prevent or treat complications.

    a. Monitor BUN and serum creatinine for increases and report significant changes.

    b. Monitor for hemorrhage and prepare the patient for surgery, as needed.

Drug Therapy

1. Volume expanders—controversy exists regarding fluid replacement. Generally, if blood loss is the cause of hypovolemia, blood should be replaced.

    Examples: Crystalloids—Ringer's, Ringer's lactate (plain Ringer's is used if the patient has a chance of returning to aerobic metabolism) and normal saline solution are commonly used

        Blood or blood products—packed red blood cells (RBCs), whole blood, autotransfusion, and synthetic blood products

    Action: Replace lost intravascular volume with caution exercised to prevent fluid overload

    Cautions: Can cause hypervolemia and pulmonary edema

        Should be used judiciously in the presence of major lung injury

2. Antibiotics

    Examples: cephalosporins

        ticarcillin (Timentin)

        ceftazidime (Fortaz)

            aminoglycosides

        gentamycin (Garamycin)

        tobramycin (Nebcin)

    Action: Bacteriocidal

        Broad-spectrum drugs that kill aerobic and anaerobic gram-negative and gram-positive bacteria

        Before the source is identified, at least a two-drug combination should be given

        When the source is identified, therapy may be tailored to the cause

Cautions: Can cause nephrotoxicity, allergic reaction, and ototoxicity

3. Opioid analgesics

Examples: morphine (Duramorph)
meperidine (Demerol)
hydromorphone (Dilaudid)

Action: Alters the perception of and response to painful stimuli by depressing the central nervous system (CNS)

Used to relieve the pain associated with renal trauma

Caution: Can cause sedation, respiratory depression, and drug dependency

4. Sedatives

Examples: lorazepam (Ativan)
diazepam (Valium)
midazolam (Versed)

Action: Depresses the CNS producing sedation and relief of anxiety

Caution: Can cause psychological dependence, tolerance, and respiratory depression

NURSING MANAGEMENT

Monitoring and Managing Clinical Problems

1. Pain
   a. Administer ordered analgesics, as indicated.
   b. Remember that opioids may cause urinary retention, so monitor for this if there is no urinary catheter.
   c. Report inability to control pain.
2. Tissue Perfusion, altered
   a. Maintain an adequate circulating volume with IV fluids.
   b. Measure hourly intake and output, and report discrepancies.
   c. Insert an arterial line or external blood pressure monitoring device, and monitor blood pressure and pulse hourly and as indicated.
   d. Check skin turgor every 4 hours and as indicated.
   e. Observe for signs and symptoms of shock, such as change in the level of consciousness, anxiety and restlessness, tachycardia, tachypnea, decreasing MAP, decreasing blood pressure, or decreasing urine output.

    f. If a flank mass is present, measure abdominal girth frequently. Do not palpate, as this may dislodge a clot and cause further bleeding.

3. Urinary Elimination: altered
    a. Measure intake and output hourly.
    b. Monitor serial BUN and serum creatinine for evidence of decreasing renal function.
    c. Observe urine color and test for the presence of blood each shift.

4. Infection: high risk for
    a. Monitor serial WBCs for increases.
    b. Record temperature every 4 hours.
    c. Inspect drainage from wounds and tubes for signs of infection.
    d. Inspect wound sites daily for redness, swelling, pain, or purulent drainage.
    e. Use aseptic technique when performing procedures.
    f. Administer ordered prophylactic antibiotics.

5. Tissue Perfusion, altered: renal
    a. Monitor intake and output hourly.
    b. Observe wound sites for fistula formation.
    c. Monitor serial WBCs, BUN, and serum creatinine for evidence of chronic pyelonephritis or renal failure.

6. Injury: high risk for
    a. Insert an arterial line or apply an external blood pressure monitoring device and monitor blood pressure for hypertension.
    b. Monitor intake and output hourly to identify fluid overload.
    c. Provide pain relief to decrease blood pressure elevation from pain.
    d. Report consistently high blood pressure readings without identifiable cause.
    e. Begin antihypertensive medication if necessary.

Monitoring, Managing, and Preventing Life-Threatening Emergencies

1. Acute tubular necrosis
    a. Prevent complications related to continued hypotension, infection, and use of nephrotoxic agents.
      1) Administer order IV fluids and medications.

2) Regulate fluid intake to achieve fluid and electrolyte balance.
3) Administer ordered buffering agents to achieve acid-base balance.
4) Closely monitor for decreasing level of consciousness and intervene quickly to preserve neurologic function.
b. Manage nutrition.
1) Restrict protein intake to maintain anabolism while limiting load on kidneys; amount varies depending on patient's weight and activity level and whether or not patient is on dialysis; protein needs to be of high biologic value.
2) Restrict dietary potassium.
3) Restrict fluids.
4) Provide adequate calories to prevent catabolism.
5) Administer ordered supplemental vitamins.
c. Administer blood transfusions to maintain adequate level of RBCs for optimum tissue oxygenation.
d. Prepare to initiate renal replacement therapy (RRT) for any of the following:
1) BUN >100 mg/dL
2) Serum creatinine >5–9 mg/dL or at lower serum creatinine levels for patients with reduced muscle mass, such as the elderly
3) Volume overload and signs of pulmonary edema
4) Pericarditis
5) Hyperkalemia that has not responded adequately to other treatment modalities
6) Uncontrollable acidosis
7) CNS dysfunction related to uremia
e. Institute RRT as ordered.
1) Hemodialysis
2) Continuous ultrafiltration or continuous RRT
3) Peritoneal dialysis
2. Hemorrhage
a. Monitor for physical findings of blood loss.
1) Tachycardia with a faint, thready pulse
2) Tachypnea
3) Hypotension in recumbent position or postural hypotension
4) Cool, pale, or cyanotic clammy skin

5) Capillary refill >3 seconds
6) Poor skin turgor with dry mucous membranes
7) Lethargy, confusion, or obtundation
8) Decreased urine output
9) Flank swelling with or without bruising

b. Monitor serial hemoglobin and hematocrit for decreasing values.

c. Monitor hemodynamic parameters for decreased central venous pressure, pulmonary artery pressure, pulmonary capillary wedge pressure, and cardiac output; report significant findings.

d. Prevent hemorrhage.
   1) Apply direct pressure over bleeding sites.
   2) Prepare patient for selective angiography with embolization or laparotomy.
   3) Leave any impaled objects in place before surgery.
   4) Apply medical antishock trousers for pelvic fracture.
   5) Administer fresh frozen plasma.

5 ENDOCRINE DISORDERS

Diabetes Insipidus

Diabetes insipidus is excessive urine excretion and thirst caused by antidiuretic hormone ([ADH], vasopressin) deficiency, the osmoreceptor function, or the kidneys' response to ADH. It frequently starts in childhood or early adulthood and is more common in male patients. The three forms are neurogenic or central, nephrogenic, and psychogenic.

Etiology/Pathophysiology

1. Neurogenic
   a. Decreased levels of ADH can be secreted by the posterior pituitary (neurohypophysis) in response to incorrect messages from osmoreceptors in the hypothalamus.
   b. Transient decreases in ADH synthesis or secretion may occur with the following:
      1) Head trauma
      2) Neurosurgery causing swelling in the area of the pituitary or the hypothalamus
      3) Central nervous system infection, such as meningitis or encephalitis
      4) Any other neuropathology that increases pressures in the area of the pituitary or hypothalamus, for example, cerebral aneurysms or cerebrovascular accidents
      5) Drugs such as alcohol, phenytoin, atropine, and clonidine
   c. Chronic decreases in ADH synthesis or secretion may occur with pituitary tumor.
2. Nephrogenic
   a. Cells of the kidney's tubules and collecting ducts do not respond to ADH's actions.
   b. Usually does not involve the massive polyuria seen with neurogenic form
   c. Two forms: familial and acquired
      1) Acquired form
         a) Metabolic disturbance such as hypokalemia or hypercalcemia
         b) Adverse response to certain drugs such as lithium, amphotericin B, methoxyflurane
         c) Diseases that may alter the kidney's ability to concentrate urine, such as obstructive nephropathy, pyelonephritis, sickle cell disease, amyloidosis, granulomatous disease, and multiple myeloma
3. Psychogenic
   a. Psychopathology leads the patient to drink excessive amounts of fluids.

b. The release of ADH is suppressed as a result of the excess quantity of fluid intake.

Assessment/Analysis

ASSESSMENT FINDINGS

Subjective

1. Excessive thirst, sometimes described as unquenchable; may include a preference for cold or iced water
2. Urinary frequency
3. Increased volume of urine
4. Nocturia
5. Fatigue
6. Weight loss and constipation if unable to drink larger quantities of fluids

Objective

1. Massive increases in volume of urine (as much as 5–10 L/d); frequency of urination
2. Dry mucous membranes; dry skin and poor skin turgor
3. Weight loss
4. Weakness and listlessness
5. Tachycardia
6. Rapid, shallow respirations
7. Hypotension

SUPPORTING TEST FINDINGS

Laboratory Tests

1. Urine electrolytes
   Abnormality: Decreased urine sodium (<20 mEq/L)
2. Urine specific gravity
   Abnormality: Very decreased (1.001–1.005)
3. Urine osmolality
   Abnormality: Decreased (50–100 mOsm/kg)
4. Serum osmolality
   Abnormality: Increased (>295 mOsm/kg)
5. Serum sodium
   Abnormality: Increased (>148 mEq/L)

Diagnostic Tests

1. Water deprivation test
   Abnormality: If neurogenic in origin, little change in urine
   concentration occurs and body weight decreases when
   water is withheld; when vasopressin (ADH) is given,
   urine osmolality increases by 50% or more
       If nephrogenic in origin, little change in urine con-
   centration occurs while water is withheld and vasopressin does not increase the urine osmolality to normal levels
2. Computed tomography scan
   Abnormality: Pituitary tumor or lesion in the area of the
   hypothalamus

Planning/Intervention

COLLABORATIVE MANAGEMENT

Procedures

1. Assist with identification of the etiology. If nephrogenic,
   identify potential drug etiology.
2. Monitor the degree of fluid and electrolyte imbalance and
   initiate a plan to correct it, if ordered.
   a. If serum sodium is initially > 160 mEq/L, initiate ther-
      apy to reach normal levels in 36–72 hours.
   b. Implement treatment to decrease plasma osmolality
      at the rate of 1 mOsm/kg per hour.
3. Monitor the patient's response to treatment by assessing
   urine volume, urine osmolality, plasma osmolality, and
   serum sodium levels routinely.

Drug Therapy

1. Hormone replacement
   Example: aqueous vasopressin injection (Pitressin)
   Action: Similar to that of the natural hormone; causes kidneys to increase water reabsorption
       Has a short duration of action and is preferred for
   management of transient or potentially transient diabetes insipidus

Caution: Cannot be given by mouth because it is destroyed by gastric acid

Excess activity of the drug can cause water intoxication; monitor for signs and symptoms of water intoxication (confusion, drowsiness, headache, weight gain)

Monitor urine volume and urine osmolality

Can increase the risk of thromboembolic disease

Causes vasoconstriction, which can increase risk for hypertension, myocardial ischemia, and related cardiac dysfunction.

Example: desmopressin (DDAVP)

Action: Causes kidneys to increase water reabsorption

Preferred for long-term management

Caution: Cannot be given by mouth because it is destroyed by gastric acid

Excess activity of the drug can cause water intoxication; monitor for signs or symptoms of water intoxication

Monitor urine volume and urine osmolality

Can increase the risk of thromboembolic disease

Causes vasoconstriction, which can increase risk for hypertension, myocardial ischemia, and related cardiac dysfunction

Teach patient on home therapy to titrate dose based on urinary frequency and output

2. Intravenous (IV) fluids

Example: hypotonic solutions (0.45% sodium chloride solution)

Action: Replaces fluids lost from the kidney's inability to reabsorb water

Hypotonic fluids are more similar to the fluid that has been lost

Caution: The volume of fluids required will change once vasopressin therapy has begun

The volume given may be approximately 1 mL of IV fluid per mL of urine output

3. Thiazide diuretics

Example: hydrochlorothiazide (HydroDIURIL)

Action: Thought to enhance kidney's responsiveness to ADH allowing greater water reabsorption

Caution: Requires sodium restriction to increase water reabsorption

NURSING MANAGEMENT

Monitoring and Managing Clinical Problems

1. Fluid Volume Excess or Deficit: high risk for
   a. Monitor for symptoms that may signal dehydration, including:
      1) Increased hourly urine output
      2) Dry mucous membranes
      3) Poor skin turgor
      4) Soft eyes
      5) Decreased central venous pressure (CVP) or pulmonary capillary wedge pressure (PCWP)
      6) Tachypnea
   b. Monitor for confusion, drowsiness, headache, and weight gain possibly indicating water intoxication.
   c. Monitor for increasing blood pressure, neck vein distention, onset or increase in peripheral edema, increased CVP or PCWP or shortness of breath possibly indicating fluid overload.
   d. Measure accurate intake and output hourly.
   e. Weigh patient daily at the same time and with the same scale.
   f. Record hourly blood pressure and heart rate; report significant findings.
   g. Assist with insertion of hemodynamic monitoring catheter and monitor readings every 2–4 hours.
   h. Promote fluid balance.
      1) Administer IV fluid replacement to balance current losses.
      2) Administer replacement hormone and monitor patient response to treatment.
      3) If the etiology is psychogenic, assist the patient to adhere to fluid intake limits.
   i. Prevent fluid imbalances.
      1) Identify patients at risk.
      2) Monitor urine output and laboratory values for early recognition of trends and changes.
2. Tissue Perfusion, altered: renal, high risk for
   a. Obtain blood specimens and monitor serum sodium levels for hyponatremia.
   b. Promote normal electrolyte balance through adequate

fluid intake and hormone replacement therapy; recognize risks and correct them.

Monitoring, Managing, and Preventing Life-Threatening Emergencies

1. Seizures
   a. Can occur if fluid and electrolyte imbalances become severe.
   b. Institute seizure precautions to protect the patient from possible injury.
      1) Pad siderails and keep them raised.
      2) Keep bed in low position.
      3) Keep equipment for airway management close by, but inconspicuous.
      4) Have supplemental oxygen available.
      5) Remove all potentially harmful objects from the patient's area.
      6) Restrict smoking.
   c. If seizure occurs:
      1) Protect the airway.
      2) Do not insert anything into the patient's mouth.
      3) Loosen restrictive clothing.
      4) Protect the patient from self-injury during the seizure.
      5) Administer ordered medications.
2. Encephalopathy
   a. Monitor level of consciousness for any sign of decrease.
   b. Obtain blood specimens and monitor for hyponatremia.
   c. Institute ordered treatment, if indicated.
   d. Prevent encephalopathy by early recognition and intervention.
3. Hypovolemic shock
   a. Monitor for and correct hemodynamic instability.
      1) Provide continuous hemodynamic monitoring.
      2) Titrate fluids and inotropic agents to maintain a systolic blood pressure of at least 80 mm Hg.
      3) Position the patient in modified Trendelenburg position (elevation of the legs at 45 degrees).
   b. Promote adequate oxygenation.
      1) Administer ordered supplemental oxygen.

2) Obtain specimens and monitor arterial blood gases and hemoglobin, and report significant changes.

3) Monitor capillary refill and skin color to assess peripheral perfusion.

c. Monitor for altered organ and tissue perfusion by doing the following:

1) Monitor for decreased urine output and elevated renal function tests, possibly indicating acute renal failure.

2) Monitor for a falling arterial oxygen concentration, suggesting adult respiratory distress syndrome.

3) Monitor for decreased or absent bowel sounds, suggesting gastroparesis, and bright-red or coffee-ground drainage from the nasogastric tube, suggesting stress ulceration.

4) Check temperature every 4 hours to monitor for hypothermia or hyperthermia.

5) Monitor for decreased alertness and attention span, drowsiness, or excessive sleeping, indicating a downward change in the level of consciousness.

d. Monitor for and correct loss of fluid volume from the vasculature.

1) Provide ordered fluid replacement.

2) Maintain accurate intake and output measurements hourly.

3) Continuously monitor blood pressure.

4) Monitor skin turgor for signs of dehydration.

5) Observe for a new onset of an S_3 heart sound, peripheral edema, and moist crackles in the lungs, indicating fluid volume overload.

6) Closely monitor serum electrolytes and osmolality, and urine studies to assess hydration status.

Syndrome of Inappropriate Secretion of Antidiuretic Hormone

The syndrome of inappropriate secretion of antidiuretic hormone (SIADH) is characterized by increased or continued release of the antidiuretic hormone (ADH). Normally, ADH is released in response to hypoxia, reduced blood pressure sensed by baroreceptors, or reduced blood volume sensed by pressure receptors in the atria and in the pulmonary artery. In SIADH, the negative feedback system that normally controls the release of ADH fails. It is one of the most common causes of hyponatremia.

Etiology/Pathophysiology

1. Etiology
   a. Although any cancer can cause SIADH, the most common cause is malignant bronchogenic oat cell carcinoma because this tumor causes ectopic production of ADH.
   b. Other causes or risks
      1) Hypoxia or other events that decrease left atrial filling pressures
         a) Positive pressure breathing with mechanical ventilation
         b) Pulmonary diseases that result in hypoxia such as pneumonia, tuberculosis, and chronic pulmonary disease
         c) Cardiac failure
      2) Central nervous system disease or injury that interferes with the negative feedback system or increases production and release of ADH
         a) Guillain-Barré syndrome
         b) Cerebrovascular disruption
         c) Head trauma
         d) Infection such as meningitis
         e) Tumors or metastatic lesions
      3) Various drugs
         a) Those that potentiate the action of ADH, such as chlorpropamide and other hypoglycemics, carbamazepine, thiazide diuretics, and some phenothiazines
         b) Those that increase tubular reabsorption of water, such as vasopressin and oxytocin
         c) Those that cause increased release of ADH, such as vincristine, cyclophosphamide, nicotine, morphine, and barbiturates
         d) Anesthetic agents
      4) Endocrine disorders that influence ADH secretion through hormonal effects, such as hypopituitarism and ectopic ADH tumors
      5) Postoperative experiences, such as stress, nausea, and hypoxia

      6) Administration of excess amounts of hypotonic fluids

2. Pathophysiology
  a. The abnormally increased or continuous secretion of ADH
     1) Increases renal tubule permeability to water allowing increased reabsorption of water without accompanying reabsorption of solutes
     2) Urine production (and output) decreases
     3) Serum osmolality decreases
     4) Blood volume increases slightly
     5) The slight increase in blood volume causes an increase in the glomerular filtration rate and an increase in urine filtrate production. However, because of the presence of ADH, the final urine product is concentrated, less in volume, and higher in sodium and other ions.
     6) Water is retained in the extracellular fluid compartment, and sodium is lost in larger-than-normal quantities because suppression of aldosterone release occurs with this process; aldosterone normally acts on kidney tubules to cause Na^+ reabsorption
  b. Onset is gradual. Symptoms are related to the water intoxication and hyponatremia. Because free water, not salt, is retained, edema is not seen.

Assessment/Analysis

ASSESSMENT FINDINGS

Subjective

1. History of use of medications that are known to be associated with development of SIADH, or a disease associated with its onset
2. Headache
3. Personality changes
4. Confusion, disorientation
5. Impaired memory
6. Irritability

7. Lethargy
8. Muscle cramps
9. Anorexia, nausea, vomiting, and diarrhea
10. Weakness, fatigue
11. Restlessness
12. Gait disturbances

Objective

1. Confusion, disorientation, decreasing level of consciousness
2. Hostility
3. Apprehension
4. Small weight gain with no edema
5. Weakness, muscle twitching
6. Diminished deep tendon reflexes
7. If severe imbalance (water load), seizures or coma could occur.

SUPPORTING TEST FINDINGS

Laboratory Tests

1. Serum sodium
   Abnormality: Decreased; <130 mEq/l
2. Serum osmolality
   Abnormality: Decreased; <280 mOsm/kg
3. Urine osmolality
   Abnormality: Abnormally increased when serum osmolality is decreased; equal to or greater than serum osmolality
4. Urine sodium
   Abnormality: Increased; >180 mEq/L
5. Urine specific gravity
   Abnormality: Increased; >1.030

Diagnostic Tests

1. Water loading test
   Abnormality: When a large volume of fluids is given, urine output is less than half of administered volume and the urinary sodium is abnormally increased

Planning/Intervention

COLLABORATIVE MANAGEMENT

Procedures

1. Assist with identifying cause and instituting ordered treatments.
2. Restore fluid balance.
   a. Restrict fluids to 300–1000 mL/d.
   b. May be only treatment if SIADH is mild.
3. Restore electrolyte balance; often this may occur without specific electrolyte therapy.

Drug Therapy

1. Diuretics
   Example: furosemide (Lasix)
   Action: Inhibits sodium and chloride reabsorption at the level of the ascending limb of the loop of Henle and thus causes a significant increase in the volume of urine
   Caution: May require potassium replacement; if given intravenously (IV), reduce risk of ototoxicity by giving slowly (no more than 4 mg/min if given in a small volume as an IV piggyback or over 1–2 minutes if given IV bolus)
2. Hypertonic sodium chloride (NaCl) solution
   Example: 3% NaCl solution IV
   Action: Replaces sodium content without adding a larger volume of water
   Caution: May precipitate fluid overload in patients with pre-existing cardiac or kidney disease
3. Osmotic diuretic
   Example: urea
   Action: Osmotic diuresis that causes free-water excretion
   Caution: Reserved for more serious imbalances (serum sodium of <125 mEq/l)
4. Drugs that decrease effectiveness of ADH at the level of the kidney tubules
   Example: demeclocycline (Declomycin)
   Action: Inhibits the action of ADH within the kidney tubules

Caution: If used by an outpatient, teach patient that drug has potential for a severe phototoxic reaction for which sunscreens are not sufficient protection

NURSING MANAGEMENT

Monitoring and Managing Clinical Problems

1. Fluid Volume Excess
   a. Monitor for trends that indicate appropriately decreasing fluid load such as:
      1) Increased urine output
      2) Accurate intake and output reflecting greater output than intake
      3) Decreasing daily weights
      4) Increasing serum osmolality levels
      5) Improvement in level of consciousness
   b. Promote decrease to a normal fluid volume.
      1) Restrict fluid intake.
      2) Teach patient and family about important fluid restriction.
2. Tissue Perfusion, altered: renal, high risk for
   a. Monitor serum sodium levels for hyponatremia.
   b. Monitor for changes in level of consciousness. Report significant changes.
   c. Promote increase to normal serum sodium levels.
      1) Restrict fluids as indicated.
      2) Administer hypertonic NaCl if patient's symptoms are severe or if having seizure activity.

Monitoring, Managing, and Preventing Life-Threatening Emergencies

1. Seizures
   a. Monitor level of consciousness.
   b. Monitor serum sodium.
   c. Restrict fluids to prevent decrease in serum sodium or increase in excessive water reabsorption.
   d. Institute seizure precautions to protect the patient from possible injury.
      1) Pad siderails and keep them raised.
      2) Keep bed in low position.
      3) Keep emergency resuscitation equipment for airway management available.

      4) Remove all potentially harmful objects from the patient's area.

      5) Restrict smoking.

  e. If seizure occurs:

      1) Protect the airway.

      2) Do not insert anything into the patient's mouth.

      3) Loosen restrictive clothing.

      4) Protect the patient from self-injury during the seizure.

      5) Administer ordered medications.

2. Encephalopathy

  a. Monitor level of consciousness for any sign of decrease.

  b. Monitor decreasing serum sodium level and changes in electrolyte balance.

  c. Institute ordered treatment as indicated.

  d. Prevent encephalopathy by early recognition and intervention.

Thyroid Storm/ Thyrotoxic Crisis

Thyroid storm (thyrotoxic crisis) is an acute manifestation of hyperthyroidism resulting from abnormally high levels of circulating thyroid hormones. It most commonly occurs in patients with pre-existing hyperthyroidism (thyrotoxicosis). (See Reviewing Hyperthyroidism, pp 423–425.) It is characterized by hyperthermia (unusually high fever), severe tachycardia (heart rate > 100 bpm), hypertension (systolic pressure > 140 mm Hg and diastolic pressure > 90 mm Hg), and an altered mental status.

Etiology/Pathophysiology

1. Patients at risk of developing thyroid storm are those who:
   a. Have poorly controlled thyrotoxicosis
   b. Do not comply with antithyroid regimen
   c. Receive excessive administration of exogenous thyroid hormone
2. Physiologic and psychological stressors that could trigger the onset of thyroid storm include:
   a. Surgery
   b. Infection/sepsis
   c. Severe emotional upset
   d. Diabetic ketoacidosis, hyperosmolar nonketotic coma, insulin-induced hypoglycemia
   e. Congestive heart failure (CHF)
   f. Myocardial infarction
   g. Burns
   h. Trauma
   i. Childbirth/toxemia of pregnancy
   j. Pulmonary embolus
   k. Bowel infarction
   l. Iodine-containing X-ray contrast
   m. Radioiodine therapy
   n. Vigorous manipulation of thyroid gland
3. Pathophysiologic alterations seen with high levels of thyroid hormone include:
   a. Increased metabolic rate of the body, especially stimulating the heart, skeletal muscle, liver, and lungs
   b. Increased heat production
   c. Increased carbohydrate and fat metabolism
   d. Increased heart rate, force of contraction (only in mild elevation of thyroid hormone), and cardiac output (CO)
   e. Increased rate and depth of respiration
   f. Increased or decreased appetite with increased gastrointestinal motility
   g. Hyperactive reaction of deep tendon reflexes
   h. Emotional instability and insomnia
   i. Other endocrine glands are stimulated to increase secretion of hormones; tissue needs and sensitivity for other hormones are increased.

    j. Increased libido and infertility
4. The exact physiologic mechanism(s) by which thyroid storm is precipitated is unknown.
    a. Serum thyroid hormone levels are not significantly higher than in a stable thyrotoxic state.
    b. May be related to a decrease in protein-bound thyroid hormone with an associated increase in levels of free fractions of thyroid hormones.
    c. Also may be an indirect stimulation of the sympathetic/adrenal systems.

Assessment/Analysis

ASSESSMENT FINDINGS

Subjective

1. Shortness of breath
2. Loose stools with increased frequency; frank diarrhea
3. Nausea, vomiting
4. Abdominal pain
5. Palpitations
6. Aggravation of angina

Objective

1. Dyspnea and increased work of breathing caused by respiratory muscle weakness
2. Extreme irritability progressing to delirium then coma
3. Extreme hyperpyrexia—38–41°C (100–106°F)
4. Severe tachycardia, even at rest
5. Loud heart sounds; may auscultate a murmur, an S_3, or an S_4
6. Severe hypertension with a wide pulse pressure progressing to circulatory collapse

SUPPORTING TEST FINDINGS

Laboratory Tests

1. Serum thyroxine (T_4), free thyroxine and free triiodothyronine, free thyroxine index, triiodothyronine (T_3) by radioimmune assay

Abnormality: Increased
2. Sensitive thyroid stimulating hormone (STSH)
   Abnormality: Usually decreased; may be increased if thyroid storm is caused by an excess secretion of STSH
3. Plasma cortisol
   Abnormality: Usually increased; may be normal
4. Serum electrolytes
   Abnormality: Increased serum calcium; decreased serum potassium; may see a decreased serum magnesium
5. Blood sugar
   Abnormality: Usually increased
6. Complete blood count
   Abnormality: Increased white blood cell (WBC) count with an increase in the number of stabs or bands; may see a microcytic (abnormally small red blood cell [RBC]) or macrocytic (abnormally large RBC) anemia
7. Liver function tests
   Abnormality: Usually increased

Diagnostic Tests

In thyroid storm, treatment is initiated based on physical findings, even before all laboratory tests have been reported. Other tests that may be done include:
1. Cardiac monitoring: electrocardiogram (ECG)
   Abnormality: Atrial fibrillation, paroxysmal supraventricular tachycardia, sinus bradycardia, heart blocks, conduction disturbances, and lethal ventricular arrhythmias
2. Radioiodine uptake scan
   Abnormality: Increased uptake of radioiodine

Planning/Intervention

COLLABORATIVE MANAGEMENT

Procedures

1. Reduce metabolic rate.
   a. Administer pharmacologic agents to prevent the production of thyroid hormone; prevent the release of thyroid hormone; and inhibit the peripheral conversion of T_4 to T_3, as ordered.

b. Institute measures to reduce body temperature (i.e., cooling blanket, ice packs, acetaminophen), as ordered.

c. AVOID ADMINISTRATION OF SALICYLATES, as they increase free thyroid hormone levels.

d. Administer ordered medications to reduce shivering and block beta activity.

e. Administer vitamins, especially B complex, as ordered.

f. Institute plasmapheresis (removal of all plasma and substances in the plasma), as ordered.

g. Monitor results of serial thyroid function tests to determine patient response to treatment.

2. Correct fluid and electrolyte imbalances.

a. Administer fluid and electrolyte replacements, as ordered.

b. Assist with insertion of a pulmonary artery catheter to monitor hemodynamic status.

c. Control CHF.

1) Monitor ECG and hemodynamic parameters, and treat dysrhythmias and fluid imbalance.

2) Administer diuretics and inotropic agents, as ordered.

3. Prevent complications and identify precipitating event.

a. Prevent stress ulcers by administering antiulcer medications, as ordered.

b. Prevent adrenal insufficiency by administering glucocorticoid hormones, as ordered.

c. Initiate work-up to identify precipitating event by obtaining specimens for culture and sensitivity (blood, urine, sputum, and other body fluid), as ordered.

d. Administer prophylactic antibiotics, as ordered.

e. Assist with gathering data to identify precipitating conditions.

Drug Therapy

1. Antithyroid drugs

Examples: propylthiouracil (PTU), methimazole (MMI [Tapazole]), lithium carbonate (Eskalith), perchlorate

Action: Prevents production of thyroid hormone

Caution: PTU and MMI can cause the development of

agranulocytosis (pronounced reduction of polymorphonuclear WBCs <500 granulocytes/mm^3).
Lithium can cause numerous side effects; blood levels should be monitored twice weekly initially. Perchlorate can cause aplastic anemia.

2. Iodine/Antithyroid drugs
   Examples: Lugol's iodine solution, saturated solution potassium iodine; sodium iodine
   Action: Prevents the release of thyroid hormone
   Caution: Iodine-containing medications are usually ordered in combination with an antithyroid medication; some physicians order the antithyroid medication to be given 1 hour before administration of the iodine-containing drug.

3. Contrast dye
   Examples: iopanoic acid (Telepaque), sodium ipodate (Oragrafin)
   Action: Inhibits the peripheral conversion of T_4 to T_3

4. Glucocorticoids
   Examples: hydrocortisone (Solu-Cortef), dexamethasone (Decadron)
   Action: Replacement of glucocorticoid due to the state of relative hypoadrenalism that occurs with an increased metabolic rate; also mildly inhibits the peripheral conversion of T_4 to T_3
   Caution: Do not abruptly discontinue drug; must taper dose to prevent adrenocortical insufficiency

5. Beta-blocking drugs
   Example: propranolol (Inderal)
   Action: Blocks sympathetic activity; has mild effect in blocking the conversion of T_4 to T_3 in the periphery
   Caution: USE WITH CAUTION IN ELDERLY PATIENTS AND IN PATIENTS WITH ASTHMA OR CHF. May cause bradycardia, hypotension, atrioventricular block, dyspnea, bronchospasm, fatigue, depression, and insomnia; can mask signs and symptoms of hypoglycemia

6. Antipyretic
   Example: acetaminophen (Tylenol)
   Action: Inhibits synthesis of prostaglandins that may act as mediators for fever
   Caution: DO NOT ADMINISTER SALICYLATES, as they increase free thyroid hormone levels.

7. Dextrose and crystalloid solutions
   Examples: 5% dextrose in normal saline, 5% dextrose in Ringer's solution
   Action: Replace lost fluid and electrolytes due to increased metabolic rate; glucose given to provide energy source
   Caution: Can cause electrolyte imbalance and fluid overload
8. Narcotic analgesic and phenothiazine
   Examples: meperidine (Demerol) and chlorpromazine (Thorazine)
   Action: Depresses central nervous system to decrease shivering from cooling blanket
   Caution: Can cause hypotension and sedation
9. Multivitamin complex
   Example: multivitamin infusion
   Action: Functions as coenzymes in many metabolic processes (i.e., carbohydrate metabolism)
   Caution: DO NOT administer undiluted intravenous (IV)
10. Thyroxine-binding globulin is being developed for clinical use.

NURSING MANAGEMENT

Monitoring and Managing Clinical Problems

1. Protection: altered
   a. Promote reduction of serum thyroid hormones by administering antithyroid medications, iodine-containing medications, beta-blockers, and glucocorticoids, as ordered.
   b. Reduce sympathetic activity and reduce hypermetabolic state by administering beta-blockers and glucocorticoids, as ordered.
   c. Monitor effectiveness of therapy.
      1) Assess for a reduction in temperature, pulse, arrhythmias, respiratory rate, diaphoresis, tremors, and serum thyroid hormone levels; report significant findings.
      2) Assess for improvement in mental status and stabilization of blood pressure and hemodynamic parameters; report significant findings.

2. Hyperthermia
   a. Promote reduction of body temperature.
      1) Administer acetaminophen and medications to prevent shivering; DO NOT ADMINISTER SALICYLATES.
      2) Provide external cooling by using devices such as ice packs to the groin and axillae, and a cooling blanket; keep environmental temperature cool.
   b. Monitor body temperature every hour or continuously with a rectal probe, urinary catheter thermistor, or pulmonary artery catheter thermistor.
      1) Monitor effectiveness of therapy.
         a) Assess for a reduction in temperature, pulse, arrhythmias, respiratory rate, diaphoresis and tremors; report significant findings.
         b) Assess for improvement in mental status and stabilization of blood pressure and hemodynamic parameters; report significant findings.
3. Fluid Volume Excess or Deficit
   a. Monitor for volume depletion.
      1) Assess for complaints of thirst, nausea, vomiting, diarrhea, weakness, and weight loss; report significant findings.
      2) Assess for abnormal physical findings, such as lethargy, confusion, obtundation, decreased skin turgor, dry mucous membranes, sunken eyeballs, tachycardia, postural hypotension, hypotension in recumbent position, oliguria, and weight loss; report significant findings.
      3) Monitor for alterations in serum sodium and potassium, increased blood urea nitrogen, increased hemoglobin and hematocrit, increased serum osmolality, and increased urine specific gravity; report significant findings.
      4) Monitor serial hemodynamic parameters for decreased central venous pressure (CVP), pulmonary artery pressure (PAP), pulmonary capillary wedge pressure (PCWP), and CO; report significant findings.
   b. Monitor for volume overload.
      1) Assess for complaints of dyspnea; report significant findings.

2) Assess for abnormal physical findings, such as jugular venous distention, crackles, dependent edema, increased blood pressure, bounding pulse, tachycardia, altered mental status, S_3 or S_4, tachypnea, weight gain, and intake greater than output; report significant findings.

3) Monitor for alterations in serum sodium and potassium, decreased hemoglobin and hematocrit, decreased total serum protein and albumin, decreased serum osmolality, and decreased urine specific gravity; report significant findings.

4) Monitor serial hemodynamic parameters for increased CVP, PAP, and PCWP; report significant findings.

c. Monitor for hypercalcemia.

1) Assess for complaints of nausea, vomiting, headache, constipation, fatigue, weakness and increased urination and thirst; report significant findings.

2) Assess for abnormal physical findings, such as lethargy, confusion, coma, emotional lability, weakness, hypotonic and flaccid muscles, and decreased deep tendon reflexes; report significant findings.

3) Assess for laboratory and cardiac findings: hypercalcemia, arrhythmias, and a short QT interval on ECG; report significant findings.

d. Monitor for hypokalemia.

1) Assess for complaints of weakness, malaise, nausea, vomiting, abdominal cramps, and anorexia; report significant findings.

2) Assess for abnormal physical findings, such as muscle weakness, paralytic ileus, diminished reflexes, hypotension, and altered mental status; report significant findings.

3) Assess for laboratory and cardiac findings, such as hypokalemia, dysrhythmias, depressed ST segments, T-wave changes, and presence of U waves on ECG; report significant findings.

e. Promote fluid and electrolyte balance by administering ordered fluids, electrolyte replacements, and diuretics.

4. Cardiac Output: decreased
   a. Monitor cardiovascular status.
   1) Monitor heart rate, rhythm (especially note atrial fibrillation with rapid ventricular response, supraventricular tachycardia, paroxysmal atrial tachycardia, sinus bradycardia, heart blocks, conduction disturbances, and lethal ventricular arrhythmias), blood pressure (supine and upright), pulse pressure, heart sounds, peripheral pulses, capillary refill, cardiac enzymes, mental status, urine output, color, and respiratory status; report significant findings.
   2) Monitor serial ECGs for changes and report significant findings.
   3) Monitor serial hemodynamic parameters including CVP, right atrial pressure, PAP, PCWP, CO, cardiac index, systemic vascular resistance, and SvO_2; report significant findings.
   4) Monitor for side effects of beta-blockers.
   b. Promote CO.
   1) Institute measures to:
      a) Reduce serum thyroid hormones
      b) Reduce sympathetic activity
      c) Reduce body temperature
      d) Promote fluid and electrolyte balance
   2) Administer beta-blocker, inotropic, antiarrhythmic, vasoactive, and diuretic medications, as ordered.

Monitoring, Managing, and Preventing Life-Threatening Emergencies

1. Cardiogenic shock
   a. Monitor for hemodynamic instability.
   1) Continuously monitor hemodynamic parameters to evaluate the cardiovascular response to treatment.
   2) Titrate fluids and inotropes to maintain a systolic blood pressure of at least 80 mm Hg.
   3) Position the patient in modified Trendelenburg position (elevation of the legs at 45 degrees).
   4) Continuously monitor blood pressure to determine the response to treatment.

     5) Monitor cardiac rhythm for tachycardia and life-threatening ventricular arrhythmias (ventricular tachycardia and/or fibrillation).

  b. Promote adequate oxygenation.

     1) Administer supplemental oxygen, as ordered.

     2) Obtain blood specimens and monitor results of serial arterial blood gases (ABGs) and hemoglobin; report abnormalities.

     3) Monitor capillary refill and monitor skin color to assess peripheral perfusion.

     4) Maintain a patent airway and adequate ventilation. Use supplemental oxygen to ensure that sufficient oxygen is delivered to the lungs.

  c. Monitor for altered organ and tissue perfusion.

     1) Monitor hourly intake and output, and renal function tests for signs of acute renal failure.

     2) Monitor ABGs for a falling arterial oxygen concentration, which is evidence of adult respiratory distress syndrome.

     3) Monitor for decreased or absent bowel sounds and bright-red or coffee-ground drainage from the nasogastric tube, which are signs of gastroparesis and stress ulceration.

     4) Check temperature every 4 hours for hypothermia or hyperthermia.

     5) Monitor for downward changes in the level of consciousness, such as decreased alertness and attention span, drowsiness, or excessive sleeping.

  d. Provide enteral or parenteral nutritional support to prevent a negative nitrogen balance.

2. Cardiopulmonary arrest

  a. Call for help.

  b. Begin cardiopulmonary resuscitation.

  c. Follow with advanced cardiac life support.

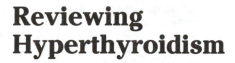

Reviewing Hyperthyroidism

Hyperthroidism is the excess of thyroid hormone in the blood. Thyroid hormone affects almost every body system, so excess hormone will increase the metabolic activity of almost all tissues, especially the heart, liver, skeletal muscle, and kidney. Increased metabolic activity results in an increased energy demand.

1. Hyperthyroidism can result from:
   a. Disorders that result in excess production and secretion of thyroid hormone from the thyroid gland such as:
      1) Graves' disease
      2) Toxic multinodular goiter
      3) Excess production of thyroid stimulating hormone
   b. Disorders that result in the abnormal storage and release of thyroid hormone such as:
      1) Chronic thyroiditis
      2) Subacute thyroiditis
   c. Disorders related to an exogenous or ectopic increase of thyroid hormone such as:

    1) Ingestion of high doses of thyroid hormones (thyrotoxicosis factitia)
    2) Ectopic production of thyroid hormone such as struma ovarii (a thyroid tumor of the ovary)

2. Presenting signs and symptoms will vary with the severity of the thyrotoxicosis and the age of the patient, and can consist of any combination of the following:

  a. Skin and appendages
    1) Fine, limp hair
    2) Early graying of hair
    3) Increased sweat production
    4) Warm, thin, soft skin
    5) Rosy complexion
    6) Easy bruising
    7) Erythema of the palms
    8) May have diffuse increased pigmentation or vitiligo (white patches of skin due to loss of pigmentation)
    9) Exophthalmos (protrusion of the eyeballs)
    10) Thyromegaly

  b. Respiratory
    1) Dyspnea
    2) Respiratory muscle weakness
    3) Increased work of breathing

  c. Metabolic
    1) Increased appetite; occasionally may have decreased appetite, especially in severe disease
    2) Intolerance to heat
    3) Weight loss, occasionally may have weight gain
    4) In older persons, weight loss and failure to thrive

  d. Gastrointestinal
    1) Loose stools with increased frequency; frank diarrhea
    2) Dysphagia
    3) Nausea, vomiting
    4) Abdominal pain, especially in severe disease
    5) Hepatomegaly with jaundice

  e. Nervous
    1) Nervousness
    2) Emotional lability
    3) Extreme irritability
    4) Insomnia

    5) Severe psychiatric disturbances
    6) Restlessness, short attention span
    7) Increased frequency of seizures in patients with a seizure disorder

f. Musculoskeletal
    1) Weakness
    2) Easy fatigability
    3) Quick, exaggerated, jerky movements
    4) Fine, rhythmic tremors of hands and tongue; lightly closed eyelids
    5) Muscle wasting; may be severe.
    6) Weakness of proximal muscles of limbs; may involve muscles of the trunk, face, and eyes.
    7) Periodic paralysis and aggravation of myasthenia gravis

g. Renal
    1) Mild polyuria

h. Reproductive
    1) Increased libido
    2) Menstrual dysfunction
    3) Infertility
    4) Spontaneous abortion
    5) Gynecomastia in men

i. Cardiovascular
    1) Palpitations
    2) Aggravation of angina
    3) Tachycardia at rest
    4) Widened pulse pressure with a low diastolic pressure
    5) Hypertension or hypotension
    6) Loud heart sounds; may auscultate a murmur, an S_3, or an S_4
    7) Decreased response to digoxin

Myxedema Coma

Myxedema coma is an extreme state of hypometabolism resulting from low levels of thyroid hormone and caused by a severe and long-standing depletion of thyroid hormone. It is characterized by hypothermia, an altered mental status ranging from slow mentation to coma, and an identifiable precipitating event.

Etiology/Pathophysiology

1. Etiology
   a. Usually seen in patients with a severe depletion of thyroid hormones, particularly primary hypothyroidism
   b. Rarely seen in patients with secondary hypothyroidism (dysfunction in the hypothalamic–anterior pituitary–thyroid axis) or in patients with hormone resistance syndromes
2. Patients at risk of developing myxedema coma are as follows:
   a. Persons with hypothyroidism who are given a sedative, narcotic, tranquilizer, or an anesthetic agent, or who may be exposed to cold
   b. Elderly women with long-standing hypothyroidism who develop an acute illness
3. Factors that may trigger the onset of myxedema coma include:
   a. Exposure to cold
   b. Infection
   c. Trauma
   d. Central nervous system depressant (sedative, narcotic, tranquilizer, anesthetic agent)
   e. Surgery
   f. Cerebral vascular accident
   g. Gastrointestinal bleed
   h. Congestive heart failure
   i. Hypercapnic narcosis
4. Pathophysiology
   a. The lack of thyroid hormone depresses the function of most body cells, resulting in:
      1) Decreased metabolic rate of the body, especially affecting the heart, skeletal muscle, liver, and kidneys
      2) Decreased heat production
      3) Decreased carbohydrate and fat metabolism
      4) Decreased heart rate, force of contraction, and cardiac output (CO)
      5) Decreased rate and depth of respiration
      6) Decreased appetite, rate of secretion of digestive juices, and gastrointestinal motility

7) Decreased mentation and reaction of deep tendon reflexes
8) Decreased muscle tone and reactivity
9) Decreased libido with a decreased reproductive function
   b. Mucinous edema results from the interstitial accumulation of hyaluronic acid and water, and occurs after a prolonged period of hypothyroidism.

Assessment/Analysis

ASSESSMENT FINDINGS

Subjective

1. Physical evidence of hypothyroidism (See Understanding Hypothyroidism, pp 436–438)
2. History of a precipitating event

Objective

1. Extreme hypothermia
2. Coma
3. Decreased respirations

SUPPORTING TEST FINDINGS

Laboratory Tests

1. Serum thyroxine (T_4)
   Abnormality: Decreased
2. Serum triiodothyronine (T_3)
   Serum reverse triiodothyronine (rT_3)
   Abnormality: Decreased or normal T_3 and rT_3
3. Sensitive thyroid stimulating hormone (STSH)
   Abnormality: Usually increased; if patient has been acutely ill for a while and/or has been unable to eat, STSH level may not increase to show severity of hypothyroid state. Pituitary hypothyroidism is suggested if the T_4 is decreased without an increased STSH
4. Arterial blood gases (ABGs)
   Abnormality: Decreased PaO_2 with an increased $PaCO_2$
5. Serum cortisol

Abnormality: Usually increased; may be normal
6. Blood sugar
   Abnormality: Decreased
7. Serum electrolytes
   Abnormality: Decreased serum sodium; increased serum potassium
8. Complete blood count with differential
   Abnormality: May have a microcytic (abnormally small red blood cells [RBCs]) or macrocytic (abnormally large RBCs) anemia
      Increased white blood cell count with an increase in the number of stabs or bands
9. Serum cholesterol
   Abnormality: Usually increased; if patient has been acutely ill for a while and/or has not been able to eat, cholesterol level may be within a normal range
10. Serum creatinine
    Abnormality: Usually increased
11. Serum cardiac enzymes
    Abnormality: Increased creatinine kinase mm band

Diagnostic Tests

1. Chest X-ray
   Abnormality: Pleural effusions
2. Electrocardiogram (ECG)
   Abnormality: Prolonged PR interval, decreased amplitude of the P wave and QRS complex, ST-segment changes, T-wave changes. May have a complete heart block
3. Echocardiogram
   Abnormality: Pericardial effusion; may see changes similar to idiopathic hypertrophic subaortic stenosis

Planning/Intervention

COLLABORATIVE MANAGEMENT

Procedures

1. Optimize function of respiratory system
   a. Promote oxygenation by assisting with intubating and providing respiratory support with mechanical ventilation.

    b. Monitor serial chest X-rays, ABGs, and pulmonary function tests; assess oxygenation status.

2. Correct metabolic dysfunction.
   a. Replace thyroid and glucocorticoid hormones, as ordered.
   b. Correct hypothermia with gradual rewarming using a regular blanket. *Avoid using active rewarming devices* because rapid rewarming may cause increased peripheral vasodilation and shock.
   c. Administer ordered glucose solutions to correct hypoglycemia, as indicated.

3. Optimize cardiovascular function.
   a. Promote fluid and electrolyte status by restricting free water to correct hyponatremia.
   b. Monitor cardiovascular status by placing patient on cardiac monitor, assisting with insertion of a pulmonary artery catheter, drawing baseline and follow-up cardiac enzymes, and following results of serial ECGs.

4. Prevent complications and identify precipitating event.
   a. Administer ordered antiulcer medications (use decreased doses) to prevent stress ulceration.
   b. Initiate work-up to identify precipitating event by obtaining specimens for cultures and sensitivity (blood, urine, sputum, and other body fluids), as ordered.
   c. Administer ordered antibiotics.
   d. Obtain specimens for evaluation of anemia.
   e. Administer ordered blood products.
   f. Assess for fecal impaction and treat as needed.
   g. Avoid administering alpha-adrenergic drugs (patients are already vasoconstricted).

Drug Therapy

1. Thyroid hormones
   Examples: levothyroxine (T_4) (Synthroid)
   liothyronine sodium (T_3) (Cytome)
   Action: Replace thyroid hormones to regulate metabolic activity of body tissues
   Caution: May cause tachycardia, arrhythmias, and cardiovascular collapse

2. Glucocorticoids
   Examples: hydrocortisone (Solu-Cortef)
   dexamethasone (Decadron)

Action: Replacement of glucocorticoid to protect patient who may have concurrent primary hypoadrenalism

Caution: Do not abruptly discontinue drug; must taper dose to prevent adrenocortical insufficiency

NURSING MANAGEMENT

Monitoring and Managing Clinical Problems

1. Spontaneous Ventilation: inability to sustain — Depressed ventilatory function requiring mechanical ventilation
   a. Monitor respiratory status.
      1) Assess chest for abnormal respiratory rate and rhythm, asymmetric chest expansion, absence of breath sounds bilaterally, crackles or rhonchi, or findings suggestive of a pleural effusion (fever, dyspnea, cough, area of involved lung dull to percussion, decreased to absent breath sounds); report significant findings.
      2) Monitor mechanical ventilator settings, such as FiO_2, tidal volume, rate, mode of ventilation, inspiratory/expiratory ratio, sigh rate, sensitivity settings, and system pressure settings. Be sure alarms are turned on and note any pressure leaks in the system.
      3) Monitor for a patent airway and for complications of the mechanical ventilator, such as barotrauma, tracheal or laryngeal damage, atelectasis, inability to wean or oxygen toxicity; report significant findings.
      4) Assess patient's readiness to wean by noting forced expiratory volume, forced vital capacity, negative inspiratory force, maximal inspiratory pressure, ABGs, and chest X-ray findings.
   b. Promote respiratory function.
      1) Administer thyroid preparations, as ordered, to increase rate and depth of respirations.
      2) Avoid the use of respiratory depressant drugs if at all possible. (If drugs that cause respiratory depression must be used, the dose is significantly reduced.)
      3) Administer ordered prophylactic antibiotics, as indicated.

4) Position patient to facilitate breathing.
5) Turn patient every 2 hours.
6) Suction as needed.
7) Be sure that mechanical ventilator is functioning properly.

2. Cardiac Output: decreased
   a. Monitor cardiovascular status.
      1) Monitor heart rate and rhythm (especially note bradycardia and conduction disturbances).
      2) Monitor heart sounds (muffled heart sounds could mean a pericardial effusion is present).
      3) Monitor blood pressure (supine and upright) and pulse pressure.
      4) Obtain blood specimens and monitor changes in cardiac enzymes.
      5) Monitor peripheral pulses.
      6) Monitor mental status.
      7) Monitor urine output hourly.
      8) Monitor skin color and capillary refill, and respiratory status.
      9) Monitor for ECG changes of a prolonged PR interval, a decreased amplitude of the P wave and QRS complex, and ST-segment and T-wave changes.
      10) Monitor results of echocardiograms.
      11) Monitor central venous pressure, right atrial pressure, pulmonary artery pressure, pulmonary capillary wedge pressure, CO, cardiac indices, systemic vascular resistance, and oxygen saturation. Report significant changes.
   b. Promote CO.
      1) Administer ordered thyroid hormone to increase cardiac function and glucocorticoid hormone replacement to protect patients who might have concurrent primary hypoadrenalism.
      2) Administer ordered intravenous (IV) fluids.
      3) Be prepared to administer emergency drugs, such as atropine, vasopressors, or inotropic agents.
      4) Have a temporary pacemaker readily accessible; be prepared to assist with a pericardiocentesis.

3. Hypothermia
   a. Monitor body temperature every hour by using a rectal probe or digital thermometer; if a glass thermome-

ter is used, be sure it is completely shaken down. (Note: patients frequently have a temperature below 35.5°C [96°F]. Use a rectal probe or digital thermometer when possible); report significant findings.

b. Promote rewarming to normal body temperature.

1) Administer ordered thyroid hormone replacement to help to increase heat production.

2) Keep environment warm; put several regular blankets and socks on patient to allow gradual rewarming.

3) DO NOT USE mechanical heating devices to rewarm the patient.

4) Monitor response to thyroid hormone replacement.

a) Obtain blood specimens and monitor results of thyroid hormone levels (especially thyroid stimulating hormone)

b) Assess for a gradual increase in temperature, heart rate, respiratory rate, and blood pressure.

c) Assess for an improvement in mental status and ECG changes.

d) Report significant findings.

4. Fluid Volume Excess or Deficit

a. Monitor fluid and electrolyte status.

1) Monitor serum sodium, potassium, chloride, bicarbonate, calcium, magnesium, albumin, and creatinine; blood urea nitrogen; hemoglobin and hematocrit; serum and urine osmolality; urinalysis; and urine electrolytes; report significant findings.

2) Monitor daily weights, intake and output every hour, and vital signs (assess for orthostatic hypotension), and measure abdominal and ankle girth daily; report significant findings.

3) Assess lethargy, confusion, stupor, coma, muscle twitching, seizures, complaints of malaise or headache, and a low serum sodium and osmolality; report significant findings suggestive of hyponatremia.

b. Promote fluid and electrolyte balance by administering ordered IV fluids and restricting free water.

5. Thought Processes: altered

a. Monitor neurologic function by assessing mental status, motor function, reflexes, and cranial nerve status. Be alert for seizure activity; report significant findings.

b. Promote normal mental status.

1) Administer ordered thyroid hormone replacement.

2) Orient patient to time, person, place, and date.

3) Avoid the use of sedatives, narcotics, and tranquilizers (if these drugs must be used, the dose should be significantly reduced).

4) Promote uninterrupted time for sleep.

5) Explain all procedures.

6) Encourage patient to ask questions and verbalize feelings.

Monitoring, Managing, and Preventing Life-Threatening Emergencies

1. Respiratory Failure — The patient may suffer irreversible damage to the respiratory centers and be ventilator dependent.

a. Monitor for increasing respiratory distress leading to increasing hypoxemia.

1) Monitor serial ABGs and report significant changes.

2) Monitor serial chest X-ray reports.

3) Auscultate lungs frequently for decreased breath sounds, crackles, and/or rhonchi.

4) Apply a pulse oximeter and continuously measure oxygen saturation.

5) Administer ordered bronchodilators.

6) Monitor for air hunger, tachypnea, restlessness, and confusion indicating increasing respiratory distress.

b. Prepare for and assist with immediate intubation, if necessary.

c. Monitor for effective ventilation while on mechanical ventilator.

1) Assess lung sounds frequently.

2) Suction, as needed, to remove sputum and promote a clear airway.

3) Measure compliance frequently and report decreases.

4) Measure peak pressures and report increases.

5) Sedate the patient, as needed, to control ventilator fighting. Paralytics also may be necessary.

6) Monitor serial ABGs for effectiveness of mechanical ventilation. Indications for positive end-expiratory pressure (PEEP):

   a) PaO_2 < 60 mm Hg on an FiO_2 > 50%

   b) pH < 7.25

   c) $PaCO$ > 45 mm Hg

7) Decrease FiO_2 to < 50% as quickly as possible to prevent oxygen toxicity.

8) If the patient is on PEEP, remember that PEEP holds alveoli open, thus increasing functional residual capacity, decreasing shunting, and decreasing hypoxemia. But, PEEP can decrease CO, increase the risk of oxygen toxicity, and cause fluid overload.

d. Monitor fluid volume status.

   1) Measure CO frequently.

   2) Measure hourly urine output and report output < 30 mL/h.

   3) Observe for signs of fluid overload (new S_3, increasing pulmonary crackles and rhonchi, edema, weight gain, intake greater than output); report significant findings.

   4) Observe for signs or dehydration (weight loss, low CO, intake less than output, tenting of skin); report positive findings

   5) Cautiously give IV fluids to prevent fluid overload but maintain adequate fluid volume.

2. Cardiopulmonary arrest

   a. Call for help.

   b. Begin cardiopulmonary resuscitation.

   c. Follow with advanced cardiac life support.

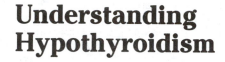

Understanding Hypothyroidism

Hypothyroidism is a metabolic disorder characterized by a deficiency of the thyroid hormones triiodothyronine or thyroxine. It is classified as either primary, when the cause is the thyroid gland itself, or secondary, when the cause is a failure to stimulate normal thyroid function or a failure of target tissues to respond to the normal blood levels of thyroid hormone. The variety of symptoms associated with this disorder reflect the systemic effect of thyroid hormone.

1. Causes of primary hypothyroidism
   a. Autoimmune thyroiditis (Hashimoto's disease)
   b. Primary idiopathic hypothyroidism
   c. Postradioiodine therapy
   d. Subtotal thyroidectomy
   e. Drug-induced (lithium, phenylbutazone, sulfonamides, para-aminosalicylic acid, resorcinol, propylthionracil, amiodarone)
   f. Defects in hormone production and activity
   g. Edemic iodine deficiency

2. Causes of secondary or central hypothyroidism
   a. Pituitary failure to produce thyroid-stimulating hormone, because of
      1) Tumors
      2) Infiltrative disease, ie, sarcoidosis
      3) Iatrogenic causes, ie, surgery or radiation
      4) Infections, ie, tuberculosis, syphilis
      5) Infarction or hemorrhage
      6) Genetic causes
   b. Hypothalmic lesions or tumors
3. Symptoms of hypothyroidism
   a. Low basal body temperature
   b. Bradycardia
   c. Muffled heart sounds
   d. May be normotensive, hypotensive, or hypertensive
   e. Coarse, dry, brittle hair
   f. Hair loss in lateral aspect of eyebrows, axillae, and pubic area
   g. Pale dry skin with coarse, scaly elbows and knees
   h. Brittle nails
   i. Yellow skin without scleral icterus
   j. Macroglossia (enlargement of the tongue)
   k. Delayed wound healing
   l. Hoarseness
   m. Thyromegaly (in some patients)
   n. Decreased sweat production
   o. Dyspnea
   p. Intolerance to cold
   q. Weight gain
   r. Ascites
   s. Nonpitting edema in extremities, eyelids, and periorbital area
   t. Constipation
   u. Decreased peristalsis to ileus
   v. Night blindness
   w. Obstructive sleep apnea
   x. Headache
   y. Syncope
   z. Memory defects
   aa. Altered mental status ranging from lethargy to frank coma

bb. Decreased intellectual function and slurred speech
cc. Depression, paranoia, or agitation
dd. Seizures
ee. Decreased auditory acuity
ff. Stiff, aching muscles
gg. Slow, clumsy movement; ataxia
hh. Delayed muscle contraction with normal strength and slight increase in mass
ii. Myoclonus may be present (clonic spasm or twitching of a muscle group)
jj. Slow deep tendon reflexes to areflexia
kk. Paresthesias in extremities
ll. Weakness, fatigue
mm. Nocturia
nn. Decreased libido
oo. Irregular menstrual bleeding, amenorrhea
pp. Infertility
qq. Spontaneous abortion
rr. Impotence

Acute Adrenocortical Insufficiency (Adrenal Crisis)

Adrenal crisis is a life-threatening event that is characterized by an absence or deficiency of glucocorticoids (cortisol) and mineralocorticoids (aldosterone).

Etiology/Pathophysiology

1. Patients at risk of developing adrenal crisis
   a. Primary adrenal insufficiency
      1) An established diagnosis of adrenal insufficiency when glucocorticoids are not or cannot be sufficiently replaced
      2) Major physiologic stressor with a coexisting undiagnosed primary adrenal insufficiency (major stressors include an acute infection, trauma, surgery, and myocardial infarction)
      3) A sudden loss of adrenal function due to hemorrhage, infection, or embolus (risk factors are anticoagulation therapy, thromboembolic disorders, coagulapathies, meningococcemia or pseudomonal septicemia, and major surgical trauma).
      4) Use of drugs that can inhibit steroid synthesis or can increase steroid metabolism in patients with diminished adrenocortical reserve. These drugs include aminoglutethimide, metyrapone, mitotane, ketoconazole, phenytoin, and rifampin.
2. Loss of mineralocorticoid activity is the primary pathophysiologic factor precipitating adrenal crisis.
   a. Aldosterone exerts its major effects in the renal tubule to promote the absorption of sodium and water and to promote the excretion of potassium and hydrogen ions.
   b. Lack of aldosterone results in the loss of sodium and water in the urine, which significantly decreases extracellular fluid volume.
   c. Hyperkalemia (serum potassium >5.5 mEq/L) and acidosis (blood has an acid excess or base deficit with pH <7.35) also develops due to the retention of potassium and hydrogen ions.
3. Glucocorticoid deficiency also contributes to the pathophysiology of adrenal crisis
   a. Increases difficulty maintaining a normal blood sugar (patient may be hypoglycemic)
   b. Decreases ability to tolerate stress
   c. Contributes to hypotension (sensitizes arterioles to the effects of norepinephrine)

4. Adrenal crisis is rarely seen in patients with chronic secondary or tertiary adrenal insufficiency, except in patients who are withdrawn from chronic glucocorticoid therapy too quickly (These patients may have developed adrenal gland and pituitary gland suppression.).

Assessment/Analysis

ASSESSMENT FINDINGS

Subjective

1. Anorexia
2. Nausea
3. Vomiting
4. Weight loss
5. Abdominal pain
6. Weakness
7. Fatigue
8. Headache
9. Thirst
10. Salt cravings

Objective

1. Lethargy
2. Confusion
3. Obtundation
4. Coma
5. Fever (may be 40.5°C or more)
6. Decreased skin turgor
7. Dry mucous membranes
8. Sunken eyeballs
9. Hyperpigmentation or vitiligo (white patches of skin due to loss of pigmentation)
10. Oliguria
11. Generalized abdominal tenderness
12. Tachycardia
13. Postural hypotension (hypotension in a recumbent position)
14. Other considerations
    a. Symptoms will vary if crisis is due to an acute, abrupt

onset of adrenal insufficiency versus a patient with chronic adrenal insufficiency who goes into crisis.

1) Patients with chronic adrenal insufficiency will present with classic signs/symptoms of Addison's disease (hyperpigmentation, weakness and fatigue, weight loss, anorexia, hypotension, nausea and vomiting, hyponatremia, hyperkalemia).

2) In acute adrenocortical insufficiency, the patient will present with magnified signs and symptoms (severe weakness, apathy and confusion, severe nausea, vomiting, anorexia, acute abdominal pain, and severe hyponatremia with hyperkalemia. Hyperpigmentation may be absent).

SUPPORTING TEST FINDINGS

Laboratory Tests

1. Serum electrolytes
   Abnormality: Decreased serum sodium
   Increased serum potassium
   Increased serum calcium
2. Serum glucose
   Abnormality: Decreased
3. Blood urea nitrogen (BUN)
   Abnormality: Increased
4. Complete blood count (CBC) with differential
   Abnormality: Decreased hemoglobin and hematocrit (in hemorrhage)
   Increased hemoglobin and hematocrit (in volume depletion)
   Increased eosinophils
5. Arterial blood gases (ABGs)
   Abnormality: Decreased pH
   Decreased bicarbonate (metabolic acidosis)
6. Plasma cortisol
   Abnormality: Decreased
7. Plasma adrenocorticotropic hormone (ACTH)
   Abnormality: Increased (in primary adrenal insufficiency)
   Decreased (in secondary adrenal insufficiency)
8. Short ACTH test
   Abnormality: Decreased baseline plasma cortisol

Decreased plasma cortisol at 30 minutes and 60 minutes after receiving intravenous (IV) ACTH

Diagnostic Tests

1. Computed tomography (CT) scan of the adrenal glands
   Abnormality: Enlarged adrenal glands or presence of calcium suggests an infectious, hemorrhagic, or metastatic process.

   Atrophied adrenal glands suggests an autioimmune process.
2. CT scan of the head
   Abnormality: A mass in the sella turcica suggests a tumor of the pituitary gland.

Planning/Intervention

COLLABORATIVE MANAGEMENT

Procedures

1. Promote fluid and electrolyte balance.
   a. Secure IV access with peripheral large-bore catheters, a central venous catheter, and/or a pulmonary artery catheter, as ordered.
   b. Resuscitate with normal saline solution, as ordered.
2. Assess for laboratory abnormalities
   a. Draw blood specimens for baseline laboratory analysis: serum electrolytes; serum glucose; BUN, CBC with differential, ABGs, plasma cortisol, and ACTH levels. (Treatment will be initiated before obtaining laboratory results.)
   b. Continuously monitor fluid and electrolyte, cardiovascular (by hemodynamic and cardiac monitoring), and blood glucose status.
   c. Perform short ACTH stimulation test at 30 and 60 minutes, as ordered.
      1) Obtain blood specimens for baseline levels of cortisol, aldosterone, and ACTH.
      2) Administer ACTH (cosyntropin) IV.
      3) Obtain repeat blood specimen for cortisol and aldosterone at 30 and 60 minutes.

    d. Initiate diagnostic work-up procedure to determine cause of adrenal insufficiency and precipitating illness, as ordered.

3. Replace glucocorticoids, as ordered.
    a. Expect to taper glucocorticoid replacement over 1 to 3 days and initiate an oral maintenance dose.
    b. Lifelong replacement of glucocorticoids and mineralocorticoids will be necessary for patients with primary adrenal insufficiency.

4. Initiate measures to maintain blood pressure, as ordered.
    a. Administer IV fluid resuscitation.
    b. Administer vasopressors (dopamine, levophed, and dobutamine).

Drug Therapy

1. Dextrose and crystalloid solutions
    Examples: 5% dextrose in normal saline solution, 5% dextrose in Ringer's solution
    Action: Replace lost fluid and electrolytes due to deficiency of mineralocorticoids
        Glucose given to provide energy source
    Caution: Electrolyte imbalance, fluid overload

2. Glucocorticoids
    Examples: dexamethasone/sodium phosphate (Decadron) hydrocortisone (Solu-Cortef)
    Action: Replacement of glucocorticoid due to adrenal insufficiency
    Caution: Do not abruptly discontinue medication
        Taper dosage over 2 to 3 days
        Mineralocorticoids may be added

NURSING MANAGEMENT

Monitoring and Managing Clinical Problems

1. Fluid Volume Deficit or Excess
    a. Monitor for volume depletion.
       1) Assess for complaints of thirst, nausea, vomiting, diarrhea, weakness, and weight loss; report significant findings.
       2) Assess for abnormal physical findings, such as lethargy, confusion, obtundation, decreased skin

turgor, dry mucous membranes, sunken eyeballs, tachycardia, postural hypotension, hypotension in recumbent position, oliguria, and weight loss; report significant findings.

3) Monitor serial laboratory values for alterations in sodium and potassium, increased BUN, increased hemoglobin and hematocrit, increased serum osmolality, and increased urine specific gravity; report significant findings.

4) Monitor serial hemodynamic parameters for decrease in central venous pressure (CVP), pulmonary artery pressure (PAP), pulmonary capillary wedge pressure (PCWP), and cardiac output (CO); report significant findings.

b. Monitor for the complication of volume overload after rapid infusion of IV fluids.

1) Assess for complaints of dyspnea; report findings.

2) Assess for signs of volume overload (jugular venous distention, crackles, dependent edema, increased blood pressure, bounding pulse, tachycardia, altered mental status, S_3 or S_4, tachypnea, weight gain, and intake greater than output) report significant findings.

3) Monitor serial laboratory values for alterations in sodium and potassium, decreased hemoglobin and hematocrit, decreased total serum protein and albumin, decreased serum osmolality, and decreased urine specific gravity; report significant findings.

4) Monitor serial hemodynamic parameters for increased CVP, PAP, and PCWP; report significant findings.

c. Monitor for hyponatremia.

1) Assess for headache, malaise, lethargy, confusion, obtundation, coma (muscle twitching and seizures may be seen); report findings.

2) Monitor laboratory values for hyponatremia; report findings.

d. Monitor for hyperkalemia.

1) Assess weakness, paralysis, paralytic ileus; report significant findings.

    2) Assess for changes in electrocardiogram of high-peaked T waves, prolongation of the PR interval, wide QRS, ventricular fibrillation, asystole; report significant findings.

    3) Monitor laboratory values for hyperkalemia; report significant findings.

  e. Promote fluid and electrolyte balance.

    1) Administer IV fluids, as ordered (usually normal saline solution or 5% dextrose in normal saline solution).

    2) Administer glucocorticoid preparations, as ordered (may be in divided doses or continuous drip).

2. Nutrition: altered, less than body requirements

  a. Monitor for hypoglycemia.

    1) Assess for headache; dizziness; lethargy; fatigue; changes in mental status (such as inability to concentrate and visual clouding); palpitations, nervousness; hunger; nausea; pallor; cool, clammy skin; tremors; tachycardia; and arrhythmias.

    2) Monitor serial laboratory values for hypoglycemia; report significant findings.

  b. Prevent/control hypoglycemia.

    1) Administer IV dextrose solutions, as ordered.

    2) Administer dexamethasone or hydrocortisone, as ordered.

3. Cardiac Output: decreased

  a. Monitor cardiovascular status.

    1) Monitor heart rate, rhythm, heart sounds, blood pressure, peripheral pulses, mental status, urine output, color, capillary refill, respiratory rate and rhythm, breath sounds, and ABGs; report significant findings.

    2) Monitor serial hemodynamic parameters of CVP, PAP, PCWP, CO, cardiac index, systemic vascular resistance, and SVo_2; report significant findings.

  b. Promote CO.

    1) Administer ordered IV fluids.

    2) Administer dexamethasone or hydrocortisone preparations, as ordered.

    3) Administer vasopressors, as needed.

Monitoring, Managing, and Preventing
Life-Threatening Emergencies

1. Hypovolemic shock
   a. Monitor for hemodynamic instability.
      1) Use continuous hemodynamic monitoring.
      2) Titrate fluids and inotropes to maintain a systolic blood pressure of at least 80 mm Hg.
      3) Position the patient in modified Trendlenburg position (elevation of the legs at 45 degrees).
   b. Promote adequate oxygenation.
      1) Administer supplemental oxygen, as ordered.
      2) Collect and monitor results of serial ABGs and hemoglobin; report abnormalities.
      3) Monitor capillary refill and monitor skin color to assess peripheral perfusion.
   c. Monitor for altered organ and tissue perfusion.
      1) Monitor for decreased urine output and elevated renal function tests, possibly indicating acute renal failure.
      2) Monitor for a falling arterial oxygen concentration, possibly indicating adult respiratory distress syndrome.
      3) Auscultate for decreased or absent bowel sounds, suggesting gastroparesis, and for bright-red or coffee-ground drainage from the nasogastric tube, possibly indicating stress ulceration.
      4) Monitor temperature every 4 hours for hypothermia or hyperthermia.
      5) Monitor for decreased alertness and attention span, drowsiness, or excessive sleeping, indicating downward changes in the level of consciousness.

Diabetic Ketoacidosis

Diabetic ketoacidosis (DKA) is an acute metabolic disorder involving lack of insulin and resulting in a significant elevation of blood sugar and metabolic changes as the body attempts to find alternate sources of energy.

Etiology/Pathophysiology

1. Etiology
   a. DKA occurs as a complication of diabetes mellitus, a disease that involves an absolute or relative lack of insulin.
   b. DKA is more likely to occur with type I, or insulin-dependent diabetes mellitus, formerly known as juvenile-onset diabetes.
   c. DKA occurs most often in a patient with diabetes who was previously undiagnosed or in a patient with known diabetes who has a disorder or condition that changes the body's metabolic balance, such as:
      1) Infection
      2) Nausea, vomiting, and/or diarrhea
      3) Trauma, including surgical trauma
      4) Pregnancy
      5) Insufficient insulin coverage
      6) Increased dietary intake without increasing insulin coverage
      7) Decreased exercise without adjusting food intake and insulin amounts
      8) Use of a medication that adversely affects glucose/insulin balance such as glucocorticoids, steroids, catecholamines (epinephrine, isoproterenol, and others that may be found in nonprescription drugs), psychotropic drugs (haloperidol, phenothiazines, tricyclic antidepressants, lithium), analgesics, anti-inflammatory agents (aspirin, acetaminophen, indomethacin).
2. Pathophysiology
   a. Inadequate amount of insulin to handle amount of glucose
   b. Cells without sufficient glucose trigger metabolic changes
      1) Increased lipolysis
      2) Increased ketogenesis
      3) Increased gluconeogenesis
   c. When glucose levels in the blood are increased:
      1) Serum osmolality changes lead to intracellular and extracellular dehydration.

2) Renal excretion of glucose increases and causes an increased renal excretion of water and sodium.
d. Metabolic changes cause:
   1) Increased production of acids and metabolic acidosis
   2) Increased production of ketones
e. Tissue hypoxia occurs and cells shift to anaerobic glycolysis (product is lactate), which adds to the acidemia.
f. Blood glucose levels can be corrected more quickly than levels of acids.

Assessment/Analysis

ASSESSMENT FINDINGS

Subjective

1. Polyuria
2. Polydipsia
3. Polyphagia, which changes to a decreased appetite as blood sugar elevates and ketonuria and ketoacidosis occur
4. Nausea/vomiting
5. Diarrhea
6. Epigastric discomfort
7. Abdominal pain, abdominal cramps
8. Leg cramps
9. Tiredness, weakness
10. Weight loss
11. Headache
12. Drowsiness progressing to stupor as condition worsens

Objective

1. Lethargic
2. Tachycardia
3. Hypotension if dehydration is severe
4. Tachypnea and possibly Kussmaul's respiration if acidosis is severe
5. Acetone or sweet, fruity odor to breath
6. Flushed color

7. Hot, dry skin
8. Dry mucous membranes
9. Poor skin turgor
10. Confusion or deteriorating level of consciousness to the level of coma
11. Decreased or absent deep tendon reflexes

Supporting Test Findings

1. Blood glucose
   Abnormality: Increased to 300–500 mg/dL; may be 1000 mg/dL or higher if severe dehydration or impaired kidney function is present
2. Urine glucose
   Abnormality: Glucose is present
3. Urinalysis
   Abnormality: Acetones present; increased specific gravity
4. Serum electrolytes
   Abnormality: Serum potassium decreased or normal in early stages and, in later stages, >5.5 mEq/L although total body deficit exists
   Serum sodium increased initially to >135 mEq/L; often hyponatremia occurs (if mild, about 130 mEq/L, if severe, <130 mEq/L
   Serum magnesium and serum phosphate may be decreased
5. Serum osmolality
   Abnormality: Mildly increased, but usually less than 330 mOsm/kg
6. Arterial blood gases (ABGs)
   Abnormality: Decreased pH (<7.20 reflecting metabolic acidosis); decreased HCO^{-3} (<10 mEq/L)
7. Serum creatinine
   Abnormality: Increased if renal dysfunction accompanies DKA
8. Blood urea nitrogen
   Abnormality: Increased if severe dehydration is present
9. Serum acetone
   Abnormality: Strongly positive
10. Anion gap
    Abnormality: Increased to >15 mmol/L; often as high as 20–40 mmol/L

Planning/Intervention

COLLABORATIVE MANAGEMENT

Procedures

1. Restore fluid balance by administering ordered intravenous (IV) solutions.
2. Return blood glucose to normal level by administering ordered insulin.
3. Improve acid-base balance by treating metabolic acidosis, as ordered.
4. Improve electrolyte balance by replacing losses and removing excesses, as ordered.
5. Identify and treat any precipitating etiologies (reduced or omitted insulin doses or infection).
6. Prevent complications such as compromised respiratory effort (possible intubation), aspiration (nasogastric intubation), and shock (monitoring of hemodynamic functions).

Drug Therapy

1. IV fluids

   Example: 0.9% sodium chloride solution

   Action: Replaces lost fluid with an isotonic saline solution

   Caution: May give as much as 1–2 L during the first hour and then 0.5–1 L each hour until hypotension is resolved and urine output stabilizes; fluids may cause hemodilution, hypotonicity, interstitial edema, or circulatory overload

   Example: dextrose 5% in 0.45% sodium chloride solution

   Action: Maintains fluid balance while adding a source of glucose when patient's blood sugar falls to a level where glucose is needed (at about 250 mg/dL)

   Caution: Serum glucose levels still need to be carefully, frequently monitored

2. Insulin

   Example: regular insulin (Humulin R)

   Action: Restores glucose levels to normal; assists glucose across cellular membranes; assists in storage of glucose as glycogen in the liver; helps prevent break-down of fats into fatty acids because inhibits enzyme lipase; promotes fatty acid synthesis; stimulates transport of amino acids into cells, assisting protein anabolism and inhibiting protein catabolism; inhibits liver glyconeogenesis (release of glycogen stores that would increase serum glucose levels)

Caution: Dosage must be individualized and success is monitored by frequent serum glucose determinations

3. Potassium replacement

Example: potassium chloride
potassium phosphate

Action: Replaces renal loss of potassium

Caution: if there is renal dysfunction, potassium must be given more carefully;

Monitoring for potassium-caused lethal dys-rhythmias

Administer diluted in IV fluids; do not administer by IV push

4. Alkalinizing agent

Example: sodium bicarbonate

Action: Replaces lost bicarbonate to help counteract metabolic acidosis

Caution: Dosage determined by ABGs

Avoid excessive amounts that may cause metabolic alkalosis; changes in acidosis affect serum potassium levels

IV administration can be irritating and may possibly cause phlebitis at injection site

NURSING MANAGEMENT

Monitoring and Managing Clinical Problems

1. Fluid Volume Deficit
   a. Monitor and report abnormalities in:
      1) Vital signs
      2) Intake and output
         a) Urine output should be about 30 mL/h.
         b) Nasogastric output if nasogastric intubation is required

3) Level of consciousness, dyspnea, jugular vein distention, and skin turgor as fluids are replaced.
4) Serial serum glucose, serum osmolality, and urine glucose values (They should decrease.)
5) Daily weights

b. Promote improved fluid balance.
1) Administer IV fluids, 1–2 L during the first hour and 0.5–1 L/h until blood pressure is stabilized.
2) Administer insulin to decrease fluid loss through osmotic diuresis. Amounts of insulin may include an initial IV bolus of 10 U and then, about 5–10 U/h or 0.1 U/kg per hour; a steady, progressive decrease in levels is desired (a decrease of 50–100 mg/dL per hour); when serum glucose reaches 250 mg/dL, glucose needs to be added to IV therapy to help prevent hypoglycemia.

c. Recognize early signs of fluid overload (shortness of breath, jugular vein distention, edema, increased blood pressure), and decrease IV fluids and administer diuretics, if necessary.

d. Obtain specimens and monitor serum electrolytes and ABGs; report significant changes and correct them, as indicated.

2. Tissue Perfusion, altered: renal, high risk for
a. Monitor for and report abnormalities in:
1) Serum potassium
a) Decreases as blood glucose levels decrease
b) Changes as acid-base balance is restored
c) Changes as renal excretion of sodium changes
2) Serum sodium
3) Serum magnesium and phosphate, which may be low in patients with DKA

b. Promote potassium balance by administering potassium in the IV fluids, beginning when the serum potassium decreases to 4.5 mEq/L; some may begin replacement immediately as long as there are no electrocardiogram (ECG) changes suggestive of hyperkalemia. Altered magnesium and phosphate levels usually do not require treatment although potassium phosphate may be ordered for potassium replacement.

Monitoring, Managing, and Preventing
Life-Threatening Emergencies

1. Seizures
    a. Can occur if fluid and electrolyte imbalances become severe or if uremia is present.
        1) Restore fluid balance with IV fluids. Avoid using hypotonic saline, which may cause too rapid a shift in fluid and increase risk of cerebral edema.
        2) Steadily and gradually reduce glucose to normal levels with insulin administration; goal is to decrease blood sugar at a rate of 50–100 mg/dL per hour.
        3) Administer sodium bicarbonate if metabolic acidosis is severe, but be careful not to change pH too quickly to avoid cerebral deterioration (related to the ease at which CO_2 penetrates cerebral spinal fluid when compared to the more difficult penetration by HCO^-_3); if pH is 7.0 or greater, do not administer.
    b. Institute seizure precautions to protect the patient from possible injury.
        1) Pad siderails and keep them raised.
        2) Keep bed in low position.
        3) Have emergency resuscitation equipment nearby.
        4) Remove all potentially harmful objects from the patient's area.
        5) Restrict smoking.
    c. If seizure occurs:
        1) Protect the airway.
        2) Do not insert anything into the patient's mouth.
        3) Loosen restrictive clothing.
        4) Protect the patient from self-injury during the seizure.
        5) Administer ordered medications.
    d. Assist with instituting dialysis, as ordered, to prevent electrolyte abnormalities or uremia that may result in seizures.
2. Serious dysrhythmias from alterations in serum potassium

a. Monitor ECG continuously until blood sugar is decreased and potassium level stabilizes.
b. Monitor urine output and serum potassium levels to assess renal function.
c. Administer supplemental potassium as blood glucose is treated with insulin.
d. Recognize renal dysfunction and alter potassium dosages, as indicated.
e. If cardiopulmonary arrest occurs:
    1) Call for help.
    2) Begin cardiopulmonary resuscitation.
    3) Follow with advanced cardiac life support.

Hyperglycemic Hyperosmolar Nonketotic Coma

Hyperglycemic hyperosmolar nonketotic coma (HHNC), an acute complication of diabetes mellitus, is a disorder of glucose metabolism in which there is insulin resistance and a relative insulin deficiency that results in severe hyperglycemia, hyperosmolality with osmotic diuresis, and minimal to absent ketonemia. The death rate is 20–50%.

Etiology/Pathophysiology

1. Patients at risk
   a. Middle-aged elderly individuals
   b. Obese individuals
   c. Sedentary individuals
   d. Type II (non–insulin-dependent) individuals
   e. Individuals with previously undiagnosed diabetes mellitus
2. Factors that may trigger the onset include:
   a. Acute illness, such as infection, burns, pancreatitis, myocardial infarction, and intracranial injury
   b. Trauma
   c. Surgery
   d. Hypothermia
   e. Chronic illness, such as renal disease
   f. Drugs, particularly propranolol, phenytoin, furosemide, thiazide diuretics, glucocorticosteroids, and diazoxide
   g. Total parenteral nutrition solution and high-calorie enteral feeding solutions
   h. Peritoneal dialysis with hypertonic glucose dialysate solutions
   i. Hemodialysis
   j. Excessive levels of thyroxine, growth hormone, or catecholamines
3. Pathophysiology
   a. A stressor precipitates the release of stress hormones (glucagon, cortisol, and epinephrine), which act to increase serum glucose.
   b. A state of insulin resistance and relative insulin deficiency exists. The lack of insulin activity and availability reduces the transport of glucose into the cell and results in hyperglycemia.
   c. Severe hyperglycemia results in cellular dehydration and an osmotic diuresis in which excess amounts of water and electrolytes are lost.
   d. Without an adequate intake, hypovolemia and hyperosmolality develop, further enhancing insulin resistance and hyperglycemia.
   e. The overall effects are severe hyperglycemia, hyper-

osmolality, severe dehydration, and electrolyte imbalance.

Assessment/Analysis

ASSESSMENT FINDINGS

Subjective

1. History of a progressive decline in mental status and fluid intake over days to weeks
2. Usually is no prior history of diabetes mellitus
3. Polyuria
4. Polydipsia
5. Polyphagia
6. Weight loss
7. Weakness, listlessness, mental fatigue
8. Headache
9. Blurred vision
10. Vaginitis
11. Skin infection, itching

Objective

1. Stuporous to comatose
2. Seizures
3. Positive Babinski's reflex
4. Asymmetric reflexes
5. Muscle fasciculations
6. Aphasia
7. Paresis
8. Low central venous pressure (CVP), pulmonary artery pressure (PAP), pulmonary capillary wedge pressure (PCWP), and cardiac output (CO)
9. Poor skin turgor, soft sunken eyeballs, longitudinal wrinkles in tongue, and oliguria or polyuria, suggesting severe dehydration
10. Normal to depressed respirations
11. Hyperthermia or hypothermia
12. Tachycardia
13. Hypotension, possibly shock

SUPPORTING TEST FINDINGS

Laboratory Tests

1. Blood sugar
   Abnormality: Usually >600 mg/dL; levels over 1000 mg/dL are common
2. Serum osmolality
   Abnormality: Usually >350 mOsm/L; may exceed 400 mOsm/L
3. Serum sodium and potassium
   Abnormality: May be decreased, normal, or increased
4. Serum phosphate and magnesium
   Abnormality: Usually increased at onset; declines with fluid replacement
5. Serum calcium
   Abnormality: Usually normal; with severe hypophosphatemia may be increased
6. Arterial blood gases (ABGs)
   Abnormality: Normal or mild acidosis
7. Serum bicarbonate
   Abnormality: Normal or mildly decreased
8. Anion gap
   Abnormality: Normal or may be increased
9. Serum ketones
   Abnormality: Normal or mildly increased
10. Serum lactate
    Abnormality: Normal or mildly increased
11. Blood urea nitrogen (BUN)
    Abnormality: Increased
12. Hemoglobin and hematocrit
    Abnormality: Increased
13. White blood cell count
    Abnormality: Increased
14. Urinalysis
    Abnormality: Positive for glucose
    Normal or slight increase in ketones
    Trace protein
    Increased specific gravity

Diagnostic Tests

1. None

Planning/Intervention

COLLABORATIVE MANAGEMENT

Procedures

1. Promote oxygenation. If the patient has altered mental status or respiratory dysfunction, assist with intubation and mechanical ventilation.
2. Monitor ABGs to assess oxygenation status.
3. Prevent aspiration by inserting a nasogastric tube and connecting to low suction.
4. Administer ordered crystalloid and colloid solutions to promote fluid balance.
5. Assist with insertion of a pulmonary artery catheter; insert an indwelling urinary catheter; monitor hourly intake and output and vital signs, daily weights, and serum osmolality to monitor fluid status.
6. Administer ordered insulin replacement and fluid resuscitation to correct hyperglycemia.
7. Monitor blood sugar hourly and periodically measure urine ketones to assess for onset of hypoglycemia. Administer 5% dextrose solution once blood sugar decreases to 250 – 300 mg/dL.
8. Administer ordered isotonic and hypotonic crystalloid solutions with potassium and phosphate to promote electrolyte balance.
9. Monitor serum sodium, potassium, chloride, calcium, magnesium, and phosphate every 1 – 2 hours to assess electrolyte status. Assess QRS and T-wave morphology on cardiac monitor every hour to evaluate effect of electrolyte imbalance.
10. Monitor serial serum lactate, venous CO_2, anion gap, arterial blood pH, and serum ketones to determine significant changes in acid-base balance.
11. Monitor CVP, PAP, PCWP, and CO every hour to determine hemodynamic status.

Drug Therapy

1. Isotonic crystalloid solutions
   Examples: normal saline solution
   Ringer's lactate
   Action: Replace water and electrolytes lost during os-

motic diuresis; expand plasma volume to correct hyperosmolar state

Caution: Carefully monitor patients with cardiovascular disease or renal failure for pulmonary edema/volume overload; patient should be monitored for a hyperchloremic metabolic acidosis and a rapid fall in blood osmolality

2. Hypotonic crystalloid solutions

Example: 0.45% sodium chloride solution

Action: Replace water and electrolytes lost during osmotic diuresis; replace lost free water

Caution: When blood sugar drops to between 250–300 mg/dL, fluid replacement should contain dextrose 5% to prevent hypoglycemia

3. Insulin

Example: regular insulin (Humulin, Novolin)

Action: Promotes the transport of glucose into cells; inhibits the release of free fatty acids

Caution: Intravenous (IV) administration of insulin is the preferred route; the subcutaneous route should NOT be used due to the possibility of hypoperfusion of tissue and unpredictable absorption; the intramuscular (IM) route may be used if IV access is a problem. Use a 1–1½-inch needle to administer IM insulin.

4. Potassium and phosphate replacement

Examples: potassium chloride and potassium phosphate

Action: Potassium helps to maintain the following: osmotic pressure; nerve impulse transmission; contraction of cardiac, skeletal, and smooth muscle; metabolism of protein and carbohydrates, and normal renal function

Phosphate is needed for carbohydrate metabolism and energy transfer, needed in maintaining calcium levels, and influential in the excretion of hydrogen ions.

Caution: Monitor rhythm strip for signs of hyperkalemia (peaked T wave and a widening QRS complex) during infusion of potassium.

DO NOT ADMINISTER POTASSIUM UNTIL INSULIN HAS BEGUN TO ACT. WITHOUT INSULIN, POTASSIUM CANNOT ENTER THE CELL AND CAN PRODUCE A SEVERE STATE OF HYPERKALEMIA.

Monitor serum potassium every 2 to 4 hours initially.
5. Bicarbonate
   Examples: Sodium bicarbonate
   Actions: An alkalizing agent that helps to maintain ion balance and osmotic pressure
   Caution: Bicarbonate is used only in severe acidosis (pH <7.0), patients with hemodynamic instability with a pH <7.1, or in patients with hyperkalemic electrocardiogram (ECG) changes.
      Routine use of bicarbonate is controversial

NURSING MANAGEMENT

Monitoring and Managing Clinical Problems

1. Fluid Volume Excess or Deficit
   a. Monitor for volume depletion.
      1) Assess for complaints of polyuria, polydipsia, weight loss, weakness, and listlessness; report significant findings.
      2) Assess for changes in level of consciousness from lethargy to coma, decreased skin turgor, soft sunken eyeballs, longitudinal wrinkles in tongue, tachycardia, hypotension, polyuria, oliguria, and weight loss. Report significant findings.
      3) Monitor for alterations in serum sodium, potassium, phosphate, magnesium, and calcium; increased BUN; increased serum osmolality; increased total serum protein and albumin; and increased urine specific gravity; report significant findings.
      4) Monitor CVP, PAP, PCWP, and CO. Report significant findings.
   b. Monitor for volume overload after rapid infusion of IV fluids.
      1) Assess for neck vein distention, crackles, dependent edema, increased blood pressure, bounding pulse, S_3 or S_4, tachypnea, dyspnea, weight gain, and intake greater than output; report significant findings.
      2) Monitor for alterations in serum sodium, potassium, phosphate, magnesium, and calcium; decreased hemoglobin and hematocrit; decreased

total serum protein and albumin; decreased serum osmolality and urine specific gravity; report significant findings.

3) Monitor for increased CVP, PAP, PWCP, and CO; report significant findings.

4) Monitor for evidence of pulmonary edema, hyperchloremic metabolic acidosis (due to replacement with 0.9% sodium chloride solution), and rapid fall in blood osmolality.

c. Monitor for hyperkalemia.

1) Assess for altered bowel function, muscle weakness, and paralysis.

2) Assess for changes in ECG: high-peaked T waves, prolongation of the PR interval, wide QRS complex, ventricular fibrillation, asystole; report significant findings.

3) Obtain blood specimens and monitor for hyperkalemia; report significant findings.

d. Monitor for hypokalemia.

1) Assess for muscle weakness, malaise, nausea, vomiting, abdominal cramps, anorexia, diminished reflexes, hypotension, and alteration in mental status; report significant findings.

2) Assess for dysrhythmias, specifically depressed ST segments, T-wave changes, presence of U waves on ECG; report significant findings.

e. Monitor for alterations in serum sodium, phosphate, calcium, and magnesium levels. Report significant findings.

f. Administer ordered hypotonic and isotonic IV fluids, electrolyte replacements, and regular insulin to promote fluid and electrolyte balance. ALWAYS ADMINISTER POTASSIUM REPLACEMENT AFTER INSULIN HAS BEGUN TO ACT.

2. Tissue Perfusion, altered: peripheral

a. Monitor for hyperglycemia/hyperosmolality.

1) Assess for dry mouth, polyuria, polydipsia, polyphagia, weight loss, weakness, headache, blurred vision, altered mental state from lethargy to coma, seizures, positive Babinski's reflex, asymmetric reflexes, fasciculations, aphasia, paresis, hypother-

mia or hyperthermia, vaginitis, and skin infection or itching.

    2) Monitor for elevated blood sugar, elevated serum osmolality, normal to mildly elevated serum ketones, and urine positive for glucose.

b. Administer ordered IV hypotonic and isotonic solutions, and IV or IM regular insulin to promote gradual reduction in hyperglycemia and hyperosmolality.

c. Monitor serial blood sugar levels. Add 5% dextrose to IV solutions once blood sugar decreases to 250–300 mg/dL, as indicated, and administer ordered insulin to prevent hypoglycemia. (DO NOT ADMINISTER INSULIN SUBCUTANEOUSLY.)

d. Carefully monitor serum osmolality and administer ordered hypotonic and isotonic IV solutions to prevent rapid drop of serum osmolality. Gradually reduce blood sugar with regular insulin.

e. Assess neurologic changes to monitor for complications of a rapid drop in serum osmolality.

3. Injury: high risk for

a. Monitor for decreased arterial blood pH with mildly decreased HCO_3, increased serum ketones, increased serum lactate, and decreased venous CO_2 to determine onset of acidosis.

b. Administer ordered hypotonic and isotonic IV solutions with potassium, sodium bicarbonate, and regular insulin, as indicated.

Monitoring, Managing, and Preventing Life-Threatening Emergencies.

1. Persistent coma

a. Monitor level of consciousness.

    1) Assess for changes in pupillary response to light, sensorimotor functions, respiratory rate and rhythm, and blood pressure.

    2) Test responses to verbal and tactile (including painful) stimuli.

    3) Observe for decerebrate or decorticate posturing or seizure activity.

b. Maintain homeostasis.

       1) Protect and manage airway. Be prepared to institute emergency intubation and mechanical ventilation if airway becomes compromised.

       2) Monitor laboratory values to determine fluid status and report significant changes.

       3) Continuously monitor cardiac rhythm and report arrhythmias.

  c. Provide adequate nutrition.

       1) Institute ordered enteral or parenteral nutrition.

       2) Weigh daily to identify weight loss.

       3) Monitor serum albumin and transferrin to identify altered nutrition.

       4) Monitor for and institute measures to prevent skin breakdown.

  d. Prepare family to accept persistent coma state, if it becomes imminent.

       1) Provide support and answer questions.

       2) Convene family conferences with multidisciplinary team members to discuss the patient.

2. Pulmonary or cerebral emboli

  a. Promote nursing actions that prevent venous stasis.

       1) Apply antiembolic stockings.

           a) Sequential compression devices provide cyclic compression and relaxation periods that closely approximate muscle contractions. They are the most effective type of antiembolic stocking for the intensive care unit (ICU) patient.

           b) Elastic hose and ace bandage wraps compress superficial veins in the legs and prevent venous stasis there. They are difficult to apply and remove in the ICU setting. They are most useful in the ambulatory patient.

       2) Assist with active and passive exercises.

       3) Avoid venipunctures in the legs.

       4) Do not forcibly irrigate clotted IV lines.

       5) Administer ordered anticoagulants.

       6) Prevent dehydration.

       7) Elevate legs to promote venous return.

       8) Instruct patient not to cross legs.

       9) Instruct patient not to keep knees bent while in bed.

   b. Assess for changes in:
     1) Pupillary response to light
     2) Sensorimotor functions
     3) Respiratory rate and rhythm
     4) Blood pressure
   c. Monitor for signs of respiratory distress.
     1) Observe for dyspnea and tachypnea.
     2) Check nailbeds for pallor or cyanosis.
     3) Observe for anxiety, apprehension, and restlessness.
     4) Be prepared to institute mechanical ventilation, if necessary.
     5) Apply pulse oximeter and continuously monitor oxygen saturation.
     6) Obtain blood specimens and monitor ABGs.
   d. Promote activities to improve ventilation.
     1) Encourage coughing and deep breathing in the non-comatose patient.
     2) Observe color and consistency of expectorated secretions. Hemoptysis may occur.
     3) Administer ordered supplemental oxygen.
     4) Observe for respiratory distress with patient care activities; interrupt care if it occurs; and space activities to prevent recurrence of respiratory distress.
     5) Elevate the head of the bed.
     6) Auscultate the lungs frequently for abnormal and adventitious sounds and report significant findings.
     7) Assist with incentive spirometry in the non-comatose patient or aerosol treatments in the comatose patient, as ordered.
   e. Institute and monitor patient for side effects of anticoagulant therapy.
     1) Assess for and prevent overt bleeding.
       a) Check injection sites for bleeding.
       b) Apply pressure to venipuncture sites until bleeding stops.
       c) Observe for bleeding from the gums following mouth care.
       d) Check for epistaxis (nosebleeds).
     2) Assess for and prevent occult bleeding.

     a) Check for blood in the urine and stool.
     b) Administer ordered antacids to prevent stress ulceration.
     c) Observe for bruising and hematomas especially at injection sites.
     d) Monitor hematocrit and hemoglobin for decrease.
   3) Keep protamine sulfate or vitamin K available for bleeding.
   4) Monitor laboratory studies to assess anticoagulation.

3. Cardiopulmonary arrest
  a. Call for help.
  b. Begin cardiopulmonary resuscitation.
  c. Follow with advanced cardiac life support.

6 HEMATOLOGIC DISORDERS

Disseminated Intravascular Coagulation

Disseminated intravascular coagulation (DIC) is a secondary disorder of widespread microvascular clotting that depletes clotting factors causing a paradoxic coexistence of both thrombosis and hemorrhage.

Septic shock, caused by every type of infection, is the primary cause of DIC and has a mortality rate of 80%. Burns and trauma are the second leading cause.

Etiology/Pathophysiology

1. Disorders that trigger an excessive consumption of the clotting factors include:
   a. Sepsis/Infection — metabolic acidosis, sluggish blood flow, release of adenosine diphosphate and phospholipids from traumatized cells, endothelial damage, and hypoxemia of cells contribute to developing DIC
   b. Burns/Trauma
   c. Massive gastrointestinal bleeding
   d. Liver trauma
   e. Severe hypoxia
   f. Abruptio placentae
   g. Sickle cell crisis
   h. Leukemia — especially acute progranulocytic leukemia
   i. Incompatible transfusion reactions
   j. Transurethral prostatectomy
2. Pathophysiology
   a. Results from an increased amount of normal clotting with a decrease in clotting factors and platelets
   b. Severe illness or injury generates an excess of thrombin with resultant fibrin formation, ischemic tissue damage and rapid consumption of clotting factors. Eventually clotting factors are consumed, and the blood loses its ability to clot.
   c. The body's fibrinolytic system, a homeostatic mechanism that limits coagulation, is triggered. Then the patient cannot form stable clots, and bleeding occurs at multiple sites throughout the body.
   d. Any organ system may be involved; however, the kidneys, lungs, central nervous system, and the gastrointestinal system are most often affected.

Assessment/Analysis

THROMBOTIC ASSESSMENT FINDINGS (Based on underlying cause and degree of organ involvement)

Subjective

1. Confusion
2. Chest pain

Objective

1. Oliguria
2. Cool extremities
3. Purpura
4. Edema
5. Generalized diaphoresis
6. Cyanosis
7. Weak or absent pulses

HEMORRHAGIC ASSESSMENT FINDINGS (Based on underlying cause and degree of organ involvement)

Subjective

1. Weakness
2. Dyspnea
3. Nausea or vomiting
4. Bone or joint pain
5. Abdominal tenderness
6. Headache
7. Vertigo
8. Visual disturbances
9. Difficulty voiding because of bladder clots or retroperitoneal hematoma

Objective

1. Bleeding from intravenous (IV) insertion sites or from body orifices such as ears, rectum, vagina, nose, lungs, and the gastrointestinal tract
2. Petechiae, purpura, or ecchymosis
3. Gingival or scleral hemorrhages
4. Hematuria
5. Hematemesis, hematochezia, hemoptysis, or melena
6. Increased abdominal girth from deep hemorrhages
7. Paresis
8. Hypoxemia

9. Decreased blood pressure
10. Narrowing pulse pressure
11. Rapid and thready pulse
12. Postural hypotension
13. Decreased breath sounds and gurgles

SUPPORTING TEST FINDINGS

Laboratory Tests

1. Platelet count
   Abnormality: Decreased
2. Bleeding time
   Abnormality: Increased bleeding time suggests decreased platelet count or severe factor deficiency.
3. Serum fibrinogen levels
   Abnormality: Decreased because of hypofibrinogenemia, fibrinolysis, severe hepatic disease, malignant processes, or obstetric trauma.
4. Prothrombin time (PT)
   Abnormality: Increased because of decreased factor I, II, VII, or X, hepatic disease, or vitamin K deficiency.
5. Partial thromboplastin time (PTT)
   Abnormality: Increased because of heparin, fibrin split products, decreased factors other than VII or XIII.
6. Fibrin split products
   Abnormality: Increased during DIC and may differentiate DIC from other coagulation disorders
7. Protamine sulfate test
   Abnormality: Positive
8. D-dimer test
   Abnormality: Increased in DIC, predictive of DIC, and a conformation test for elevated fibrin degradation product
9. Serum bilirubin
   Abnormality: Increased as it measures the extent of red blood cell (RBC) destruction or ability of the liver to excrete
10. Serum creatinine phosphokinase
    Abnormality: Increased
11. Serum lactate
    Abnormality: Increased

12. Reticulocyte count
    Abnormality: Increased

Diagnostic Tests

1. There are no specific diagnostic tests for DIC.
2. Appropriate examination of organ suspected of causing the disorder may be performed.

Planning/Intervention

COLLABORATIVE MANAGEMENT

Procedures

1. Assist with treatment of the underlying cause, such as surgical debridement of necrotic tissue or abscess or antibiotic treatment of pathogenic organisms.
2. Administer heparin therapy, blood component therapy, and antithrombin therapy to stop the vicious cycle of thrombosis-hemorrhage.
3. Maintain patient on strict bed rest.
4. Correct hemostatic deficiencies that compromise the clotting mechanisms with drug therapy, as ordered.
5. Administer ordered IV fluids to correct hypovolemia, hypotension, and tissue ischemia.

Drug Therapy

1. Anticoagulant therapy
   Example: sodium heparin (Heparin)
   Action: Inhibits the formation of new clots that will slow down the consumption of clotting factors. Prevents thrombus formation and extension of existing thrombi.
   Caution: Do not use if bleeding
        Heparin is not helpful in sepsis
        Can cause hepatitis, bleeding thrombocytopenia, rashes, urticaria, hypersensitivity, and fever
2. Antifibrinolytic therapy
   Examples: aminocaproic acid (Amicar)
   Action: Interrupts the fibrinolytic process through inhibition of plasmin

Caution: Has potential for large-vessel thrombosis
   Never administer without first treating with blood products and heparin

3. Blood replacement therapy (in order of priority)
   a. Administer platelets, fresh frozen plasma, cryoprecipitates, and RBCs given for severe depletion of platelets and coagulation factors.
   b. Replace platelet transfusions if platelet count falls below 50,000/mm^3.
      1) Infuse platelets rapidly to prevent clumping.
      2) Obtain a blood specimen for a platelet count 1 hour after transfusion to determine patient response to treatment.
   c. Administer fresh frozen plasma that contains clotting factors V, VIII, XIII, and antithrombin III for volume expansion.
   d. Administer cryoprecipitates, which contain factors VIII, XIII, and fibrinogen, for severe hypofibrinogenemia. As many as thirty 20-mL bags may be needed.
   e. Administer RBCs to replace hemoglobin.

NURSING MANAGEMENT

Monitoring and Managing Clinical Problems

1. Injury: high risk for
   a. Treat sepsis—administer fluids and antibiotics.
   b. Treat shock—administer IV fluids, inotropes, and vaso- pressors.
2. Tissue Perfusion, altered: cardiopulmonary
   a. Monitor vital signs for the following:
      1) Heart rate >100 bpm
      2) Systolic blood pressure <90 mm Hg
      3) Central venous pressure (CVP) <5 cm H_2O
      4) Mean arterial pressure <60 mm Hg
      5) Check pulses for adequate extremity perfusion.
   b. Report significant findings
3. Gas Exchange: impaired
   a. Assess breath sounds.
   b. Monitor for abnormal arterial blood gases (ABGs), dyspnea, cyanosis, and hypoxemia.
   c. Institute pulse oximetry to monitor PaO_2.

    d. Administer oxygen, as ordered.

    e. Monitor mental status for oxygenation problems.

    f. Prevent atelectasis by turning, coughing, and deep breathing.

    g. Administer bronchodilators and fluid replacement, as ordered.

    h. Implement positive end-expiratory pressure (PEEP), sedation, and paralysis, as ordered.

4. Urinary Elimination: altered

    a. Monitor hourly intake and output noting decreased urinary output, which may indicate hypovolemia or renal microemboli.

    b. Monitor urine specific gravity noting an increase, which may indicate hypovolemia or renal microemboli.

    c. Decreased urinary output may indicate fluid retention.

5. Fluid Volume Excess

    a. Assess heart and lung sounds for signs of volume overload.

    b. Monitor cardiac output (CO) and pulmonary artery pressure (PAP).

    c. Record hourly intake of IV and oral fluids.

6. Skin Integrity: impaired, high risk for

    a. Monitor and manage skin and mucous membranes for bleeding, cyanosis, and lesions resulting from hypovolemia and ischemia.

    b. Prevent skin breakdown by:

        1) Perform frequent mouth care.

        2) For oral care, use a mild solution of peroxide.

        3) Avoid mouthwashes containing alcohol.

        4) Suction trachea, as needed, using low pressure to prevent damage to the tracheal mucosa.

        5) Keep the skin moist and intact by applying lotions to the skin and lubricants to the lips.

        6) Note extremity warmth, color, and pulses.

        7) Check emesis, nasogastric tube drainage, and stool for occult blood.

7. Pain

    a. Reposition every 2 hours for comfort and proper alignment.

    b. Rate pain level 0–10 every 1–2 hours.

    c. Administer pain medication promptly.

    d. Use noninvasive pain relief measures such as relaxation techniques.

    e. Prepare patient for all treatments and procedures.

    f. Perform gentle range of motion every 2 hours.

8. Nutrition: altered, less than body requirements

    a. Monitor hourly intake and output.

    b. Avoid offering hot fluids that will irritate the oral mucosa and gingival bleeding.

    c. Weight daily and maintain body weight within 10% of normal weight.

    d. Assess bowel sounds for presence of paralytic ileus.

    e. Monitor hyperalimentation, if ordered.

Monitoring, Managing, and Preventing Life-Threatening Emergencies

1. Hemorrhage

    a. Treat the underlying cause.

    b. Monitor the following organ systems every 2 hours:

        1) Neurologic system for pupil constriction, headache, and weakness

        2) Respiratory system for dyspnea, hemoptysis, and chest pain

        3) Renal system for clots in urine and bladder spasms

        4) Gastrointestinal system for occult blood in stool and abdominal pain

    c. Monitor the amount of bleeding and record to determine significant change.

    d. Observe for oozing of blood at multiple sites and presence of petechiae, purpura, ecchymoses, and hemorrhagic gingivitis.

    e. Test all drainage for occult blood.

    f. Measure all blood loss: emesis, nasogastric drainage, hemoptysis, wound drainage, drains, and hematochezia.

    g. Weigh all bandages.

    h. Measure abdominal girth or other body parts where bleeding may occur for example in the arm after ABGs are drawn.

    i. Monitor for changes in blood pressure.

    j. Administer IV fluids and medications to maintain a normal blood pressure.

k. Limit using a blood pressure cuff to avoid rupture of superficial capillaries.
l. Avoid having the patient dangle limbs or be in Trendelenburg position since gravitational pressure can cause bleeding or ecchymoses.
m. Administer heparin, as ordered, and monitor the PTT so that a therapeutic blood level may be maintained.
n. Monitor all coagulation values: PT, PTT, fibrinogen levels, and factors V and VIII.
o. Administer transfusion therapy, as ordered, to replace depleted products such as RBCs, fresh frozen plasma, and cryoprecipitate.
   1) Institute blood administration.
      a) Use at least a 20-gauge needle.
      b) Start all transfusions at a slow rate.
      c) Do not infuse any fluids or medications in the same line.
      d) When administering large amounts of blood, use a warming device.
   2) Monitor any transfusion reactions:
      a) Hives
      b) Chills
      c) Fever
      d) Chest pain
      e) Shortness of breath
      f) Headaches
      g) Altered level of consciousness
      h) Nausea and vomiting
      i) Low back pain
   3) Monitor vital signs and urine output.
   4) Treat transfusion reactions as needed by:
      a) Infusing large volumes of IV fluids to prevent renal damage.
      b) Administering diuretics such as furosemide of at least 100 mL/h
      c) Prepare patient for dialysis, if needed.
p. To prevent bruising, observe safety precautions, such as padding the siderails and using an electric razor.
q. Avoid needle stick or use a very small-gauge needle and apply pressure to the venipuncture site for 10 minutes.
r. Avoid the use of rectal temperatures, vaginal or rectal

suppositories, enemas, and digital examinations of the rectum and vagina.
- s. Avoid use of aspirin and steroids that compromise hematologic and immunologic functions leading to potential bleeding and infection.
- t. Avoid the Valsalva maneuver.
- u. Administer histamine-2 receptor antagonists, as ordered.
2. Thrombosis
   - a. Results in tissue ischemia and necrosis.
   - b. Monitor the following organ systems every 2 hours:
     1) Renal system — May cause acute tubular necrosis.
        - a) Monitor hourly fluid intake and urine output.
        - b) Assess for fluid retention and electrolyte disturbances.
     2) Neurologic system
        - a) Monitor level of consciousness.
        - b) Check pupil reaction to light and accommodation.
        - c) Monitor for paresthesias, numbness, and tingling.
        - d) Assess for headaches, behavioral changes, lethargy, confusion dizziness, focal changes, weakness, and inequality in motor strength.
     3) Gastrointestinal system
        - a) Auscultate bowel sounds.
        - b) Palpate for abdominal distention and tenderness.
     4) Cardiovascular system
        - a) Monitor blood pressure.
        - b) Auscultate heart sounds for gallop rhythms and murmurs.
        - c) Monitor for dysrhythmias.
        - d) Monitor hemodynamic status by measuring CVP, PAP, pulmonary capillary wedge pressure, and CO.
        - e) Assess peripheral pulses, capillary refill, and dependent edema.
        - f) Observe for angina and signs of myocardial infarction.

    5) Respiratory system
      a) Monitor respiratory patterns.
      b) Auscultate breath sounds.
  c. Monitor for hypoxemia and acidosis.
    1) Monitor ABGs, respirations, and skin color.
    2) Check serum lactate, as ordered.
    3) Administer O_2, PEEP, or mechanical ventilation, as ordered.

Organ Transplantation

Transplantation is the removal of a normal functioning organ from one body and placement of it into another body. Kidney, heart, and liver are the most commonly transplanted organs.

Etiology/Pathophysiology

1. Kidney transplantation is performed for end-stage renal diseases such as glomerulonephritis (the leading cause of renal failure), anatomic defects, trauma, or diabetes. Transplantation is usually not performed until the patient with end-stage renal failure has been stabilized on hemodialysis.
2. Heart transplantation is performed for organ failure and end-stage diseases, such as cardiomyopathy, coronary artery disease, valvular disease, congenital heart disease, and myocarditis.
3. Liver transplantation is performed for end-stage liver disease, such as chronic active hepatitis, acute fulminant hepatitis, sclerosing cholangitis, autoimmune cirrhosis, biliary tract carcinoma, and Budd-Chiari syndrome.

Assessment/Analysis

ASSESSMENT FINDINGS AFTER TRANSPLANTATION

KIDNEY TRANSPLANTATION

Subjective

1. Pain
2. Feelings of apprehension

Objective

1. Low-grade fever
2. Dehydration
3. Blood and urine drainage from abdominal dressing
4. Mouth ulcerations
5. Hypertension
6. Signs of electrolyte imbalance

HEART TRANSPLANTATION

Subjective

1. Pain

2. Anxiety

Objective

1. Arrhythmias
2. Bleeding
3. Dehydration
4. Fever

LIVER TRANSPLANTATION

Subjective

1. Pain
2. Anxiety

Objective

1. Seizures
2. Signs of thrombosis at the anastomosis site
3. Hypothermia
4. Dehydration
5. Signs of biliary obstruction
6. Fever

SUPPORTING TEST FINDINGS
AFTER TRANSPLANTATION

KIDNEY

Laboratory Tests

1. Blood urea nitrogen (BUN) and serum creatinine
   Abnormality: Increased
2. Beta$_2$-microglobin test
   Abnormality: Increased
3. Serum potassium
   Abnormality: Increased

Diagnostic Tests

1. Renal scan
   Abnormality: Decreased renal perfusion
2. Technetium diethylenetriamine penta-acetic acid (DPTA) scan of the kidney
   Abnormality: Decreased renal vascular supply

Tests Ordered for Suspected Transplant Rejection

Sequential multiple analysis-20
Complete blood count with differential
Prothrombin time (PT)
Partial thromboplastin time (PTT)
Serum cyclosporine trough level
Bacterial cultures of bile, urine, and throat
Serum amylase, ammonia, and magnesium levels

HEART

Laboratory Tests

1. Serum potassium
   Abnormality: Decreased when patient is experiencing unstable myocardial conduction
2. Serum cholesterol and lipids
   Abnormality: Increased with related atherosclerosis

LIVER

Laboratory Tests

1. Serum glutamic oxaloacetic transaminase (SGOT) serum glutamic pyruvic transaminase (SGPT) and bilirubin
   Abnormality: Increased in hepatic failure
2. Blood glucose
   Abnormality: Decreased in hepatic failure
3. PT, PTT, fibrinogen
   Abnormality: Increased PT in hepatic failure
   Decreased fibrinogen levels in hepatic failure
4. Serum liver enzymes and alkaline phosphatase
   Abnormality: Increased with rejection, obstruction, and cell destruction

Planning/Intervention

COLLABORATIVE MANAGEMENT OF THE RENAL TRANSPLANT PATIENT

1. Organ transplantation
   a. Monitor/assess graft function.

    b. Monitor/assess fluid and electrolyte status.
        1) Maintain patency and functioning of central line to ensure accurate monitoring of fluid status.
        2) Maintain patency of urinary drainage catheter.
        3) Maintain patency of nasogastric tube.
    c. Administer ordered immunosuppressive and pain medications.
    d. Monitor/assess for rejection, infection, and bleeding.
    e. Prepare patient for hemodialysis, as ordered.
    f. Do continuous cardiac monitoring.
2. Drug therapy
    a. Corticosteroids
       Example: prednisone (Deltasone)
       Action: Reduces accumulation of macrophages and leukocytes
          Inhibits phagocytosis and lysosomal enzyme release
          Reduces T lymphocytes, monocytes, and eosinophils
       Caution: Can cause osteoporosis, hyperglycemia, infection, bleeding, delayed healing, steroid psychosis, fluid retention, and hypertension
    b. Antimetabolites
       Example: azathioprine (Imuran)
       Action: Inhibits deoxyribonucleic acid (DNA), ribonucleic acid (RNA), and protein synthesis that limits proliferation of T or B lymphocytes; once T-cell recognition of graft occurs, drug should be discontinued
       Caution: Before each dose, the hematocrit, white blood cell (WBC) count and differential, and platelet count are studied to determine if changes in dosage are needed; any evidence of the following requires a dosage change or discontinuation of drug: decreased leukocyte count, decreased platelet count, liver dysfunction, skin eruption, and evidence of infection; can cause infection, hepatotoxicity, pancreatitis, leukopenia, anemia, or thrombocytopenia
    c. Fungal cyclic peptide
       Example: cyclosporine (Cyclosporin A)
       Action: Prevents early T-cell activation; suppresses T-

lymphocyte proliferation; affects humoral and cell-mediated immunity

Caution: Can cause nephrotoxicity, tremors, seizures, coma, hirsutism, hypertension, hyperkalemia, hepatotoxicity, and lymphomas

d. Immunoglobulin and lymphocyte immunosuppressant

Example: antihymocyte globulin (ATG)

Action: Prevents or delays onset or reverses acute renal allograft rejection

Caution: Can cause seizures, tachycardia, dyspnea, laryngospasm, and pulmonary edema

e. Murine monoclonal antibody

Example: orthoclone (OKT3)

Action: Interferes with normal T-cell function causing immunosuppression

Caution: Can cause severe pulmonary edema, chest pain, fever, and chills

f. Alkylating agent

Example: cyclophosphamide (Cytoxan)

Action: Blocks DNA, RNA, and protein to provide pronounced immunosuppressive activity

Caution: Can cause leukopenia, pulmonary emboli, interstitial pulmonary fibrosis, and hemorrhagic cystitis

g. Antimetabolite and folic acid antagonist

Example: methotrexate (Mexate)

Action: Interferes with folic acid metabolism inhibiting DNA synthesis and cell reproduction; causes immunosuppression

Caution: Can cause hepatotoxicity, hepatic cirrhosis, aplastic bone marrow, pneumonitis, marked myelosuppression, and ulcerative stomatitis

NURSING MANAGEMENT OF THE RENAL TRANSPLANT PATIENT

Monitoring and Managing Clinical Problems

1. Fluid Volume Excess: high risk for
   a. Monitor vital signs. Take blood pressure on the extremity that does not have a functioning vascular access site.

    b. Monitor for increased central venous pressure (CVP).

    c. Monitor for changes in level of consciousness.

    d. Monitor level of pain and response to pain medication.

    e. Monitor abdominal dressing for drainage.

    f. Monitor nasogastric drainage for coffee-ground or bloody drainage.

    g. Weigh and measure abdominal girth daily.

    h. Check patency of urinary drainage systems and ureteral catheters.

    i. Check the vascular access site and determine patency by placing a stethoscope over the access site and listening for a loud pulsating bruit.

    j. Assess breath sounds for crackles.

    k. Monitor for signs of dependent edema.

2. Urinary Elimination: altered

    a. Remember the amount of urine produced is dependent on the length of time the donor kidney was ischemic.

    b. Monitor fluctuations in urine output that could be attributed to clotted or kinked catheter tubing:

        1) Pain

        2) Urgency to void

        3) Bloody leakage around catheter

    c. If clotting occurs, gently irrigate with small amounts of preservative-free normal saline solution irrigant using strict aseptic technique.

    d. Monitor for urinary leakage on the abdominal dressing and from the ureteral anastomosis site.

    e. Monitor for and report severe abdominal flank pain or decreased urinary output, which may indicate loss of graft function.

    f. Administer ordered diuretics to maintain diuresis.

    g. Monitor for evidence of lymphocele and prepare to intervene.

        1) Monitor for genital edema, ipsilateral lower extremity edema, decreased urine output, increased BUN, and increased serum creatinine.

        2) Prepare patient for percutaneous drainage.

    h. Monitor for evidence of ureter obstruction and prepare to intervene.

        1) Monitor for decreased urine output and increased BUN.

    2) Prepare patient for surgical repair.
  i. Monitor for evidence of renal venous thrombosis and prepare to intervene.
    1) Monitor for graft swelling, oliguria, and lower extremity edema.
    2) Prepare patient for thrombectomy and initiate ordered anticoagulant therapy.
  j. Monitor for hypertension caused by steroids, sodium and water retention caused by cyclosporine, and increased renin secretion, and institute appropriate interventions.
    1) Monitor for hypertension and increased weight gain. Immediately postoperative hypertension is common.
    2) Restrict salt; teach patient the importance of weight reduction and healthy heart living.
3. Fluid Volume Excess or Deficit
  a. Monitor hourly urine output for <60 mL/h.
    1) Anuria is caused by acute tubular necrosis, acute rejection, urinary tract obstruction, and renal arterial thrombosis.
    2) Prepare patient for hemodialysis, as needed.
  b. Monitor for high urine output and institute appropriate interventions.
    1) When urine output is high, diuresis replacement will be large. While in anuric state, replacement will be small.
    2) Give intravenous (IV) fluid replacement. Usually administer normal saline solution, 5% dextrose in water, or 0.5% normal saline solution.
    3) Monitor for hyperkalemia, the most frequent electrolyte imbalance. It may result from dextrose-containing IV fluids or steroid-induced diabetes. Substitute normal saline IV fluids to correct problem or administer sodium polystyrene sulfonate (Kayexelate) and ion-exchange resin.

Monitoring, Managing, and Preventing Life-Threatening Emergencies After Renal Transplant

1. Hyperacute rejection
  a. Occurs within minutes to hours after transplantation as a result of humoral immunity.

    b. There is no treatment. Results in loss of graft.

2. Acute rejection

    a. Monitor for signs and symptoms of acute rejection such as:

      1) Fever

      2) Hypertension (one of the first signs of renal rejection

      3) Tenderness at site of transplant

      4) Decreased urinary output

      5) Increased serum transaminases

      6) Decreased cardiac output (CO)

      7) Weight gain

      8) General malaise

    b. Monitor laboratory test findings for evidence of non-functioning kidney.

      1) Increased serum BUN and creatinine; decreased creatinine clearance and urine sodium.

      2) Leukocytosis

      3) Decreased renal perfusion on technetium DPTA scan

      4) Increase in the size of the transplanted kidney on ultrasound

    c. Administer methylprednisolone therapy (Solu-Medrol) 1 g IV daily 3–5 days for signs of rejection. Monitor for signs of:

      1) Muscle weakness

      2) Easy bruising

      3) Cushing's syndrome

      4) Negative nitrogen balance

      5) Emotional lability

3. Infection

    a. Originating site may be:

      1) Blood (septicemia)

      2) Single organ such as liver, lungs, or pancreas

      3) Systemic such as disseminated infection

      4) IV lines, indwelling urethral catheters, wounds, or from postoperative pneumonia

    b. Prevent the development of monilial infections that are common after renal transplantation, assessing the mouth daily and administering of an oral antifungal agent such as nystatin, as needed.

    c. If fungal infection is suspected, be prepared to administer an antifungal agent such as amphotericin B.

4. Gastrointestinal bleeding
    a. Chronic steroid therapy increases the risk of peptic ulceration and erosive gastritis because it increases the secretion of hydrochloric acid and pepsinogen.
    b. Administer a histamine$_2$-receptor antagonist, such as cimetidine to prevent gastric ulceration.
    c. Administer saline lavage if bleeding occurs.
    d. Replaced lost volume with crystalloids and colloids.
    e. Assist with endoscopy and measures to stop bleeding (sclerotherapy, vasopressin administration, or banding).

5. Hypertension
    a. If the causative agent of hypertension is steroid induced, monitor for electrolyte imbalances especially hyponatremia and hypokalemia.
    b. Monitor the patient's weight because of rapid diuresis that may follow steroid therapy.
    c. Auscultate abdomen for the sudden appearance of a bruit or an increase in an abdominal bruit, which would indicate renal artery stenosis.
    d. If renal artery stenosis causes hypertension, prepare the patient for surgical repair or balloon angioplasty, as indicated.
    e. If the patient is given metoprolol tartrate (Lopresor) or propranolol (Inderal) to treat renin-dependent hypertension, monitor for congestive heart failure.
    f. If the patient is on any antihypertensive drugs, monitor for orthostatic hypotension.

NURSING MANAGEMENT OF THE HEART TRANSPLANT PATIENT

Monitoring and Managing Clinical Problems

1. Injury: high risk for
    a. Monitor for signs of humoral rejection such as: hyperlipidemia, hypercholesterolemia, silent myocardial infarction, arrhythmias, and congestive heart failure.
    b. Prepare patient for bypass surgery, angioplasty, or retransplantation.

    c. Administer dipyridamole and warfarin therapy, as ordered.

    d. Teach patient about coronary artery disease.

2. Cardiac Output: decreased
   a. Monitor electrocardiogram (ECG) for ischemia.
   b. Monitor for arrhythmias.
   c. Monitor for peripheral edema.
   d. Reduce myocardial oxygen demands by limiting activity and spacing nursing care to allow for adequate rest periods.
   e. Monitor for increased emotional stress.
   f. Monitor hemodynamic monitoring catheter readings for decreased CO and increased pulmonary capillary wedge pressure indicating congestive heart failure.

3. Fluid Volume Deficit
   a. Monitor vital signs and check for orthostatic hypotension.
   b. Weigh daily and maintain accurate intake and output.
   c. Administer ordered blood and IV fluids.
   d. Monitor for signs of dehydration (thirst, dry mucous membranes, poor skin turgor, alterations in level of consciousness).
   e. Monitor ECG for signs of arrhythmias or ischemia.
   f. Monitor pulmonary artery pressures (PAPs) for decreases.

4. Body Image Disturbance
   a. Allow the patient to express any concerns regarding the death of the donor.
   b. Encourage the patient to communicate with a psychiatrist, clergy, or other transplant recipients.

Monitoring, Managing, and Preventing Life-Threatening Emergencies After Heart Transplant

1. Ventricular failure
   a. Monitor hemodynamics parameters and note any changes from baseline.
   b. Administer ordered inotropic and afterload-reducing agents.
   c. Assist with insertion of intra-aortic balloon pump to support ventricular function.

    d. Reduce myocardial oxygen demands by limiting activity and spacing nursing care to allow for adequate rest periods.

2. Unstable myocardial conduction
    a. Monitor for bradycardia, premature atrial or ventricular beats, and ectopic beats that can occur from edema from suture lines, manipulation of the myocardium, or ischemia.
    b. Administer a lidocaine drip, as ordered (usually 2 mg/min).
    c. Monitor serum potassium levels and administer potassium for hypokalemia.
    d. Provide adequate oxygenation.
    e. Monitor serial arterial blood gases and maintain acid-base balance through hyperventilation or medication.

3. Infection
    a. Assess surgical incisions, invasive catheters, and procedure sites for evidence of infection.
    b. Administer ordered prophylactic antibiotics.

4. Rejection
    a. Administer ordered immunosuppressive drugs.
    b. Hyperacute rejection can be minimized by screening the recipient for cytotoxic antibodies before transplantation and confirming the donor's ABO blood group type with the recipient before transplantation.
    c. Monitor for signs and symptoms of rejection, such as:
      1) Malaise, secondary to necrosis of the myocardial tissue
      2) Weight gain
      3) S_3 or S_4 heart sounds
      4) Signs of heart failure, particularly right ventricular failure
      5) Vague chest discomfort
      6) Fever
    d. As needed, prepare the patient for endomyocardial biopsy, the only reliable indicator of rejection.
    e. Assist with management to reverse attempts of acute rejection.
      1) Assist with placement of an intra-aortic balloon pump for maintenance of blood pressure.
      2) Provide inotropic support using dopamine hydro-

chloride, dobutamine hydrochloride, and epinephrine.
3) Administer orthoklone along with azathioprine,
prednisone, and cyclosporine.
4) Prepare patient for daily plasmapheresis to prevent antibody resynthesis.
5) Administer rabbit antihymnocyte globulin (RATG)
to treat acute rejection episodes resistant to high-
dose corticosteroid therapy.

NURSING MANAGEMENT OF THE LIVER TRANSPLANT PATIENT

Monitoring and Managing Clinical Problems

1. Tissue Perfusion, altered: cardiopulmonary
   a. Assist with insertion of peripheral and central catheters, and monitor arterial and PAPs.
   b. Measure output of urine and abdominal drains.
   c. Replace blood losses with crystalloids or colloids, as
   ordered.
   d. Prepare patient for mechanical ventilation (usually
   for 24–48 hours postoperatively) and monitor ventilator parameters.
   e. Monitor serum glucose for initial increases followed
   by decreases if liver rejected.
2. Injury: high risk for
   a. Monitor for signs and symptoms of liver failure from
   hepatic vein thrombosis including increased liver
   enzymes, sepsis, bile leak, and coagulopathies.
   b. Prepare patient for retransplantation, if needed.
3. Injury: high risk for
   a. Monitor for signs and symptoms of partial vein
   thrombosis including abdominal distention, increased ascites, and portal hypertension.
   b. Prepare patient for retransplantation, if needed.
4. Tissue Perfusion, altered: hepatic
   a. Monitor for signs and symptoms of biliary obstruction including decreased bile production, jaundice,
   increased liver enzymes, and fever.
   b. Prepare patient for surgical placement of a T tube.
5. Fluid Volume Deficit
   a. Monitor serum electrolytes for abnormalities.

b. Monitor hemodynamic stability by frequent hemodynamic catheter readings to assess for decreased
   CO, CVP, and PAP.
c. Maintain accurate intake and output.
d. Monitor for dehydration by:
   1) Assessing skin turgor
   2) Auscultating breath sounds
   3) Measuring blood pressure and checking for or-
      thostatic hypotension
   4) Checking for decreased CVP and PAPs
e. Weigh daily.
f. Monitor immunosuppressive drug levels and renal
   function.
g. Be prepared to administer blood transfusion, fluids,
   vasopressors, dialysis, or continuous fresh frozen
   plasma.

6. Protection: altered
   a. Maintain strict handwashing technique to prevent
      nosocomial infection.
   b. Monitor serum drug levels to maintain the therapeu-
      tic range.
   c. Monitor for infection by monitoring serial WBCs and
      taking temperature every 4 hours.
   d. Monitor liver enzymes and alkaline phosphatase for
      increase, which may indicate rejection, obstruction,
      and cell destruction.

7. Hypothermia
   a. Monitor for shivering.
   b. Keep patient warm with blankets, warming lights,
      and warm inspired oxygen; administer fluid through
      blood warmer.
   c. Monitor temperature with a pulmonary artery
      catheter.

8. Injury: high risk for
   a. Observe bile drainage from T tube every hour; bile
      should be thick and golden brown.
   b. Monitor serum bilirubin, liver enzymes, and tem-
      perature.
   c. Observe for signs of infection by monitoring serial
      WBCs and taking temperature every 4 hours.
   d. Clean the T-tube site and keep dressing dry and in-
      tact changing, as needed.

 e. Assist patient with cholangiogram, if necessary.

 f. Observe for jaundice and right upper quadrant abdominal pain.

 g. Administer lipids with caution.

9. Tissue Perfusion, altered: hepatic

 a. Monitor for increase in serum transaminases (SGOT, SGPT) and bilirubin

 b. If liver function tests are elevated, prepare the patient for a Doppler ultrasound to assess for patent hepatic artery and portal vein.

 c. If Doppler ultrasound reveals an occlusion of the hepatic artery or the portal vein, prepare the patient for angiography.

 d. Prepare the patient for percutaneous dilatation or retransplantation if there is stricture or thrombosis.

10. Injury: high risk for

 a. Monitor for seizures, which are usually due to side effects of immunosuppressive medication, including OKT3 and cytoxan.

 b. Protect the patient from injury if a seizure occurs.

Monitoring, Managing, and Preventing Life-Threatening Emergencies After Liver Transplant

1. Infection

 a. Viral infection

  1) Monitor for fever, malaise, and arthralgias.

  2) Monitor for abdominal pain, nausea, vomiting gastrointestinal hemorrhage, diarrhea, pulmonary infiltration, elevated serum transaminases, decreased platelets, and decreased WBCs.

 b. Bacterial infections

  1) Administer broad-spectrum antibiotics, as ordered.

  2) Assure that the patient receives adequate caloric intake daily. Preventing malnutrition can reduce susceptibility of bacterial infections. A major source of bacterial infections is manipulation of the gastrointestinal tract during surgery, which leaks bacteria from the gut to the tissues and circulation.

 c. Fungal infections

  1) Administer low-dose amphotericin B, as ordered.

2. Hyperacute rejection
   a. Rare in liver transplantation
   b. Monitor for signs of total hepatic failure, such as:
      1) Depressed mental status (the most important indicator of early function); the patient should be awake and alert within 12 hours after surgery.
      2) Abnormal liver function
      3) Uncorrectable coagulopathy
      4) Hypothermia
      5) Thin, watery bile
      6) Hypoglycemia
   c. If this rare occurrence happens, immediate retransplantation is required.
3. Subacute rejection
   a. May occur 2–4 days after transplantation
   b. Monitor for signs of:
      1) Fever
      2) Jaundice
      3) Clay-colored stools
      4) Dark tea-colored urine
      5) Bile changes from golden brown to a colorless fluid
      6) Malaise
      7) Fluid retention
   c. Prepare patient for a biopsy, which is needed to confirm the diagnosis.
   d. Increased dosages of immunosuppressive drugs will be needed; administer higher doses, as ordered.
4. Acute rejection
   a. Remember this usually occurs 7–10 days after transplantation.
   b. Monitor for signs of rejection such as:
      1) Fever
      2) Jaundice
      3) Clay-colored stools
      4) Dark tea-colored urine
      5) Bile changes from golden brown to colorless fluid
      6) Altered liver function
   c. Monitor laboratory results for indications of rejection (increased liver function tests, increased WBC, evidence of altered coagulation studies, hyperglycemia).
   d. Be prepared to treat the patient with corticosteroids and monoclonal antibody (OKT3).

5. Fever
   a. May be a sign of rejection or infection in any transplant patient
   b. Evaluate the fever thoroughly before treatment
   c. Assess the following areas:
      1) Assess the lungs, urinary tract, and surgical incision first since these are the most common areas of infection.
      2) Assess for bacterial infection.
      3) Assess for fungal, viral, and protozoan infections.
6. Pulmonary edema
   a. Observe for increased circulating volume.
   b. Measure pulmonary vascular pressures.
   c. When edema occurs, administer O_2 and mechanical ventilation with positive end-expiratory pressure therapy
   d. Administer ordered diuretics.
   e. Observe for adequate ventilation, which can be compromised with fluid retention.

7 GASTRO-INTESTINAL DISORDERS

Acute Pancreatitis

Acute pancreatitis is an acute pancreatic inflammation. It may present in the following two ways: it may occur as an isolated event, or it may be one in a series of repeated attacks.

Etiology/Pathophysiology

1. Etiology
   a. Ninety percent of all cases are caused by ethanol abuse or cholelithiasis or are idiopathic.
   b. Other causes include:
      1) Abdominal surgery
      2) Trauma
      3) Injection into pancreatic duct (endoscopic retrograde (cholangiopancreatography)
      4) Hyperlipidemia
      5) Hypercalcemia
      6) Organ transplantation
      7) Peptic ulcer
      8) Outflow obstruction (i.e., sphincter of Oddi dysfunction
      9) Pregnancy
      10) Hereditary
      11) End-stage renal failure
      12) Scorpion bite
      13) Viral infections
      14) Parasite invasion of biliary ducts
      15) Hypoperfusion
      16) Drug-induced, particularly by azathioprine, thiazide diuretics, furosemide, estrogen, sulfonamides, tetracyclines, valproic acid, corticosteroids, and L-asparaginase
   c. In acute pancreatitis, a stimulus triggers the conversion of trypsinogen to activated trypsin within pancreatic tissue or within the intrapancreatic ducts. Activated trypsin then converts pancreatic proenzymes to active enzymes, converts kallikreininogen to kallikrein, and activates thrombolytic and thrombotic factors.
   d. Consequences of prematurely activated trypsin include:
      1) Active pancreatic enzymes
         a) Trypsin and chymotrypsin digests proteins and directly damages blood vessel walls.
         b) Lipase and phospholipase A cause fat necrosis and destruction of pancreatic cell membranes.

    c) Elastase dissolves elastic fibers of blood vessels, resulting in necrosis, erosion, and hemorrhage.

    d) Overall effect is the autodigestion of the pancreas with edema, vascular damage, hemorrhage, and necrosis. Fat digestion in the peritoneum allows calcium to sequester in the areas of necrosis, leading to hypocalcemia. Collections of tissue debris, blood, pancreatic juice and fat may form pseudocysts.

    e) The inflammatory process may extend to the duodenum, bile ducts, spleen, omentum, mediastinum, diaphragm, and perarenal spaces (this occurs because the pancreas has no capsule).

    f) A chemical peritonitis may occur, resulting in pancreatic ascites and abscess formation. Pleural effusions and pneumonitis may occur as a result of the spread of the inflammatory process via the diaphragmatic lymphatics. Distal lesions of fat necrosis may occur in the bone marrow, skin, mediastinum, pleural tissue, and nervous system due to circulating pancreatic lipase.

2) Kallikrein is converted to bradykinin and kallidin. This results in the following:

    a) Vasodilation

    b) Increased capillary permeability

    c) Leukocyte accumulation

    d) May decrease myocardial contractility

    e) Overall effects are stimulation of the inflammatory process causing pain, leaking of albumin into the interstitial space, third spacing of fluid, and the potentiation of shock.

3) Activated thrombolytic and thrombotic factors

    a) Trypsin encourages the conversion of plasminogen to plasmin, thereby promoting clot lysis.

    b) Trypsin promotes the conversion of prothrombin to thrombin, thereby encouraging clot formation.

    c) Overall effect is to promote the development of disseminated intravascular coagulation (DIC).

Stages of Pancreatitis

Acute Edematous Pancreatitis
- Interstitial edema
- Leukocyte infiltration
- Dilated capillaries and lymphatics

Necrotizing Pancreatitis
- Acinar cell death
- Necrosis of surrounding fatty tissue

Hemorrhagic Pancreatitis
- Collection of blood around and within the pancreas due to hemorrhage from ruptured blood vessels

2. Criteria to determine patients at high risk for a complicated course and increased mortality
   a. Increasing age
   b. Leukocytosis
   c. Hyperglycemia
   d. Elevated serum lactic dehydrogenase (LDH) and serum aspartate aminotransferase (AST) (serum glutamic oxaloacetic transminase [SGOT])
   e. Low hematocrit or significant drop in hematocrit with hydration
   f. Increased blood urea nitrogen (BUN)
   g. PaO_2 <60 mm Hg and other abnormal pulmonary findings
   h. Base deficit
   i. Hypotension
   j. Decreased serum calcium
   k. Serum albumin level <3.5 g/100 mL
   l. Need for massive fluid and colloid replacement
   m. Abdominal mass
   n. Hemorrhagic or discolored peritoneal fluid
   o. First episode of pancreatitis

Assessment/Analysis

ASSESSMENT FINDINGS

Subjective

1. Mild to severe incapacitating pain in the epigastrium or periumbilical area
   a. Dull and steady
   b. May radiate to the back, chest, flanks, or lower abdomen
   c. Intensified in a supine position
   d. Relieved by sitting in a knee-chest position
   e. May be referred to the shoulder or pleuritic pain if there is pulmonary involvement
2. Nausea
3. Vomiting
4. Hiccups

Objective

1. Acute overt distress
2. Anxiety
3. Mild abdominal distention
4. Tachypnea
5. Febrile 37.8–38.3°C (100–101°F)
6. Grey Turner's sign
7. Cullen's sign
8. Erythematous skin nodules primarily in the extremities
9. Jaundice (rarely)
10. Cool, pale, clammy skin
11. Oliguria
12. Coma
13. Confusion due to autotoxemia (toxic psychosis)
14. Hiccups
15. Diminished bowel sounds; may be absent
16. Basilar crackles, atelectasis, pleural effusions, if pulmonary involvement
17. Tachycardia
18. Hypotension or mild hypertension
19. Abdomen soft with no abdominal wall rigidity or rebound tenderness on initial examination

20. Intense localized epigastric tenderness to deep palpation

SUPPORTING TEST FINDINGS

Laboratory Tests

1. Serum amylase
   Abnormality: Increased 2–12 hours after onset of symptoms
   Returns to normal in 3–5 days
   May stay normal in some cases
   Magnitude of elevation gives no clue to prognosis
2. Serum lipase
   Abnormality: Increased 24 hours after onset of symptoms
   Returns to normal in 7–14 days
3. Pancreatic amylase isoenzyme
   Abnormality: Pancreatic/salivary ratio is >0.7
   Returns to normal in 7–14 days
4. Urine amylase/creatinine clearance ratio
   Abnormality: Increased to >4% (rises earlier and stays elevated longer than serum amylase)
5. Ascitic or pleural fluid amylase
   Abnormality: Increased levels that may be many times higher than serum values
6. Serum immunoreactive trypsinogen/trypsin
   Abnormality: Increased
7. Serum AST or SGOT
   Abnormality: Increased
8. Serum alanine aminotransferase (ALS) or serum glutamic pyruvic transaminase (SGPT)
   Abnormality: Increased in biliary tract disease
9. Serum alkaline phosphatase
   Abnormality: Increased in biliary tract disease
10. Serum LDH
    Abnormality: Increased
11. Serum bilirubin
    Abnormality: Increased (returns to normal in 4–7 days; may be associated with the presence of biliary stones)
12. Serum methemalbumin
    Abnormality: Increased

13. Blood sugar
    Abnormality: Increased, usually transiently
14. Serum calcium
    Abnormality: Decreased
15. Serum albumin
    Abnormality: Decreased
16. Hemoglobin and hematocrit
    Abnormality: Increased and will correct with volume replacement
17. White blood cell (WBC) count
    Abnormality: Increased
18. Serum triglycerides
    Abnormality: Increased
19. BUN
    Abnormality: Increased
20. Arterial PaO$_2$
    Abnormality: Decreased
21. Serum C-reactive protein
    Abnormality: Increased

Other Tests Proposed as Clinical Markers for Pancreatitis

1. Serum ribonuclease
2. Elastase-1
3. Phospholipase A2

Diagnostic Tests

1. Plain film of the abdomen
   Abnormality: Presence of free intraperitoneal air caused by perforation; may see dilated intestinal loops and/or edema or "thumb-printing" in intestinal infarction
2. Chest X-ray
   Abnormality: Fluffy infiltrates denoting pulmonary edema; may also see pleural effusions
3. Upper gastrointestinal contrast studies
   Abnormality: Evidence of pancreatic enlargement and parapancreatic inflammation; delayed gastric emptying
4. Abdominal ultrasound
   Abnormality: Presence of stones and dilation in the biliary

tree; can diagnose acute cholecystitis and development of a pseudocyst
5. Computed tomography scan of the abdomen
   Abnormality: Diffuse enlargement of the pancreas with irregular borders and patchy densities; may see poorly encapsulated fluid collections
6. Selective angiography
   Abnormality: Bleeding from the pancreatic duct

Planning/Intervention

COLLABORATIVE MANAGEMENT

Procedures

1. Supportive care
   a. Promote fluid and electrolyte balance by keeping patient NPO and administering ordered fluid resuscitation with crystalloids and colloids.
   b. Assist with insertion of a central venous or pulmonary artery catheter, as indicated. Monitor hemodynamic parameters and report significant changes. Institute appropriate interventions to correct alterations in fluid balance.
   c. Insert an indwelling urinary catheter as indicated. Measure intake and output hourly and intervene as appropriate.
   d. Monitor fluid and electrolyte status by monitoring serial serum chemistry levels; urine electrolytes and osmolality; daily weights; hourly vital signs; daily measurement of abdominal girth.
   e. Assist with insertion of central line and monitor central venous pressure (CVP) or pulmonary artery pressure (PAP). Report significant changes.
   f. Prepare patient for peritoneal lavage, sump drainage of necrotic pancreas, partial or complete pancreatectomy (excision of pancreas), or sphincterotomy (incision into sphincter of Oddi to enlarge it), as indicated.
   g. Monitor gastrointestinal status by following serial pancreatic enzymes, liver and pancreatic function tests, WBCs, serum triglycerides, and blood sugars.
   h. Insert nasogastric tube, attach to low suction, and keep patient NPO to promote gastrointestinal healing.

i. Administer ordered antacids and/or histamine$_2$-receptor antagonists.

j. Promote pain relief by administering ordered analgesics.

k. Monitor nutritional status by following serial laboratory tests, assessing for changes in physical exam, and resting metabolic expenditure.

l. Promote nutritional status by administering ordered total parenteral nutrition.

2. Monitor for complications.

a. Gastrointestinal
   1) Pancreatic phlegm, abscess, pseudocyst, fistula, ascites
   2) Acute intra-abdominal hemorrhage
   3) Acute cholangitis (inflammation of bile duct)
   4) Small bowel, duodenal, or transverse colon involvement with obstruction, necrosis, perforation, or fistula formation
   5) Splenic abscess, infarction, or hemorrhage; development of gastric fundic varices (enlarged engorged veins)

b. Pulmonary
   1) Pleural effusion
   2) Pneumonitis
   3) Atelectasis
   4) Adult respiratory distress syndrome (ARDS)

c. Cardiovascular
   1) Hypotension
   2) Sudden death
   3) Pericardial effusion
   4) Shock

d. Metabolic complications
   1) Hyperglycemia
   2) Hypertriglyceridemia
   3) Hypocalcemia
   4) Toxic psychosis
   5) Fat necrosis—arthritis, bone, skin, mediastinal, pleural, and nervous system lesions

Drug Therapy

1. Opioid analgesics
   Example: meperidine (Demerol)

Action: Reduces pain; causes less rise in pressure in the common bile duct than morphine

Caution: Somewhat increases pressure in the biliary tree, respiratory depression, nausea, vomiting, dizziness, constipation

2. Colloid solutions

Example: Human albumin (Albuminar — 5% and 25%)

Action: Expands blood volume; raises serum protein levels

   Used to replace sequestered proteins

Caution: May cause circulatory failure, hypertension, pulmonary edema, fluid overload

3. Crystalloid solutions

Example: Lactated Ringer's solution

   Normal saline solution

Action: Expand blood volume; replaces fluid and electrolytes lost in vomiting, and third spacing

Caution: May cause electrolyte imbalance, circulatory overload

4. Histamine $_2$-receptor antagonists

Example: cimetidine (Tagamet)

   ranitidine (Zantac)

   famotidine (Pepcid)

Action: Inhibits gastric acid secretion; prevents gastric bleeding and ulceration

Caution: Can cause diarrhea, headache, dizziness, nausea, myalgia (muscle pain), skin rashes

5. Antibiotics

Example: Piperacillin and gentamycin used in combination

Action: Provides coverage for gram-negative rods, gram-positive cocci, and anaerobic pathogens

Caution: Piperacillin can cause seizures, rashes, hypokalemia, phlebitis at intravenous (IV) site, anaphylaxis

   Gentamycin can cause ototoxicity and nephrotoxicity

6. Antacids

Example: magnesium hydroxide/aluminum hydroxide (Maalox, Mylanta)

Action: Neutralize gastric acid to prevent gastric bleeding

Caution: Can cause constipation, diarrhea, hypermagnesemia, hypophosphatemia

Investigational Drugs

These drugs may be used to treat pancreatitis; however, there is no conclusive evidence that they are effective.
- anticholinergics
- prophylactic antibiotics
- histamine $_2$-blocking agents
- glucagon
- aprotinin
- calcitonin
- indomethacin
- somatostatin

NURSING MANAGEMENT

Monitoring and Managing Clinical Problems

1. Pain
   a. Note location, characteristics, severity, frequency, radiation, and any simultaneously occurring symptoms.
   b. Administer ordered meperidine and assess effectiveness.
   c. Assist patient to find a position of comfort; this is usually a knee-chest position with head elevated (supine position enhances pain).
   d. Use a calm, reassuring approach with the patient.
   e. Institute all measures to promote gastrointestinal function.
   f. Report any significant changes in pain status.
2. Fluid Volume Deficit or Excess
   a. Monitor fluid and electrolyte status.
      1) Monitor serum sodium, potassium, chloride, bicarbonate, calcium, magnesium, creatinine, and albumin; hemoglobin and hematocrit; serum and urine osmolality, urinalysis; and urine electrolytes; report any significant findings.
      2) Monitor daily weights, hourly intake and output, and vital signs (assess for orthostatic hypotension); measure abdominal girth daily; report any significant findings.
      3) Assess lethargy, tremors, paresthesia, tetany, la-

ryngospasm, convulsions, positive Chvostek's sign and Trousseau's sign, flat prolonged ST segment, prolonged QT interval and dysrhythmias suggesting hypocalcemia.

    4) Assess for fluid and electrolyte imbalances.

    5) Monitor CVP or pulmonary capillary wedge pressure (PCWP), PAP, right atrial pressure, cardiac output (CO), cardiac index, systemic vascular resistance, and oxygen saturation; report any significant findings.

b. Administer ordered crystalloid and colloid solutions, blood and electrolyte replacements to promote fluid and electrolyte balance; assess effectiveness.

c. Monitor for shock, dehydration, electrolyte disturbances, hypoalbuminemia, ascites, pulmonary edema, or congestive heart failure.

3. Diarrhea or Constipation

  a. Monitor bowel function

    1) Assess abdomen for softness, rigidity, rebound tenderness, presence of bowel sounds, distention, tympany or dullness to percussion, a palpable mass and presence of Cullen's or Grey Turner's signs; report any significant findings.

    2) Monitor for nausea, vomiting, altered bowel pattern, jaundice, hematemesis, melena ascites, hiccups, and gastric pH; report any significant findings.

  b. Promote gastrointestinal healing/function.

    1) Keep patient NPO.

    2) Insert a nasogastric tube and attach to low suction. Check placement and patency every 2 hours.

    3) Administer ordered medications, such as antacids, histamine $_2$-receptor antagonist.

    4) Assist with peritoneal lavage.

    5) Maintain patency of sump drainage devices.

    6) Prepare patient for endoscopy or laparotomy.

  c. Assess for gastrointestinal complications.

    1) Pancreatic phlegmon, abscess, pseudocyst, or fistula.

      a) Abdominal pain

      b) Elevated temperature

    c) Increased WBC count

    d) Nausea, vomiting, anorexia

    e) Absent bowel sounds

    f) Palpable abdominal mass

  2) Ascites

    a) Increasing abdominal girth

    b) Dullness to percussion over flank area

  3) Acute intra-abdominal hemorrhage

    a) Abdominal pain

    b) Hypotension

    c) Nausea, vomiting

    d) Elevated temperature

    e) Increased WBC count

  4) Acute cholangitis

    a) Right upper quadrant abdominal pain

    b) Jaundice

    c) Elevated temperature

    d) Increased liver function tests and bilirubin

  5) Inflammation of the large or small bowel, duodenum or spleen

    a) Abdominal pain

    b) Melena

    c) Hematemesis

    d) Nausea, vomiting, anorexia

    e) Elevated temperature

    f) Increased WBC count

4. Nutrition: altered, less than body requirements

  a. Monitor nutritional status.

    1) Monitor serum sodium, potassium, chloride, phosphate, bicarbonate, calcium, magnesium, trace elements, ferritin, transferrin, albumin, thyroid binding prealbumin, and retinal binding protein; hemoglobin and hematocrit; total absolute lymphocyte count; blood sugar; vitamin levels; creatinine/height ratio and urine urea/creatinine levels; report significant findings.

    2) Assess height and weight, skin, hair, nails, eyes head, mouth, heart, abdomen, extremities, nervous system; note results of anthropometric measures; and follow results of resting metabolic expenditure.

   b. Promote nutritional status.
      1) Administer ordered total parenteral nutrition and monitor patient response to treatment.
5. Tissue Perfusion, altered: peripheral
   a. Provide antiembolism hose and sequential compression device.
   b. Heparin may be contraindicated.
   c. Provide range-of-motion exercises.
6. Skin Integrity: impaired, high risk for
   a. Perform frequent position changes and skin assessment.
   b. May use pressure reduction or pressure relief devices.
   c. Provide range-of-motion exercises, as tolerated.
7. Gas Exchange: impaired risk, high risk for
   a. Turn every 2 hours
   b. Encourage deep breathing frequently
   c. Provide incentive spirometry and chest physiotherapy
   d. Institute measures to promote fluid balance
   e. Reduce pain and anxiety
   f. Institute measures to promote gastrointestinal function/healing
8. Injury: high risk for
   a. Monitor for dyspnea, cough, chest pain, dullness over lungs, egophony, and splinting of chest possibly indicating pleural effusion.
   b. Note hypoxemia, tachypnea, crackles or decreased breath sounds, and infiltrates on chest X-ray suggesting pneumonitis or atelectasis.
   c. Monitor for hypotension, nonspecific ST-T wave changes, muffled heart sounds, friction rub, absent apical impulse, reduced QRS voltage, cardiac silhouette enlargement on chest X-ray, and relatively echo-free space between the pericardium and the myocardial epicardium suggesting pericardial effusion.
   d. Monitor for hyperglycemia, hypertriglyceridemia, confusion, agitation, lethargy, anger, and anxiety suggesting metabolic alterations.
   e. Note results of candida and trichophyton skin tests to assess for decreased immune system response.

Monitoring, Managing, and Preventing
Life-Threatening Emergencies

1. Hemorrhagic shock
   a. Monitor for tachycardia; tachypnea; hypotension; cool, pale or cyanotic skin; capillary refill > 3 seconds; poor skin turgor with dry mucous membranes; mental status changes; decreased urine output; increasing abdominal girth; rigid abdomen; and guaiac-positive drainage from the gastrointestinal or genitourinary tracts indicating blood loss.
   b. Monitor hemoglobin and hematocrit for decreasing values.
   c. Monitor CVP, PAP, PCWP, and CO; report significant findings.
2. ARDS
   a. Monitor for increasing respiratory distress leading to increasing hypoxemia.
      1) Monitor chest X-rays and arterial blood gases (ABGs); report significant changes.
      2) Auscultate lungs frequently for decreased breath sounds, crackles, and/or rhonchi.
      3) Apply pulse oximeter and continuously measure oxygen saturation.
      4) Administer ordered bronchodilators.
      5) Monitor for air hunger, tachypnea, restlessness, and confusion indicating increasing respiratory distress.
   b. Have emergency resuscitation equipment available for immediate intubation, if necessary.
   c. Monitor for effective ventilation while on mechanical ventilator.
      1) Reassess lung sounds frequently.
      2) Suction, as needed, to remove sputum and promote a clear airway.
      3) Measure compliance frequently and report decreases.
      4) Measure peak pressures and report increases.
      5) Sedate the patient, as needed, to control ventilator fighting. Paralytics may be necessary also.
      6) Monitor serial ABGs for effectiveness of mechani-

cal ventilation. Indications for positive end-expiratory pressure (PEEP):
   a) PaO_2 <60 mm Hg on an FiO_2 >50%
   b) pH <7.25
   c) $PaCO_2$ >45 mm Hg
7) Decrease FiO_2 to <50% as quickly as possible to prevent oxygen toxicity.
8) If the patient is on PEEP, remember PEEP holds alveoli open thus increasing functional residual capacity, decreasing shunting, and decreasing hypoxemia. But, PEEP can decrease CO and increase risk of oxygen toxicity and fluid overload.
   d. Monitor fluid volume status.
      1) Measure CO and report significant changes.
      2) Measure hourly urine output and report output <30 mL/h.
      3) Observe for presence of a new S_3, increasing pulmonary crackles and rhonchi, edema, weight gain, and intake greater than output, suggesting fluid overload; report significant findings.
      4) Observe for weight loss, low CO, decreased urine output, and tenting of skin suggesting dehydration; report significant findings.
      5) Administer ordered IV fluids cautiously to prevent fluid overload, but maintain adequate fluid volume.
3. DIC
   a. Assist with treatment of the underlying cause.
   b. Administer heparin therapy, blood component therapy, and antithrombin therapy to stop the vicious cycle of thrombosis-hemorrhage.
   c. Keep patient on strict bed rest.
   d. Correct hemostatic deficiencies that compromise the clotting mechanisms with drug therapy, as ordered.
   e. Administer ordered IV fluids to correct hypovolemia, hypotension, and tissue ischemia.
   f. Monitor tachycardia, hypotension, CVP <5 mm Hg, mean arterial pressure <60 mm Hg, and decreased intensity of peripheral pulses.
   g. Assess breath sounds; note presence of dyspnea and cyanosis; and monitor for significant changes in ABGs and oxygen saturation to determine adequacy of oxy-

genation and acid-base balance. As indicated, administer ordered supplemental oxygen.

h. Prevent atelectases by having the patient turn, cough, and deep breathe.

i. Monitor for decreased urine output and increased specific gravity to assess for hypovolemia and fluid retention.

j. Monitor heart and lung sounds, CO, PAP, and intake and output for fluid overload, which can lead to pulmonary edema or pleural effusion.

k. Monitor and manage skin and mucous membranes for ischemia, bleeding, cyanosis, and lesions.

l. Monitor and manage comfort level. Reposition patient and provide gentle range-of-motion exercises every 2 hours and assess comfort level. As indicated, provide pain medication.

m. Monitor and manage nutrition.
   1) Maintain strict intake and output.
   2) Monitor ordered total parenteral nutrition.
   3) Avoid the use of hot fluids that will irritate the oral mucosa and gingival bleeding.
   4) Weigh daily and maintain body weight within 10% of normal weight.
   5) Assess for absent bowel sounds indicating paralytic ileus.

4. Acute renal failure

   a. Prevent complications related to continued hypotension, infection, and use of nephrotoxic agents by administering ordered IV fluids and medications.

   b. Regulate fluid intake to achieve fluid and electrolyte balance.

   c. Administer ordered buffering agents to achieve acid-base balance.

   d. Closely observe level of consciousness and intervene quickly as indicated to preserve neurologic function.

   e. Manage nutrition.
      1) Enforce protein restriction to maintain anabolism while limiting load on kidneys; amount varies depending on patient's weight and activity level and whether or not patient is on dialysis; protein needs to be high biologic value.
      2) Restrict dietary potassium.

    3) Restrict fluids.

    4) Provide adequate calories to prevent catabolism.

    5) Administer ordered supplemental vitamins.

  f. Administer ordered blood transfusion to maintain adequate level of red blood cells for optimum tissue oxygenation.

  g. Initiate renal replacement therapy when signs/symptoms indicate.

    1) BUN >100 mg/dL

    2) Serum creatinine exceeds 5–9 mg/dL or lower serum creatinine levels for patients with reduced muscle mass such as the elderly.

    3) Volume overload and signs of pulmonary edema

    4) Pericarditis

    5) Hyperkalemia that has not responded adequately to other treatment modalities

    6) Uncontrollable acidosis

    7) Central nervous system dysfunction related to uremia

5. Septic shock

  a. Continuously monitor hemodynamic parameters to evaluate the cardiovascular response to treatment.

  b. Continuously monitor urinary output via catheter to evaluate renal function.

  c. Monitor cardiac rhythm for tachycardia and life-threatening ventricular arrhythmias.

  d. Maintain a patent airway and adequate ventilation. Use supplemental oxygen to ensure that sufficient oxygen is delivered to the lungs.

  e. Provide enteral or parenteral nutritional support to prevent a negative nitrogen balance.

  f. Promote treatment of sepsis.

    1) Administer ordered antibiotics.

    2) Obtain specimen of all potential infection sites for culture and sensitivity testing.

    3) Monitor WBC counts.

    4) Monitor temperature every four hours and treat as needed with medications or external cooling devices.

6. Multisystem organ failure

  a. Monitor patients at risk and recognize onset during the early phases

1) Assess for risk factors
2) Monitor for changes in body temperature, increasing heart rate, tachypnea, increased or decreased WBC count, and subtle changes in the level of consciousness, early warning signals for multisystem organ failure

b. Prevent organ injury
   1) Provide ventilatory support through intubation and mechanical ventilation
   2) Control body temperature to adjust for hyperthermia or hypothermia
   3) Reverse acidosis
   4) Monitor for subtle changes in assessment findings which may indicate deterioration from the hyperdynamic phase to the hypodynamic phase. Measure hemodynamic parameters frequently and report changes.
   5) Assess the patient frequently paying particular attention to findings that indicate deterioration in previously uninvolved organ systems.
   6) Monitor patient responses to medications and treatments and report significant findings

c. Provide supportive care
   1) Control the infection
      a) Obtain a specimen of all secretions for culture and sensitivity testing
      b) Prepare the patient for surgical intervention to remove sources of infection
      c) Promote an aseptic environment to prevent nosocomial infections

d. Arrest and reverse the progress of the syndrome
   1) Prevent translocation of bacteria from the gut with enteral feeding of glutamine, an immunonutrient which maintains gut integrity and stimulates the immune system
   2) Prepare for continuous arteriovenous hemodiafiltration (CAVHD) which has been used successfully in trauma patients
   3) Recognize complications
      a) Skin breakdown
      b) Third spacing of fluid
   4) Provide metabolic support

a) Measure oxygen consumption with increased flow until lactic acid level returns to normal
b) Provide adequate nutrition. Enteral route is preferred over parenteral using a formula that is high in protein and has medium chain triglycerides for lipids

Fulminant and Chronic Hepatic Failure

Fulminant hepatic failure is the development of hepatic encephalopathy (syndrome of neurologic and psychiatric dysfunction that occurs in liver failure), usually within 8 weeks of the onset of liver-related symptoms. The syndrome results from massive necrosis of liver cells or a severe and sudden reduction of liver function, usually in patients with no previous liver disease; however, it may occur in patients with previously compensated liver disease.

Chronic hepatic failure denotes the slow, gradual, progressive degeneration of liver cells, resulting in diminished liver function and ultimately liver failure.

Etiology/Pathophysiology

1. Etiology of fulminant hepatic failure
   a. Infection
      1) Hepatitis virus A, B, C, D, and E
      2) Herpes simplex
      3) Cytomegalovirus
      4) Adenoviruses
   b. Toxins
      1) Amanita phalloides (mushroom poisoning)
      2) Fluorinated hydrocarbons (i.e., carbon tetra-chloride)
   c. Drug reaction
      1) Acetaminophen overdose
      2) Antidepressants
      3) Nonsteroidal anti-inflammatory drugs
      4) Anticonvulsants (i.e., valproic acid, phenytoin)
      5) Isoniazid
      6) Halothane
      7) Sulfonamides
      8) Disulfiram
      9) Amiodarone
      10) Propylthiouracil
      11) Trimethoprim and sulfamethoxazole combina-tion
   d. Ischemia
      1) Cardiac failure
      2) Hepatic vascular occlusions
      3) Shock, hypertension, hypoxemia
   e. Miscellaneous metabolic disorders
      1) Acute fatty liver of pregnancy
      2) Wilson's disease
      3) Reye's syndrome
2. Etiology of chronic hepatic failure
   a. Cirrhosis
      1) Alcoholic
      2) Postnecrotic
      3) Biliary
      4) Cardiac
   b. Chronic active hepatitis
   c. Hepatic vein thrombosis (Budd-Chiari syndrome)

    d. Nodular regenerative hyperplasia

3. Common pathophysiologic alterations

    a. Hepatic encephalopathy

      1) Physiologic alterations

        a) Decreased function of hepatocytes

        b) Shunting of blood from portal system via the development of "collateral" circulation and/or shunting of blood through the damaged liver

      2) Some mechanisms believed to cause encephalopathy

        a) Liver blocks the degradation of ammonia into urea, resulting in high blood levels of ammonia. Ammonia is neurotoxic.

        b) Several neurotoxic agents may work synergistically to impair transmission of neurologic signals (i.e., ammonia, phenols, short-chain fatty acids, mercaptans).

        c) Normal neurotransmitters may be displaced by false neurotransmitters (i.e., octopamine, gamma-aminobutyric acid).

    b. Coagulopathy

      1) Reduced production of clotting factors II, V, VII, IX, and X

      2) Activation of Hageman factor and inadequate clearance of activated factors

      3) Abnormal platelet production and function

    c. Increased susceptibility to infection

      1) Impaired function of Kupffer cells and polymorphonuclear (leukocytes) function

      2) Impaired cell-mediated and humoral immunity

      3) Bacteria could enter bloodstream via collateral shunting and/or poor liver filtration

    d. Jaundice

      1) Inability of the liver to metabolize bilirubin

      2) Decreased survival of erythrocytes

    e. Fetor hepaticus

      1) Increased levels of mercaptans formed by bacterial action in the gut

      2) Injured liver is unable to process the mercaptans.

      3) Seen in patients with extensive collateral circulation

    f. Cardiovascular changes

      1) Vasodilation with a decreased systemic vascular resistance and hypotension

      2) Hypovolemia

      3) Increased cardiac output (CO), cardiac index, and interstitial edema

      4) Stimulation of the sympathetic nervous system

  g. Pulmonary changes

      1) Intrapulmonary shunting

      2) Ventilation-perfusion mismatching

      3) Decreased diffusing capacity

      4) Hypoxemia, clubbing, and occasionally cyanosis

  h. Abnormal ratio of aromatic amino acids to branch-chained amino acids

      1) Increased tissue protein breakdown and decreased hepatic oxidation results in elevated levels of tyrosine.

      2) Increased plasma levels of aromatic amino acids (i.e., tyrosine, methionine), with decreased levels of branched-chained amino acids, may lead to altered neurotransmission and encephalopathy.

  i. Hepato-renal failure

      1) Extreme peripheral vasodilation results in decreased blood flow to the kidney.

      2) Marked renal vasoconstriction occurs in response to increased levels of renin, aldosterone, antidiuretic hormone, and norepinephrine.

      3) Decreased levels of renal vasodilating prostaglandins and increased levels of renal vasoconstricting prostaglandins

      4) May also develop acute tubular necrosis.

4. Pathophysiologic alterations seen in fulminant hepatic failure

  a. Cerebral edema

      1) Vasogenic edema—due to alterations in permeability of blood–brain barrier

      2) Cytotoxic edema—due to loss of cell membrane transport, resulting in swelling of astrocytes

  b. Hypoglycemia

      1) Injured liver has defective gluconeogenesis

      2) Elevated plasma levels of insulin due to inadequate uptake

      3) Depletion of glycogen

   c. Lactic acidosis
      1) Inadequate tissue perfusion due to arteriovenous shunting
      2) Injured liver cannot metabolize lactate.
   d. Hypokalemia, hyponatremia, hypophosphatemia
      1) Hypokalemia due to urinary losses, high glucose feedings, poor intake, and metabolic alkalosis
      2) Hyponatremia due to serum dilution
      3) Hypophosphatemia etiology unknown

5. Pathophysiologic alterations in chronic hepatic failure
   a. Portal hypertension
      1) Any disorder in the liver, portal system, or vena cava that obstructs blood flow results in high pressure in the portal system.
      2) Increased pressure in the portal system causes collateral vessels to open between the portal vein and the spleen, stomach, esophagus, bowel, and rectum.
      3) The formation of collateral circulation may result in gastric/esophageal varices (enlarged tortuous veins), splenomegaly, ascites, and hepatic encephalopathy.
   b. Vascular spiders (angioma with a central red body and several branching legs), palmar erythema, gynecomastia (excessive development of the male mammary glands), testicular atrophy, menstrual irregularities
      1) Normal plasma levels of estrogen with decreased plasma levels of free testosterone
      2) May be due to decreased rate of hormone metabolism, decreased hepatic blood flow, shunting of blood around liver, or increased levels of sex hormone–binding globulin.
   c. Overall state of poor health and hypoalbuminemia (serum albumin <3.8 g/dL).
      1) Loss of tissue and low levels of plasma albumin due to injured liver's inability to synthesize protein
      2) Anorexia with poor dietary intake

Assessment/Analysis

ASSESSMENT FINDINGS

Subjective

FULMINANT

1. Headache, dizziness, nightmares
2. Jaundice
3. Vomiting

CHRONIC

1. Malaise, weakness, fatigue
2. Anorexia, nausea, vomiting
3. Weight loss
4. Easy bruising
5. Jaundice

Objective

FULMINANT

1. Altered mental status with agitation, uncooperative or violent behavior, delirium, mania, somnolence, and coma (abrupt onset)
2. Asterixis
3. Fetor hepaticus
5. Small liver
6. Decerebrate rigidity and posturing in late stages
7. Abnormal pupil reflexes (usually dilated in late stages)
8. Hypotension, tachycardia, arrhythmias, cardiac failure
9. Tachypnea, respiratory arrest
10. Elevated temperature

CHRONIC

1. Emaciated, malnourished patient
2. Vascular spiders, palmar erythema (liver palms)
3. Enlarged abdomen (ascites), peripheral edema
4. Flushed extremities with clubbing and cyanosis
5. Altered mental status
6. Asterixis

7. Low-grade fever
8. Gynecomastia with soft small testes in men
9. Tachypnea
10. Hypotension, tachycardia
11. Increased, decreased, or normal liver size with or without tenderness
12. Splenomegaly
13. Fetor hepaticus
14. Patient may present with a gastrointestinal hemorrhage, spontaneous bacterial peritonitis, hepato-renal syndrome, alcohol intoxication, or electrolyte imbalance.

SUPPORTING TEST FINDINGS

Laboratory Tests

1. Blood sugar
   Abnormality: Decreased level (hypoglycemia) usually present; may be severe and intractable in fulminant liver failure.
   Increased level (hyperglycemia) may be seen in chronic liver failure
2. Serum electrolytes
   Abnormality: Decreased potassium, decreased sodium, decreased phosphate
3. Blood urea nitrogen (BUN)
   Abnormality: Decreased
4. Coagulation profile
   Abnormality: Increased prothrombin time (PT) and partial thromboplastin time (PTT).
   Normal to decreased platelet count
   A lysis time of <1 hour means abnormal fibrinolysis occurring (occurs in fulminant failure); increased levels of fibrin split products or fibrin degradation products (occurs in fulminant failure)
5. Hepatitis screening profile for hepatitis A, B, C, and D
   Abnormality: Screen is positive with viral hepatitis
6. Serum bilirubin
   Abnormality: Usually increased (level >23 mg is a good predictor of mortality)
7. Liver function tests
   Abnormality: Increased serum aspartate transaminase, serum alanine aminotransferase, and alkaline phos-

phatase levels that fall as liver function deteriorates in fulminant failure and stay increased in chronic liver failure

8. Serum albumin
   Abnormality: May be normal initially; decreases with progressive liver dysfunction in fulminant failure and in chronic liver failure

9. Serum alpha fetoprotein
   Abnormality: Decreased initially
   Increases with liver regeneration in fulminant liver failure

10. C_3 component of complement
    Abnormality: Decreased serum level; falls progressively in fulminant liver failure

11. Culture and sensitivity testing
    Abnormality: Positive blood, urine, stool, and sputum cultures in fulminant liver failure are frequently found

12. Complete blood count (CBC)
    Abnormality: White blood cells (WBCs) may be normal, increased or decreased; red blood cells (RBCs), hemoglobin, and hematocrit may be normal or decreased

13. Serum ammonia
    Abnormality: Increased

14. Serum lactic acid
    Abnormality: Increased in fulminant liver failure

15. Arterial blood gases (ABGs)
    Abnormality: Decreased PaO_2
    Decreased pH with metabolic acidosis in fulminant liver failure
    Increased, decreased, or normal pH with metabolic alkalosis or acidosis or normal pH in chronic liver failure

16. Drug screen
    Abnormality: Increased or toxic levels of alcohol or other hepatotoxic drugs may be found in fulminant liver failure

17. Twenty-four-hour urine test for creatinine clearance
    Abnormality: Decreased creatinine clearance

18. Urinalysis, urine electrolytes, and osmolality
    Abnormality: Decreased urine sodium, increased protein, increased granular casts, blood present, increased specific gravity, increased osmolality

19. Serum amylase
    Abnormality: Increased if pancreatitis is present

Diagnostic Tests

1. Electroencephalogram (EEG)
   Abnormality: Increasing amplitude with decreasing frequency and the development of triphasic waves in late stages of coma
2. Electrocardiogram (ECG)
   Abnormality: Increased rate, arrhythmias
3. Chest X-ray
   Abnormality: Pulmonary edema, aspiration pneumonia, lobar collapse, adult respiratory distress syndrome in fulminant liver failure
4. Computed tomography (CT) scan of liver
   Abnormality: Decreased size with areas of necrosis in fulminant liver failure
5. CT of the brain
   Abnormality: Cerebral atrophy in chronic liver failure
   Cerebral edema in fulminant liver failure
6. Percutaneous needle biopsy of the liver
   Abnormality: Hepatocellular necrosis in drug-induced or viral hepatitis; microvesicular steatosis in fatty liver of pregnancy, tetracycline toxicity, or Reye's syndrome; fibrosis with formation of regenerative nodules in cirrhosis
7. Hepatic ultrasonography
   Abnormality: Extrahepatic biliary obstruction and abnormal size of liver in chronic and fulminant liver failure
8. Cerebral blood flow (CBF)
   Abnormality: Increased or decreased blood flow (as measured with inhaled xenon during a CT scan of the head or at bedside with xenon 133) in fulminant liver failure
9. Cerebral venous blood oxygen content
   Abnormality: Decreased jugular venous oxygen content (JVO_2) as measured with a catheter placed in the jugular bulb is seen in fulminant liver failure
10. Cerebral oxygen consumption ($CMRO_2$)
    Abnormality: $CMRO_2$ is calculated by multiplying CBF times the difference between arterial and jugular venous oxygen content ($A\text{-}JVO_2$ gradient).

Constant $CMRO_2$ and widening $A\text{-}JVO_2$ gradient suggest cerebral ischemia

Constant $CMRO_2$ with narrowing of the $A\text{-}JVO_2$ gradient suggests cerebral swelling

Planning/Intervention

COLLABORATIVE MANAGEMENT

Procedures for Fulminant Liver Failure

1. Reduce and monitor for cerebral edema.
   a. Assist with insertion of an extradural pressure transducer to monitor intracranial pressure, as indicated.
   b. *Do not* elevate the head of the bed > 20 degrees.
   c. *Do not* turn head from side to side or flex neck.
   d. Hyperventilate patient with an oxygen mask before assisting with the insertion of an endotracheal tube.
   e. Monitor serial EEGs and CT scans.
   f. Prepare patient for ordered continuous hemofiltration if patient is in renal failure, as indicated.
   g. Institute ordered $CMRO_2$ monitoring, as indicated.
   h. Administer ordered osmotic diuretics and thiopental sodium.
2. Monitor for hepatic encephalopathy and institute appropriate interventions.
   a. Restrict protein intake.
   b. Administer ordered phosphate enemas.
   c. Insert a nasogastric tube and connect to low suction to remove blood from the gut, as indicated (blood in the gut is broken down into ammonia).
   d. Avoid administering sedation.
   e. Perform neurologic checks and vital signs every hour or as indicated.
   f. Assess liver size by performing percussion of liver daily and following results of serial liver ultrasound.
   g. Note routine serum ammonia levels and report significant changes.
   h. Assess for fetor hepaticus daily.
   i. Administer ordered lactulose, neomycin, or benzodiazepine antagonist.

3. Control and monitor for hypoglycemia and improve nutrition.
   a. If blood glucose is <100 mg/dL, give 100 mL 50% glucose intravenously (IV) or by mouth.
   b. Check blood glucose every hour or as indicated.
   c. Administer ordered 10% glucose with potassium chloride, ascorbic acid, and multiple vitamins continuously up to 3 L/d.
   d. If patient needs to be transported to another facility, infuse ordered 20% glucose solution.
   e. Administer ordered IV branched-chain amino acids to prevent encephalopathy. This is controversial.
4. Monitor for coagulopathy and bleeding, and institute appropriate interventions.
   a. Assist with intubation via mouth, not nose, to prevent epistaxis (nosebleed).
   b. Avoid arterial punctures.
   c. Monitor results of coagulation profiles and report significant changes.
   d. Administer ordered vitamin K, fresh frozen plasma, and platelet packs.
5. Monitor for infection and institute interventions to prevent it.
   a. Obtain specimens of blood, urine, sputum, stool, and catheter tips for culture and sensitivity testing, as ordered.
   b. When infection is identified, start ordered antibiotics.
   c. Monitor results of serial CBC with WBC count and differential and hepatitis screening profile; report significant changes.
6. Monitor for and institute interventions to prevent respiratory failure.
   a. Assist with intubation of the patient and place on mechanical ventilation, as indicated.
   b. Assess for pulmonary edema and volume overload.
   c. Monitor results of serial ABGs and chest X-rays; report significant changes.
7. Maintain and monitor blood pressure and CO.
   a. Assist with insertion of a central venous catheter or pulmonary artery catheter.
   b. Monitor hemodynamic parameters and report significant changes.

   c. Monitor results of serial ECGs and serum lactic acid levels; report significant changes.

   d. Administer ordered inotropic agents, as indicated.

8. Monitor for hepato-renal failure and institute appropriate interventions.

   a. Insert an indwelling urinary catheter and connect to urometer.

   b. Monitor intake and output hourly.

   c. Monitor results of serial serum electrolytes and creatinine and BUN.

   d. Collect ordered 24-hour urine for creatinine clearance and urea.

   e. Collect specimens and monitor urinalysis, urine electrolytes, and urine osmolality results; report significant changes.

   f. Maintain dietary sodium restriction of 250 mg/d or as ordered.

   g. Assist with paracentesis removing small volumes of ascitic fluid.

   h. Prepare patient for insertion of a peritoneovenous shunt (LeVeen/Denver/Minnesota) to drain ascitic fluid from the abdominal cavity into the superior vena cava, if needed.

   i. Prepare patient for hemodialysis, if ordered, or continuous arteriovenous hemofiltration (which uses a hemofilter to remove water, electrolytes, and small- to medium-sized molecular weight molecules from blood while leaving protein substances).

   j. Avoid using nephrotoxic drugs.

   k. Administer ordered loop and potassium-sparing diuretics.

9. Provide artificial support for liver function.

   a. Prepare patient for charcoal hemoperfusion or orthotopic liver transplant, as ordered.

   b. Administer ordered acetylcysteine (Mucomyst) orally for acetaminophen overdose.

Experimental Treatments

Several new treatments are being tried to treat hepatic failure.
- Extracorporeal liver assist device
- Liver cell transplantation using micro carriers into the abdomen
- Auxiliary partial liver transplants
- Benzodiazepine antagonists
- Prostacyclin
- Prostaglandin E_1
- Hepatocyte growth factors

10. Monitor liver function by monitoring results of laboratory and diagnostic tests; report significant changes.

Procedures for Chronic Liver Failure

1. Monitor for hepatic encephalopathy and institute appropriate interventions.
   a. Administer ordered phosphate enemas.
   b. Insert a nasogastric tube and connect to low suction to remove blood from the stomach.
   c. Perform neurologic checks and vital signs every hour or as indicated.
   d. Obtain specimens and monitor serum ammonia levels; report significant changes.
   e. Assess for fetor hepaticus daily.
   f. As liver function stabilizes and encephalopathy subsides, begin feeding 20 g of protein every other day; otherwise, administer ordered 20–40% glucose solutions for calories.
   g. Enforce restriction of protein to 40–60 g daily.
   h. If ordered, administer a high-protein diet to patients in chronic failure who may need an intake of 80–100 g/d.
   i. Avoid administering benzodiazepines, morphine, paraldehyde, and barbiturates.
   j. Prevent intake of alcohol or hepatotoxins.
   k. Prevent dehydration and avoid using diuretics aggressively.

   l. Treat low serum potassium levels and high blood pH to avoid hypokalemia and alkalosis.
   m. Institute measures to prevent gastrointestinal bleeding, systemic infection, spontaneous bacterial peritonitis, diarrhea, and constipation, as ordered.
   n. Administer ordered lactulose, neomycin, and benzodiazepine antagonist.
2. Improve nutrition.
   a. Encourage intake of full amount of daily allowance of protein as tolerated by patient.
   b. In encephalopathy, administer ordered IV glucose for nutrition.
   c. Add ordered branched chain amino acids to feedings, as indicated.
   d. Administer ordered amino acids, thiamine, folate, and vitamin K, as indicated.
3. Monitor for coagulopathy and institute appropriate interventions.
   a. Monitor results of coagulation studies; report significant changes.
   b. Administer ordered vitamin K, fresh frozen plasma, and/or platelet packs.
4. Monitor for and prevent infection.
   a. Monitor results of CBCs with WBC count and differential and hepatitis screening profile; report significant changes.
   b. Obtain specimens of ascitic fluid, blood, urine, sputum, stool, and catheter tips for ordered culture and sensitivity testing.
   c. Assess for peritonitis.
   d. Administer ordered antibiotics.
5. Assess for gastrointestinal bleeding suggesting esophageal/gastric varices, splenomegaly, ascites, and alterations in level of consciousness suggesting hepatic encephalopathy.
6. Reduce portal hypertension.
   a. Prepare patient for surgery to create a portal-systemic shunt, as indicated.
   b. Initiate measures to promote liver healing.
7. Control/prevent bleeding from varices.
   a. Administer ordered IV infusion of vasopressin into the superior mesenteric artery.

   b. Administer ordered sublingual, transdermal, or IV nitroglycerin concurrently with vasopressin.

   c. Prepare patient for endoscopic variceal sclerotherapy or endoscopic variceal band ligation of bleeding sites.

   d. Assist with insertion of tamponade tubes (Sengstaken-Blakemore or Minnesota tube).

   e. Prepare patient for surgery to stop bleeding (portacaval shunt, mesocaval shunt, splenorenal shunt, or esophageal and gastric devascularization with an esophageal transection), as indicated.

   f. Prepare patient for percutaneous obliteration of varices or transjugular intrahepatic portacaval shunt, as indicated.

8. Monitor for and institute interventions to reduce ascites.

   a. Assess daily weight, abdominal girth, shifting dullness, and presence of a fluid wave.

   b. Monitor results of abdominal ultrasound and report significant changes.

   c. Induce weight loss of 0.5 kg/d by administering ordered diuretics.

   d. Institute ordered fluid restriction of 1500 mL/d.

   e. Maintain strict bed rest, if ordered.

   f. Institute and enforce sodium restriction of 800 mg/d or per orders.

   g. Prepare patient for portacaval shunt or peritoneovenous shunt, as indicated.

   h. Administer ordered albumin.

9. Prepare patient for ordered charcoal hemoperfusion or orthotopic liver transplant.

10. Monitor liver function by following results of ordered laboratory and diagnostic tests.

Drug Therapy

1. Osmotic diuretics

   Example: mannitol (Osmitrol)

   Action: Reduces the pressure and volume of cerebrospinal fluid by increasing the plasma osmolality, thereby promoting the diffusion of water into the plasma

Used to reduce cerebral edema in fulminant liver failure

Caution: May give mannitol as long as serum osmolality does not exceed 320 mOsm

2. Laxatives

Example: lactulose (Cephulac)

Action: Increases the osmotic pressure in the gut, causing the accumulation of water in the intestinal lumen.

It also reduces production and increases utilization of ammonia by bacteria in the gut, therefore decreasing blood levels of ammonia that can cause hepatic encephalopathy in fulminant and chronic hepatic failure

Caution: Can cause hyperglycemia; will cause diarrhea

3. Aminoglycoside antibiotics

Example: neomycin sulfate (Mycifradin)

Action: Broad-spectrum antibiotic effective against gram-negative and gram-positive bacteria normally found in the gut; sterilize the gut, thus decreasing digestion of protein and, subsequently, ammonia production to prevent or reduce hepatic encephalopathy

Caution: May cause hypersensitivity reaction, renal damage, and loss of hearing

4. Vitamin replacements

Example: thiamine hydrochloride (Betalin S)

Action: Vitamin B complex functions as a co-enzyme in carbohydrate metabolism. Prevents alcoholic neuritis or Wernicke-Korsakoff syndrome in patients who are still drinking

Caution: All alcoholics should routinely be given 50–100 mg of thiamine IV *before* receiving any glucose-containing solution

Example: folic acid (Folvite)

Action: Promotes normal synthesis of deoxyribonucleic acid, especially in the hematopoietic system

Example: phytonadione (AquaMEPHYTON)

Action: Vitamin K—promotes the synthesis of clotting factors (II, VII, IX, and X) by the liver

Caution: Rash, pain, and swelling at injection sites; allergic reactions

5. Blood replacement

Example: Fresh frozen plasma

Action: Replaces clotting factors V and VIII

Caution: Can cause volume overload; carries risk of viral transmission

Example: Platelets

Action: Replaces platelets in patients who are thrombocytopenic (platelet count < 150,000 mm^3)

Caution: May sensitize patients to leukocyte and RBC antigens. ABO-incompatible plasma in platelet packs may cause a positive direct antiglobulin test and hemolysis. Also may see chills, fever, allergic reactions, and transmission of hepatitis and human immunodeficiency virus

6. Histamine $_2$-receptor antagonists

   Example: cimetidine (Tagamet)

   ranitidine (Zantac)

   famotidine (Pepcid)

   Action: Inhibits gastric acid secretion; want to keep gastric pH > 5 to attempt to prevent gastric bleeding

   Caution: Diarrhea, headache, dizziness, nausea, myalgia, and skin rashes

7. Barbiturates

   Example: thiopental sodium (Pentothal)

   Action: Produces central nervous system depression at all levels and raises the seizure threshold; used in fulminant liver failure to control cerebral edema when mannitol and ultrafiltration are not effective

   Caution: Can cause respiratory and cardiac depression and anaphylaxis; use of this drug is controversial as it may decrease cerebral blood flow

8. Inotropic agent

   Example: dopamine hydrochloride (Intropin)

   Action: Increases blood pressure; low dose (0.5–2 μg/kg per minute) stimulates dopaminergic receptors, inducing renal vasodilation; higher dose (2–10 μg/kg per minute) stimulates dopaminergic and beta$_1$ receptors, inducing renal dilation and cardiac stimulation

9. Potassium-sparing diuretic

   Example: spironolactone (Aldactone)

   Action: Antagonizes the action of aldosterone, causing

the retention of potassium and excretion of sodium and water to reduce ascites and improve output in renal failure

Caution: Hyperkalemia and gastrointestinal upset may occur

10. Loop diuretic

Example: furosemide (Lasix)

Action: Inhibits electrolyte reabsorption in the ascending loop of Henle, causing the excretion of sodium, chloride, potassium, and water, thus reducing ascites and improving output in renal failure

Caution: Can cause severe fluid and electrolyte imbalance, deafness, metabolic alkalosis, and hypovolemia

11. Volume expander

Example: human albumin (Albuminar)

Action: Replaces albumin, normalizes plasma osmolality, and expands blood volume; reabsorbs fluid accumulation in ascites

Caution: Can cause pulmonary edema

12. Antidote for acetaminophen overdose

Example: acetycysteine (Mucomyst)

Action: Prevents liver damage by reducing hepatotoxic metabolites after acetaminophen overdose

Caution: This drug is recommended if <24 hours has elapsed since ingestion of acetaminophen

NURSING MANAGEMENT

Monitoring and Managing Clinical Problems

1. Thought Processes: altered
   a. Monitor for encephalopathy.
      1) Assess neurologic status for and report changes in the following:
         a) Level of consciousness
         b) Orientation
         c) Mood and behavior
         d) Judgment
         e) Personality changes
         f) Ability to perform simple calculations
         g) Remote and recent memory
         h) Status of speech
         i) Motor function

        j) Deep tendon reflexes
        k) Response to painful stimuli
        l) Pupillary responses
        m) Positioning
        n) Asterixis
    2) Assess for stage of encephalopathy:
        a) Grade 1 — Confused with altered mood or behavior and changes in mental status
        b) Grade 2 — Drowsy with inappropriate behavior
        c) Grade 3 — Inarticulate speech, but able to follow simple commands; stuporous with marked confusion
        d) Grade 4 — Coma, unarousable; document state of coma
    3) Monitor results of serial EEGs, blood ammonia levels, and liver ultrasound; report significant findings.
    4) Assess for fetor hepaticus; report findings.
  b. Promote reduction in encephalopathy.
    1) Reduce blood levels of ammonia by administering ordered phosphate enemas, lactulose, neomycin, and branch-chained amino acids.
    2) Decrease intake of protein to ordered amounts.
    3) Administer ordered benzodiazepine antagonists
    4) Institute measures to prevent gastrointestinal bleeding; administer antacids, histamine$_2$-receptor antagonists, and sucralfate; monitor gastric pH and maintain at pH of 4.0–5.0.
    5) Avoid administering sedatives, morphine, paraldehyde, and barbiturates.
    6) Prevent intake of alcohol and other hepatotoxins.
    7) Institute measures to remove blood from gastrointestinal system; connect nasogastric tube to low suction and administer ordered laxatives and enemas.
  c. Monitor for precipitants of acute encephalopathy such as infection, gastrointestinal hemorrhage, electrolyte imbalance (hypokalemia), constipation, a large protein meal, or alcohol withdrawal.
  d. Prevent encephalopathy.
    1) Administer ordered antibiotics, histamine$_2$-receptor antagonists, antacids, sucralfate, potassium

replacements, stool softeners, and low-dose diuretics.
   2) Use aseptic technique to prevent infection.
   3) Reduce intake of protein to ordered amounts.
2. Injury, high risk for
   a. Monitor for bleeding.
      1) Assess for bleeding or oozing from wounds, drains, puncture sites, gums, nose, urinary tract, and gastrointestinal tract.
      2) Assess for presence of petechiae, purpura, ecchymoses, abdominal distention, and swelling in joints.
      3) Monitor for changes in blood pressure (orthostatic hypotension), tachycardia, decreased peripheral pulses, and tachypnea.
      4) Monitor all excrement for occult blood.
      5) Monitor laboratory values for decreased hemoglobin, hematocrit, and platelet count; prolonged PT and PTT; presence of fibrin split products or fibrin degradation products; and a euglobulin lysis time <1 hour.
   b. Prevent bleeding.
      1) Administer ordered vitamin K, fresh frozen plasma, blood, and platelets.
      2) Avoid arterial puncture, intramuscular injections, nasotracheal intubation, and use of razor blade for shaving.
      3) Have patient use a soft toothbrush, electric razor, padding for bedrails, and small-gauge needles for subcutaneous injections and venipunctures.
      4) Apply pressure for 5–10 minutes over puncture sites.
3. Infection: high risk for
   a. Monitor for signs/symptoms of infection.
      1) Assess for spontaneous peritonitis by noting the following:
         a) Abdominal pain, distention, and rigidity
         b) Nausea and vomiting
         c) Abrupt onset of fever and chills
         d) Cloudy ascitic fluid
         e) Elevated WBC and positive bacterial cultures
      2) Assess for urinary tract infection by noting the following:

      a) Cloudy or bloody urine with a foul odor
      b) Complaints of pain on urination, with or without frequency
      c) Fever and chills
      d) Abnormal urinalysis with bacteriuria, WBCs, and positive leukocyte esterase
      e) Elevated WBC and positive bacterial cultures

    3) Assess for respiratory tract infection by noting the following:
      a) Dyspnea
      b) Cough
      c) Sputum production that has a color
      d) Fever and chills
      e) Tachypnea or orthopnea
      f) Areas of dullness to percussion in thoracic cavity
      g) Adventitious breath sounds
      h) Elevated WBCs and positive bacterial cultures
      i) Changes in chest X-ray and oxygen saturation

    4) Monitor results of hepatitis screening profile.

  b. Prevent/treat infection.
    1) Obtain specimens for ordered culture and sensitivity tests of blood, urine, sputum, stool, catheter tips, and ascitic fluid sensitivity testing.
    2) When infection is suspected or identified, administer ordered antibiotics.
    3) Use aseptic technique.
    4) Prevent urinary tract infection.
      a) Avoid using urinary catheter, when possible.
      b) If urinary catheter is used, give meticulous catheter care.
    5) Prevent respiratory infection.
      a) Encourage turning, coughing, deep breathing, and use of incentive spirometer every 2 hours.
      b) Assess for gag reflex.
      c) Perform nasotracheal or pharyngeal suctioning, as needed.
      d) Position patient with head of bed >45-degree angle.
      e) Administer chest physiotherapy every 2 hours.
      f) Keep staff, visitors, or other patients with an upper respiratory infection away from patient.

4. Tissue Perfusion, altered: hepato-renal

a. Monitor for hepato-renal failure.
   1) Monitor intake and output every hour and report urine output of <30 mL/h.
   2) Monitor urinalysis, urine electrolytes, and 24-hour urine test for creatinine clearance and urea; report the following findings:
      a) Specific gravity >1.015
      b) Mild proteinuria and hematuria
      c) Presence of granular casts
      d) Osmolality >400 Osm/kg H_2O
      e) Urine sodium <10 mmol/L
      f) Decreased creatinine clearance
   3) Monitor laboratory values for altered serum electrolytes (elevated potassium and phosphate); increased or decreased BUN; and increased creatinine.
   4) Monitor serial daily weights, noting fluctuation (1 L of fluid weighs 2.2 lb) and presence of peripheral edema.
b. Promote improved renal function.
   1) Encourage sodium intake restriction.
   2) Administer ordered low-dose dopamine and potassium-sparing or loop diuretics.
   3) Prepare patient for paracentesis; assist physician in procedure.
   4) Prepare patient for insertion of a peritoneovenous shunt (LeVeen, Denver, or Minnesota), as needed.
   5) Prepare patient for hemodialysis or continuous arteriovenous hemofiltration.
   6) Avoid administration of nephrotoxic drugs.
c. Monitor for precipitants of hepato-renal failure such as abdominal paracentesis with removal of >1 L of ascitic fluid and loss of fluid volume due to hemorrhage or aggressive diuretic therapy.
5. Fluid Volume Excess or Deficit
   a. Monitor fluid and electrolyte status.
      1) Monitor ordered laboratory and diagnostics test results and report significant changes.
      2) Monitor daily weights, hourly intake and output, vital signs (assess for orthostatic hypotension), daily abdominal and ankle girth, changes in amount of bulging in the flanks and displacement

of the umbilicus, and changes in shifting dullness and fluid wave in abdomen.

3) Monitor for fatigue, malaise, nausea, vomiting, diarrhea, abdominal cramps, anorexia, muscle weakness, decreased reflexes, and cardiac arrhythmias suggesting hypokalemia.

4) Monitor for and report significant changes in hemodynamic parameters.

b. Promote adequate fluid and electrolyte status.

1) Encourage intake of sodium restricted diet (usually 250–500 mg/d).

2) Restrict fluids to 1000–1500 mL/d as ordered.

3) Administer ordered potassium-sparing and loop diuretics, low-dose dopamine, and IV salt-poor albumin.

4) Provide protein intake, usually 20–40 g/d initially and building up to as much as 100 g/d. May use branched-chain amino acids per physician order.

5) Prepare patient and assist with paracentesis.

6) Prepare patient for hemodialysis or continuous arteriovenous hemofiltration.

7) Prepare patient for insertion of peritoneovenous shunt.

6. Nutrition: altered, less than body requirements

a. Monitor nutritional status.

1) Monitor laboratory and diagnostic test findings and report significant changes.

2) Assess height and weight, skin, hair, nails, eyes, head, mouth, heart, abdomen, extremities, and nervous system; note results of anthropometric measures, candida and trichophyton skin tests, and resting metabolic expenditure.

3) If patient is in fulminant liver failure, monitor for hypoglycemia.

b. Promote nutritional status.

1) Administer ordered dextrose solutions (10%, 20%, or 50%) to maintain blood sugar >100 mg/dL.

2) Administer ordered branched-chain amino acids IV or orally.

3) Administer ordered thiamine, folic acid, vitamin K, trace elements, and lipid supplements.

4) Encourage intake of protein in diet, usually 20–100

g. If patient has encephalopathy, protein will be restricted and glucose used for energy source.
5) Encourage intake of dietary sodium, usually 250–500 mg/d.
6) Restrict fluid intake, usually 1000–1500 mL/d.

Factors for Nutrition Assessment

1. Serum electrolytes
2. Trace elements
3. Hemoglobin and hematocrit
4. Ferritin
5. Transferrin
6. Albumin
7. Cholesterol
8. Thyroxine binding prealbumin
9. Retinal binding protein
10. Total abolute lymphocyte count
11. Glucose
12. Vitamin levels
13. Urine urea/creatinine ratio

---

7. Skin Integrity: impaired, high risk for
   a. Monitor for impaired skin integrity over bony prominences and in areas of edematous tissue every 2–4 hours.
   b. Prevent skin breakdown.
      1) Put patient on pressure-relief device (i.e., a 4-in-thick corrugated mattress, special beds).
      2) Provide gentle massage of back and hips with moisturizing cream or lotion.
      3) Maintain meticulous personal hygiene.
      4) Control pruritus by administering cholestyramine (Questran) or phenobarbital; applying emollient creams, menthol, phenol, camphor lotions; topical anesthetic agents; bathing with baking soda; and avoiding extremes of temperature, conditions that dry the skin, and exposure to wool.

Monitoring, Managing, and Preventing
Life-Threatening Emergencies
1. Multisystem organ failure

a. Monitor patients at risk and recognize of onset during the early phases.
   1) Assess for risk factors
   2) Be alert for early warning signals, such as:
      a) Increased or decreased temperature
      b) Increasing heart rate
      c) Increasing respiratory rate
      d) Increased or decreased WBC count
      e) Subtle changes in sensorium
   3) Report findings consistent with the development of systemic inflammatory response syndrome.
b. Prevent organ injury.
   1) Provide ventilatory support through intubation and mechanical ventilation.
   2) Control body temperature to adjust for hyperthermia or hypothermia.
   3) Reverse acidosis.
   4) Monitor for progression.
      a) Monitor for subtle changes in assessment findings, which may indicate deterioration from the hyperdynamic phase to the hypodynamic phase.
      b) Measure hemodynamic parameters frequently and report changes.
      c) Assess the patient frequently, paying particular attention to serial findings to identify deterioration in previously uninvolved organ systems.
      d) Analyze changes in laboratory values to determine deterioration of multiple organs.
      e) Monitor patient responses to medications and treatments, and report significant findings.
c. Provide supportive care.
   1) Control the infection.
      a) Obtain a specimen of all secretions for culture and sensitivity testing.
      b) Prepare the patient for surgical intervention to remove sources of infection.
      c) Promote an aseptic environment to prevent nosocomial infections.
   2) Arrest and reverse the progress of the syndrome.
      a) Prevent translocation of bacteria from the gut with enteral feeding of glutamine, an immuno-

nutrient that maintains gut integrity and stimulates the immune system.

b) Prepare for continuous arteriovenous hemodiafiltration, which has been used successfully in trauma patients.

c) Recognize complications, including skin breakdown and third spacing of fluid.

3) Provide metabolic support.

a) Measure oxygen consumption with increased flow until lactic acid level returns to normal.

b) Provide adequate nutrition. Enteral route is preferred over parenteral using a formula that is high in protein and has medium-chain triglycerides for lipids.

2. Cerebral edema

a. Monitor for increased intracranial pressure (ICP).

1) Assess for changes in level of consciousness, pupillary response to light, sensorimotor functions, respiratory rate and rhythm, and blood pressure.

2) Assess ICP via an extradural pressure transducer and calculate cerebral perfusion pressures (CPP). (CPP = mean arterial pressure − ICP).

3) Assist in determining CBF, measured by inhaled xenon during a CT scan of the head or at bedside with xenon 133.

4) Assist in determining cerebral venous blood oxygen content by collecting blood from a catheter placed in the jugular bulb.

5) Calculate cerebral oxygen consumption ($CMRO_2$), which equals the product of CBF and the difference between arterial and jugular venous oxygen content (A-JVO_2 gradient). If $CMRO_2$ remains constant, widening of the A-JVO_2 gradient suggests cerebral ischemia; narrowing suggests cerebral hyperemia (brain swelling); notify physician of findings.

Acute Intestinal Ischemia/Bowel Infarction

Acute intestinal ischemia/bowel infarction is an acute or chronic, arterial or venous disorder caused by a complete occlusion or narrowing of mesenteric vessels. This results in a decreased perfusion and delivery of oxygen to intestinal tissue, which could culminate in the transmural (involving the full thickness) necrosis of bowel wall.

Etiology/Pathophysiology

1. Caused by any mechanism that compromises sufficient blood flow to meet the oxygen demands of intestinal tissue and results in cellular dysfunction and cell death
2. Types of intestinal ischemic disorders
   a. Arterial
      1) Superior mesenteric artery (SMA) embolus — occlusion of a blood vessel due to a free-floating plug of blood clot, bacteria, or other foreign material
      2) SMA thrombosis — occlusion of a blood vessel
      3) Nonocclusive mesenteric ischemia — diminished blood supply due to narrowing of the arteries
      4) Arteritis — inflammation of an artery
      5) Ischemic colitis — inflammation of the colon
      6) Segmental ischemia caused by strangulation
   b. Venous
      1) Mesenteric venous thrombosis
      2) Segmental ischemia caused by strangulation or local venous thrombosis
3. Predisposing factors
   a. SMA embolus
      1) Emboli from left atrium or ventricle dislodged during an arrhythmia
      2) Bacterial endocarditis
      3) Valvular prosthesis
      4) Existence of multiple emboli in other arteries
      5) History of peripheral artery embolus
      6) Atrial myxoma (cardiac neoplasm)
   b. SMA thrombosis
      1) Severe atherosclerotic narrowing
      2) Acute ischemic episode coupled with chronic ischemia
      3) Oral contraceptive use
      4) Arterial vasculitis (polyarteritis nodosa, systemic lupus erythematosus, rheumatoid arthritis)
      5) Fibromuscular hyperplasia
      6) Hypercoagulable states (antithrombin III deficiency or polycythemia vera)
      7) Amyloidosis

   c. Nonocclusive mesenteric ischemia
     1) Splanchnic vasoconstriction caused by vasoactive medications or periods of decreased cardiac output (congestive heart failure [CHF], hypovolemia, myocardial infarction [MI])
     2) Digoxin use
     3) Dissecting abdominal aortic aneurysm
     4) Postoperative abdominal aortic aneurysm repair or abdominal-perineum resection
     5) Moderate-to-severe mesenteric atherosclerosis
   d. Mesenteric venous thrombosis
     1) Stasis in mesenteric venous bed (portal hypertension, CHF)
     2) Abdominal malignancy
     3) Intra-abdominal inflammation (peritonitis, inflammatory bowel disease, abscess)
     4) Abdominal surgery or trauma
     5) Hypercoagulable state
     6) Oral contraceptive use
     7) Sclerotherapy for esophageal varices
   e. Other
     1) Intestinal adhesions
     2) Small-bowel obstruction
     3) Chronic heart disease or CHF with arrhythmias in patients older than 50 years of age, recent MI, or hypotension
4. Pathophysiology
   a. Ischemic changes begin in intestinal mucosal cells within 5 minutes. This begins the process of increased capillary permeability, loss of capillary integrity, and vasospasm.
   b. The ischemic process results in edema and hemorrhage of the submucosa, ulceration of the mucosa, secondary bacterial contamination, bowel paralysis and distention, third spacing of fluid, and ultimately perforation of the intestinal wall with peritonitis and septic shock.
   c. The degree of intestinal damage depends on the metabolic needs of the tissue, the amount of collateral circulation, the number of mesenteric vessels involved, the length of time of compromised blood flow, the overall condition of the systemic circulation, and the response of the vascular bed to hypoperfusion.

Assessment/Analysis

ASSESSMENT FINDINGS

Subjective

1. Pain that varies in severity, location, and nature
2. Weight loss with fear of eating (ingestion of food precipitates abdominal pain)
3. Nausea, vomiting
4. Diarrhea or constipation
5. Abdominal distention
6. Low-grade fever
7. History of risk factors for embolic, thrombotic, or nonocclusive intestinal ischemia

Objective

1. Pain out of proportion to physical findings in a patient at risk for ischemic bowel disease
2. Cachexia
3. Abdominal distention
4. Serosanguinous ascitic fluid (accumulation of fluid in the peritoneal cavity)
5. Bloody drainage from a nasogastric tube or the rectum
6. Mental confusion in elderly patients
7. Tachypnea
8. Cool, pale, clammy skin
9. Anxiety progressing to lethargy
10. Oliguria
11. Abdominal guarding with tenderness progressing to frank pain on palpation
12. Signs of peripheral emboli (loss of pulse in extremity; blue, dusky color to extremity; cool skin)
13. Tachycardia, hypotension
14. Absent to hyperactive bowel sounds

SUPPORTING TEST FINDINGS

Laboratory Tests

1. Complete blood count
   Abnormality: Increased white blood cell (WBC) count

with a left shift (an increase in immature neutrophils or "bands" as occurs in an infection)
Increased hemoglobin and hematocrit

2. Serum lactate
   Abnormality: Increased
3. Arterial blood gases
   Abnormality: Metabolic acidosis
4. Serum amylase and phosphate
   Abnormality: Increased
5. Serum aspartate aminotransferase and lactic dehydrogenase
   Abnormality: Increased 6–12 hours after intestinal infarction
6. Serum creatine phosphokinase
   Abnormality: Increased
7. Serum intestinal alkaline phosphatase and N-acetyl-hexosaminidase
   Abnormality: Increased
8. Peritoneal fluid for intestinal alkaline phosphatase, inorganic phosphorus, and blood
   Abnormality: Increased and positive for blood

Diagnostic Tests

1. Abdominal X-ray
   Abnormality: Dilation of intestinal loops and/or edema or "thumb printing"
2. Arteriography of the aorta and mesenteric branches
   Abnormality: Vessels with diminished blood flow; vasodilators or thrombolytic agents can be infused into vessels as needed; usually done after hemodynamic stability is achieved; must stop all vasoconstricting drugs before procedure
3. Barium enema (should not be done first if angiography is planned)
   Abnormality: Thumb printing, which represents edema and submucosal hemorrhage in ischemic colitis
4. Computed tomography scan of the abdomen
   Abnormality: May be used to rule out conditions that mimic intestinal ischemia (i.e., acute pancreatitis, perforated viscus; may show areas of intestinal edema, ascites and mesenteric thrombosis)
5. Magnetic resonance imaging

Abnormality: Mesenteric thrombosis

6. Abdominal ultrasonography

   Abnormality: None; used to rule out conditions that mimic intestinal ischemia (i.e., acute pancreatitis, perforated viscus; may show areas of intestinal edema, ascites, and mesenteric thromboses

7. Doppler ultrasound

   Abnormality: Vessels with decreased velocity and/or turbulent blood flow

8. Colonoscopy

   Abnormality: In ischemic colitis, may see red, edematous, friable mucosa alternating with areas of blanching; ulcerations also may be present

9. Esophagogastroduodenoscopy and laparoscopy

   Abnormality: Edema and diffuse superficial ulceration. (May be performed in patients who cannot undergo angiography)

Planning/Intervention

COLLABORATIVE MANAGEMENT

Procedures

Diagnosis and treatment must be started within the first 24 hours of onset to ensure a 60% survival rate; survival rate drops below 30% if treatment is started later than 24 hours after onset.

1. Provide supportive care.
   a. Insert a nasogastric tube and attach to low suction to promote bowel decompression.
   b. Administer ordered crystalloids and colloids to promote fluid and electrolyte balance.
   c. Obtain specimens for culture and sensitivity testing and administer ordered broad-spectrum antibiotics to prevent or arrest infection.
   d. Assist with treatment of any underlying medical problem (i.e., CHF).
   e. Assist with insertion of a pulmonary artery catheter and monitor hemodynamic status.
   f. Insert an indwelling urinary catheter and monitor urinary output.

g. Infuse ordered papaverine into superior mesenteric artery at 30–60 mg/min to reduce vasopasm.
2. Assist with interventions to correct underlying injury.
   a. Assist with angioplasty (percutaneous transluminal angioplasty or laser angioplasty) to promote vessel patency.
   b. Infuse ordered thrombolytic agents through inserted catheters to promote blood clot lysis.
   c. Administer ordered heparin to reduce blood clotting.
   d. Prepare patient for laparotomy, as ordered.
      1) Direct arteriotomy or catheter embolectomy
      2) Surgical revascularization with aortomesenteric bypass or endarterectomy
      3) Resection of infarcted bowel
   e. Assist with assessment of bowel viability intraoperatively via clinical judgment, Doppler ultrasound or fluorescein injection, and inspection of bowel with Wood light, as ordered.
3. Monitor postoperative status.
   a. Prepare patient for postoperative angiography to assess vessel patency, as ordered.
   b. Prepare patient for a "second look" laparotomy 24 hours after bowel resection to assess bowel viability, as ordered.

Drug Therapy

1. Crystalloid solutions
   Examples: Lactated Ringer's solution
   normal saline solution
   Action: Expand blood volume; replace fluid and electrolytes lost in vomiting, diarrhea, and third spacing
   Caution: Can cause electrolyte imbalance and circulatory overload
2. Colloid solutions
   Example: Human albumin (Albuminar—5% and 25%)
   Action: Expands blood volume; raises serum protein levels
   Used to replace sequestered proteins
   Caution: Can cause circulatory failure, hypertension, pulmonary edema, and fluid overload
3. Antibiotics
   Example: cefoxitin (Mefoxin)

clindamycin (Cleocin)
gentamycin (Garamycin)

Action: Provides coverage for a broad spectrum of gram-positive and gram-negative aerobes and anaerobes

Caution: Cefoxitan can cause pseudomembranous colitis, rashes, and gastrointestinal upset

Clindamycin can cause pseudomembranous colitis and diarrhea

Gentamycin can cause nephrotoxicity and ototoxicity

4. Vasodilator

Example: papaverine hydrochloride

Action: Infused directly into specific mesenteric arteries to relax smooth muscle of blood vessels and improve blood flow to the intestine

Caution: Can cause visual changes, headache, hypotension, slight hypertension, arrhythmias, flushing, and respiratory depression

5. Thrombolytics

Example: streptokinase (Streptase)

Action: Infused directly into specific mesenteric arteries to dissolve blood clots in acute embolus; may require therapy for 36 hours to dissolve clot

Caution: Allergic reactions, bleeding

6. Anticoagulants

Example: heparin (Lipohepin)

Action: Prevents the growth of existing blood clots and the formation of new clots; used postoperatively in cases of mesenteric venous thrombosis; may be used postoperatively in other situations (use of heparin is controversial as it may cause intestinal hemorrhage)

Caution: Can cause bleeding, thrombocytopenia, and allergic reactions

---

Nursing Alert

Avoid using vasopressors (except for low-dose dopamine) and digitalis preparations whenever possible because they produce splanchnic vasoconstriction.

NURSING MANAGEMENT

Monitoring and Managing Clinical Problems

1. Pain
   a. Monitor pain status. Note location, characteristics, severity, frequency, duration, restlessness, splinting, guarding, facial grimacing, and shallow respirations; report significant changes in pain status.
   b. Promote pain relief.
      1) Assist patient in finding a comfortable position.
      2) Administer ordered analgesics.
      3) Provide physical treatments, such as back rubs; relaxation techniques; and a restful, quiet environment to reduce anxiety and pain.
      4) Use a calm, reassuring approach with patient.
      5) Institute all measures to promote gastrointestinal function.
      6) Assist with insertion and monitor epidural catheter analgesics.
2. Infection: high risk for
   a. Monitor bowel function and for signs and symptoms of peritonitis.
      1) Assess for hypoactive or hyperactive bowel sounds; alterations in vital signs, especially temperature; abdominal distention and increased girth measurement; softness, rigidity, guarding, or rebound tenderness; tympany or dullness to percussion; abnormal nasogastric drainage and stools; report significant findings.
      2) Monitor results of laboratory and diagnostic tests, and report significant changes.
   b. Promote gastrointestinal healing/function.
      1) Maintain NPO status; keep nasogastric tube patent and connected to low suction, and assess nasogastric tube placement every 2 hours.
      2) Administer ordered papaverine, thrombolytic agents, heparin, and intravenous fluids.
      3) Optimize cardiovascular function.
      4) Prepare patient for diagnostic tests and laparotomy.
   c. Prevent peritonitis.

   1) Follow universal precautions and encourage the use of sterile technique during invasive procedures.
   2) Administer ordered antibiotics.
3. Fluid Volume Deficit: high risk for
   a. Monitor fluid and electrolyte status.
      1) Monitor serial laboratory values and report significant findings.
      2) Monitor daily weights, hourly intake and output, and vital signs (assess for orthostatic hypotension), and daily abdominal girth; report significant findings.
      3) Monitor hemodynamic parameters and report significant changes.
   b. Promote fluid and electrolyte balance by administering crystalloids, colloids, and electrolytes, as ordered; assess effectiveness of therapy.
4. Injury: high risk for
   a. Transient acute tubular necrosis
      1) Monitor hourly urine output and report output of <30 mL/h
      2) Monitor serial serum creatinine and blood urea nitrogen for increased levels.
      3) Note color and clarity of urine hourly.
      4) Obtain specimens and monitor results of ordered urine laboratory studies.
      5) Monitor for hypertension, peripheral edema, new onset of third heart sound suggesting volume overload.
      6) Monitor serum electrolyte levels closely to identify abnormalities, especially hyperkalemia.
   b. Occlusion of artery by arterial catheter
      1) Monitor for ischemic changes.
      2) Assess for pain.
   c. Catheter dislodgement
      1) Observe for sudden drop in blood pressure.
      2) Monitor for tachycardia and other arrhythmias.
      3) If catheter dislodgement is suspected, replace papaverine with normal saline until catheter placement can be confirmed.
   d. Hematomas at insertion site
      1) Inspect insertion site routinely.

2) Apply direct pressure to site if bleeding is suspected.

e. Thrombosis of catheter
1) Monitor for decreased flow of infusion.
2) Do not forcefully irrigate catheter.
3) Discontinue infusion and notify physician if thrombosis is suspected.

f. Liver abscesses
1) Observe for increased temperature.
2) Assess for right upper quadrant pain.
3) Palpate and percuss for enlarged liver.
4) Monitor for increased WBCs and abnormal liver function tests.

g. Intra-abdominal abscess
1) Monitor for increased temperature and chills.
2) Assess for tachycardia.
3) Auscultate bowel sounds to identify paralytic ileus.
4) Note abdominal distention.
5) Assess for anorexia.

h. Peritonitis
1) Monitor for increased temperature.
2) Monitor for increased WBCs.
3) Assess for abdominal pain with guarding.
4) Note abdominal distention, nausea, and vomiting.
5) Monitor for anorexia.

i. Pneumonia
1) Monitor for increased temperature.
2) Monitor for increased WBCs.
3) Assess for cough with sputum production; note hemoptysis.
4) Assess for dyspnea and pleuritic chest pain.

Monitoring, Managing, and Preventing Life-Threatening Emergencies

1. Septic shock
   a. Continuously monitor hemodynamic parameters to evaluate the cardiovascular response to treatment.
   b. Continuously monitor urinary output via catheter to evaluate renal function.
   c. Monitor cardiac rhythm for tachycardia and life-threatening ventricular arrhythmias (ventricular tachycardia and/or fibrillation).

d. Maintain a patent airway and adequate ventilation. Use supplemental oxygen to ensure that sufficient oxygen is delivered to the lungs.

e. Provide enteral or parenteral nutritional support to prevent a negative nitrogen balance.

f. Promote treatment of sepsis

1) Administer ordered antibiotics.

2) Obtain specimens of all potential infection sites for culture and sensitivity testing.

3) Monitor serial WBC counts and peak and trough levels of antibiotics for effectiveness of treatment.

4) Monitor temperature every 4 hours and treat, as needed, with medications or external cooling devices.

Abdominal Trauma

Injury to the structures located between the diaphragm and the pelvis via blunt or penetrating forces is known as abdominal trauma. Organs at risk include the large and small bowel, spleen, duodenum, pancreas, kidneys, and urinary bladder.

Etiology/Pathophysiology

1. Etiology of blunt trauma
   a. Motor vehicle accident
   b. Physical assault
   c. Falls
      1) <15 feet
      2) ≥15 feet
2. Etiology of penetrating trauma
   a. Stab wounds
   b. Gunshot wounds
      1) High-energy gunshot wounds (hunting rifles, assault weapons, shotgun blasts at close range)
      2) Medium-energy gunshot wounds (most handguns)
   c. Impalement
3. Pathophysiology of blunt trauma
   a. The severity of the injury is related to the impact's force and duration, the size of the patient, and the amount of surface area in contact with the force. Multiple injuries are common.
   b. In a direct impact injury there is a sudden significant increase in intra-abdominal pressure created by the transfer of energy from an external source to the underlying structures, resulting in the rupture of a hollow viscus or bursting of a solid organ.
   c. In crush injuries, abdominal viscera become compressed between the abdominal wall and the spine or the thoracic cage, resulting in extensive soft-tissue damage and visceral rupture.
   d. In deceleration injury, the organs continue to move forward although the body has come to a complete stop. This results in the tearing of tissue and vessels from their attachment points.
4. Pathophysiology of penetrating trauma
   a. The severity of the injury is related to the type of missile used, the amount of tissue penetration, and the velocity of the missile. Multiple organ injury is common.
   b. In penetrating injuries, crush occurs as the missile impacts tissue and stretch occurs as the energy exchange results in the development of a temporary cavity.

   c. Low-velocity missiles tend to result in tissue injury of limited proportion.

   d. High-velocity missiles result in significant tissue damage as the trajectory is variable and multiple organs as well as surrounding tissue may be damaged by dissipation of kinetic energy by the missile.

Assessment/Analysis

ASSESSMENT FINDINGS

Subjective

1. History of injury
2. May be asymptomatic
3. Diffuse or localized abdominal tenderness, severe pain
4. Pain at tip of left shoulder (Kehr's sign) may signify splenic rupture or irritation of the diaphragm with blood or fecal material.

Objective

1. Involuntary guarding, muscle rigidity
2. Abnormal abdominal contour
3. Abrasions, hematomas, multiple bruises from injury source such as tires or seat belts
4. Ecchymoses in flank areas (Grey Turner's sign) may indicate retroperitoneal bleeding.
5. Bluish color around umbilicus (Cullen's sign) may indicate retroperitoneal bleeding.
6. Presence of entrance and exit wounds on anterior and posterior abdomen.
7. Ecchymosis on scrotum or labia (Coopernail's sign) may indicate fractured pelvis.
8. Cool, pale clammy skin
9. Tachypnea, shallow labored breathing
10. Pale palmar creases when fingers are forcibly extended
11. Anxiety progressing to lethargy
12. Oliguria with urine output <30 mL/h
13. Protruding or visible foreign objects
14. Abnormal nasogastric drainage and stool

15. Hypotension, orthostatic hypotension (positive tilt test)
16. Tachycardia
17. Bowel sounds heard in chest on auscultation
18. Hyperactive, diminished, or absent bowel sounds
19. Presence of bruit, venous hums, or friction rubs
20. Shifting dullness, loss of gastric tympany, or decreased or absent liver dullness
21. Abnormal rectal exam noting presence of blood, pain, or high-riding prostate
22. Palpable masses or pulsations
23. Abdominal pain or rebound tenderness on palpation
24. Pain over lower ribs on palpation
25. Pain over symphysis pubis and iliac crest on palpation
26. Pain on palpation of the iliac crest

SUPPORTING TEST FINDINGS

Laboratory Tests

1. Renal function tests (blood urea nitrogen [BUN] and creatinine)
   Abnormality: Increased BUN and creatinine may reflect renal trauma
2. Complete blood count, hemoglobin and hematocrit, white blood cell (WBC) count
   Abnormality: Reflects blood loss, after the first few hours of injury, and hemodilution due to administration of crystalloid solutions (for every unit of blood lost, hemoglobin drops 1 g and hematocrit drops 3%); WBC count elevates initially and is a nonspecific finding
3. Serum amylase
   Abnormality: Increased value indicates pancreatic injury
4. Arterial blood gases (ABGs)
   Abnormality: Decreased PaO_2
   Increased, normal, or decreased $PaCO_2$
   Metabolic acidosis (blood has an acid excess or base deficit with a pH <7.35)
   Alkalosis (blood has an acid deficit or base excess with a pH >7.45)
5. Urinalysis
   Abnormality: Gross or microscopic blood indicates renal or bladder injury

Myoglobin following crush injury reflects muscle damage

Diagnostic Tests

1. Anteroposterior chest X-ray
   Abnormality: Performed before peritoneal lavage, it shows free air in intraperitoneal or retroperitoneal space (indicates a gastric, duodenal, small-bowel, or colon perforation)

   Malposition of nasogastric tube (indicates rupture of left diaphragm)

2. X-ray of the abdomen (flat plate)
   Abnormality: Performed before peritoneal lavage, it shows air under the diaphragm (indicates perforation of the gastrointestinal tract), location of a missile

   Presence of a large mass in the left upper quadrant (indicates rupture of the spleen or a hematoma)

   Bony injuries of lower rib cage

3. Diagnostic peritoneal lavage
   Abnormality: Blood >10 mL, bile, urine, or enteric contents

   Lavage fluid exits a chest tube or indwelling urinary catheter

   Lavage fluid contains red blood cells (RBCs) >100,000/mm^3; WBCs >500/mm^3; or amylase >20 IU/L with alkaline phosphatase >3 IU

   Unable to read newsprint through intravenous tubing containing lavage fluid (this is a gross screening test)

4. Laparotomy
   Abnormality: Injury to specific abdominal organs

5. Upper gastrointestinal tract series with water-soluble contrast (performed on stable patients only)
   Abnormality: May identify duodenal perforation

6. Computed tomography of the abdomen
   Abnormality: Intraperitoneal and retroperitoneal hemorrhage

7. Abdominal ultrasound
   Abnormality: Free intraperitoneal fluid and identify areas of solid organ hematomas

8. Hepatosplenic technetium sulfur colloid scanning (performed no sooner than 12 hours after injury)

Abnormality: Abnormal size and shape of liver (areas of impaired blood flow and decreased reticulo-endothelial function result in decreased or patchy uptake of radiocolloid)

9. Abdominal aortography, splanchnic angiography, and pelvic angiography

   Abnormality: Vascular injuries and bleeding vessels

Planning/Intervention

COLLABORATIVE MANAGEMENT

Procedures

1. Patient stabilization
   a. Assist with establishing and maintaining airway and breathing (i.e., intubation and mechanical ventilation, as needed).
   b. Assist with establishing and maintaining circulation (i.e., fluid resuscitation, direct pressure to bleeding site and use of military antishock trousers (MAST) with retroperitoneal bleeding associated with pelvic and/or long bone fractures).
   c. Assist with insertion of a central venous or pulmonary artery catheter.
   d. Obtain laboratory specimens, as ordered.
   e. Obtain ordered chest X-ray and flat plate of the abdomen before peritoneal lavage.
   f. Evaluate chest for thoracic injuries.
   g. Decompress stomach with a nasogastric tube.
   h. Assist with diagnostic peritoneal lavage.
   i. Assist with stab wound exploration, as needed.
2. Surgical intervention
   a. Prepare patients for emergency surgery with any of the following findings:
      1) Hemorrhagic shock
      2) Gunshot wound
      3) Evisceration
      4) Impaled foreign object
      5) Blood in rectum or stomach
      6) Peritonitis
      7) Positive diagnostic peritoneal lavage

   b. Patients who are stable and have a negative diagnostic peritoneal lavage may have other diagnostic tests performed to determine presence of more subtle injuries.

   c. Prepare patient for selective angiography with embolization, as needed, to control bleeding.

   d. Prepare patient for surgical repair of damage and transport patient to intensive care unit.

Drug Therapy

1. Crystalloid solutions
   Examples: Lactated Ringer's solution
           normal saline solution
   Action: Expand blood volume; replace fluid and electrolytes lost in hemorrhage
   Caution: Electrolyte imbalance, circulatory overload

2. Blood
   Example: Packed RBCs or whole blood
   Action: Replace RBCs lost during hemorrhage to improve the oxygen-carrying capacity of blood
   Caution: Massive blood transfusion can result in hypothermia, volume overload, hypocalcemia (serum calcium <8.5 mEq/100 mL), metabolic alkalosis, thrombocytopenia (platelet count $<150,000/mm^3$); coagulopathy, hyperkalemia (serum potassium >5.5 mEq/L), a tighter binding of oxygen to hemoglobin, and transfusion reactions

3. Blood products
   Example: Fresh frozen plasma
   Action: Replaces clotting factors V and VIII in patients receiving massive transfusions
   Caution: Volume overload; carries risk of viral transmission

4. Antibiotics
   Examples: cefoxitin (Mefoxin)
           clindamycin (Cleocin)
           gentamycin (Garamycin)
   Action: Provides coverage for gram-positive and gram-negative aerobes as well as anaerobes
   Caution: Cefoxitin can cause pseudomembranous colitis, rashes, and gastrointestinal upset
       Clindamycin can cause pseudomembranous colitis and diarrhea

Gentamycin can cause nephrotoxicity and oto-toxicity

5. Vaccines

Examples: Tetanus immune globulin (TIG) and tetanus toxoid

Action: TIG is an antitoxin that neutralizes circulating toxin and unbound toxin found in wounds

Tetanus toxoid stimulates active immunity

Caution: TIG should be given before manipulating wounds

TIG and tetanus toxoid should be administered at separate sites in separate syringes

NURSING MANAGEMENT

Monitoring and Managing Clinical Problems

1. Breathing Pattern: ineffective
   a. Monitor respiratory status.
      1) Assess chest for abnormalities in respiratory rate and rhythm, symmetry of chest expansion, presence of breath sounds bilaterally, presence of adventitious sounds, pain, paradoxic chest wall movement, crepitus, and thoracic deformity; report significant findings.
      2) Assess for cyanosis and dyspnea.
      3) Monitor results of ABGs for decreased PaO_2 and increased $PaCO_2$.
      4) Apply pulse oximeter and monitor continuously for O_2 saturation of $<95\%$
   b. Promote patent airway and oxygenation.
      1) Administer O_2, as ordered.
      2) Observe for obstructed airway.
         a) Implement use of airways.
         b) Suction, as needed.
      3) Assist with intubation and insertion of chest tubes, as needed.
2. Cardiac Output: decreased — high risk for
   a. Monitor cardiovascular status.
      1) Monitor heart rate and rhythm.
      2) Note distant or muffled heart sounds (could mean cardiac tamponade).
      3) Assess for murmur (could mean valvular injury).

4) Take blood pressure in both arms and at least one leg (a 10–20 mm Hg difference in systolic and diastolic pressure is normal between arm and leg pressures; a pressure > 20 mm Hg may mean injury to the aorta).

5) Assess quality of peripheral pulses and note rate of capillary return.

6) Assist with insertion of a central venous pressure (CVP) monitor or a pulmonary artery catheter, and monitor readings.

3. Tissue Perfusion, altered: cerebral — high risk for
   a. Monitor neurologic status
   1) Assess for changes in level of consciousness, pupillary response to light, sensorimotor functions, respiratory rate and rhythm, and blood pressure.
   2) Monitor results of cervical and any other spine X-rays.
   b. Prevent cervical spine injury by leaving cervical collar in place until C-spine X-rays have ruled out an injury.

4. Trauma: high risk for
   a. Monitor for abdominal injury.
   1) Remove all clothing and log roll patient to quickly assess anterior and posterior body surfaces for impaled objects, exit/entry wounds, hematomas, and other signs of injury; report significant findings.
   2) Evaluate abdominal injury by:
      a) Inspecting for shallow, labored breathing; chest and abdominal wall integrity; hematomas, abrasions, masses, pulsations, protruding organs, or foreign objects; bullet, puncture, or stab wounds; powder burns; abnormal contour; Grey Turner's sign; Cullen's sign; Coppernail's sign; and abnormal nasogastric drainage and stool every 4 hours. Report significant findings.
      b) Palpating for painful areas, rebound tenderness, rigidity and guarding, pain while compressing the iliac crest, and rectal tenderness or fullness every 4 hours; report significant findings.
      c) Percussing for increased or loss of gastric tympany, decreased or absent liver dullness, and

shifting dullness in the flanks every 4 hours; report significant findings.

   d) Auscultating for hypoactive, hyperactive, or absent bowel sounds and bruits; venous hums or friction rubs; report significant findings.

  3) Monitor results of repeated diagnostic tests.

b. Prepare patient for diagnostic peritoneal lavage or tap.

  1) Preprocedure

   a) Explain procedure and rationale to patient.

   b) Insert nasogastric tube and indwelling urinary catheter before tap.

   c) Monitor vital signs.

  2) During procedure

   a) Assist with insertion of peritoneal trocar or catheter.

   b) Gently roll patient from side to side so fluid can reach all intra-abdominal areas.

   c) Allow fluid to drain by gravity and assess color and characteristics of fluid.

   d) Monitor vital signs.

  3) Postprocedure

   a) Send sample of lavage fluid for blood count, bile, amylase, culture or gram stain, as ordered.

   b) Apply antibiotic ointment and sterile dressing over puncture site.

   c) Monitor patient for signs of perforated bladder or bowel after lavage.

   d) Monitor vital signs.

c. Stabilize all impaled objects before surgery.

d. Administer antibiotics and/or tetanus immunizations, as ordered.

e. Restore blood volume with crystalloids and/or colloid solutions, as ordered.

5. Fluid Volume Deficit

a. Promote restoration of blood volume.

  1) Administer crystalloid solutions, whole blood or packed RBCs, and fresh frozen plasma, as ordered.

  2) Position patient with legs elevated unless contraindicated by injury.

  3) Apply MAST garment (controversial).

  4) Prevent complications of MAST garment:

a) Pad all pressure points before inflation.
b) Insert a nasogastric tube and indwelling urinary catheter before inflation.
c) Insure that garment does not inflate over lower thorax.
d) Release each compartment sequentially beginning with the abdomen.
   5) Monitor for complications of MAST garment
      a) Compromised respiratory function
      b) Compartmental syndrome
      c) Vomiting
6. Infection: high risk for
   a. Prevent infection.
      1) Administer antibiotics and tetanus immunizations.
      2) Irrigate wounds with normal saline solutions or antibiotic solution.
      3) Cover wounds with sterile dressings.
      4) Stabilize all impaled objects.
      5) Use aseptic technique in wound care.
      6) Wash hands frequently.
      7) Avoid autotransfusion.
   b. Monitor for infection.
      1) Assess for temperature increase.
      2) Monitor for increasing WBCs.
      3) Observe for increasing abdominal pain, tenderness, and rigidity.
7. Pain
   a. Administer ordered analgesics.
   b. Assist the patient to find a position of comfort.
   c. Assist with insertion of and monitor epidural catheter analgesia.
   d. Monitor response to pain interventions and alter regimen, as needed.

Monitoring, Managing, and Preventing Life-Threatening Emergencies

1. Hemorrhage
   a. Monitor for physical findings of blood loss:
      1) Tachycardia with a faint, thready pulse
      2) Tachypnea
      3) Hypotension in recumbent position or postural hypotension

    4) Cool, pale, or cyanotic, clammy skin
    5) Capillary refill >3 seconds
    6) Poor skin turgor with dry mucous membranes
    7) Lethargy, confusion, or obtundation
    8) Decreased urine output
    9) Increasing abdominal girth
   10) Rigid abdomen
   11) Guaiac-positive stools or nasogastric drainage, and blood per rectum, vagina, urinary meatus, emesis, or peritoneal lavage

  b. Monitor serial hemoglobin and hematocrit for decreasing values.

  c. Monitor serial hemodynamic parameters for decreased CVP, pulmonary artery pressure, pulmonary capillary wedge pressure, and cardiac output; report significant findings.

  d. Prevent hemorrhage by:
    1) Applying direct pressure over bleeding sites
    2) Preparing patient for selective angiography with embolization or laparotomy
    3) Not removing impaled objects before surgery
    4) Applying MAST for pelvic fracture
    5) Administering fresh frozen plasma

2. Septic shock

  a. Continuously monitor hemodynamic parameters and blood pressure to evaluate the cardiovascular response to treatment.

  b. Continuously monitor urinary output via catheter to evaluate renal function.

  c. Monitor cardiac rhythm for tachycardia and life-threatening ventricular arrhythmias.

  d. Maintain a patent airway and adequate ventilation. Use supplemental oxygen to ensure that sufficient oxygen is delivered to the lungs.

  e. Provide enteral or parenteral nutritional support to prevent a negative nitrogen balance.

  f. Promote treatment of sepsis.
    1) Administer ordered antibiotics.
    2) Obtain culture specimens of potential infection sites.
    3) Monitor serial WBC count, and peak and trough levels of antibiotics for effectiveness of treatment.

      4) Monitor temperature every 4 hours and treat, as needed, with medications or external cooling devices.

3. Multisystem organ failure
  a. Monitor patients at risk and recognize onset during the early phases.
    1) Assess for risk factors.
    2) Be alert for early warning signals, such as:
      a) Increased or decreased temperature
      b) Increasing heart rate
      c) Tachypnea
      d) Increased or decreased WBCs
      e) Subtle changes in sensorium
    3) Report findings consistent with the development of multisystem organ failure.
  b. Prevent organ injury.
    1) Provide ventilatory support through intubation and mechanical ventilation.
    2) Control body temperature to adjust for hyperthermia or hypothermia.
    3) Reverse acidosis.
    4) Monitor for progression.
      a) Monitor for subtle changes in assessment findings, which may indicate deterioration from the hyperdynamic phase to the hypodynamic phase.
      b) Measure hemodynamic parameters frequently and report changes.
      c) Assess the patient frequently, paying particular attention to serial findings to identify deterioration in previously uninvolved organ systems.
      d) Analyze changes in laboratory values to determine deterioration of multiple organs.
      e) Monitor patient's responses to medications and treatments and report significant findings.
  c. Provide supportive care.
    1) Control the infection.
      a) Obtain a specimen of all secretions for culture testing.
      b) Prepare the patient for surgical intervention to remove source of infection.

c) Promote an aseptic environment to prevent nosocomial infections.
   1] Use aseptic technique when providing care.
   2] Monitor invasive tube sites for signs and symptoms of infection.
   3] Wash hands frequently.
   4] Monitor serial WBCs for signs of infection.
   5] Culture suspicious secretions from the patient.
   6] Immediately report signs and symptoms of infection.
   7] Monitor the patient's temperature every 4 hours and more frequently if fever develops.
   8] Administer medications ordered to prevent or fight infection and monitor patient's response to them.
2) Arrest and reverse the progress of the syndrome.
   a) Prevent translocation of bacteria from the gut with enteral feeding of glutamine, an immuno-nutrient that maintains gut integrity and stimulates the immune system.
   b) Prepare for continuous arteriovenous hemodiafiltration, which has been used successfully in trauma patients.
   c) Recognize complications, such as:
      1] Skin breakdown
         a] Use pressure-relieving devices (pads, mattresses, specialty beds) to prevent breakdown.
         b] Turn the patient every 2 hours, if possible.
         c] Assess the skin every 4 hours to identify and intervene in the early stages of break-
            down.
         d] Consult the enterostomal therapy nurse for definitive treatment of skin breakdown.
      2] Third spacing of fluid
         a] Assess the patient every 4 hours for edema, ascites, or anasarca.
         b] Weigh the patient daily and report significant increases.

      c] Accurately measure intake and output, and report significant disparities.

      d] Monitor lung sounds every 4 hours and report changes.

      e] Administer diuretics, as ordered, to increase urine output.

3) Provide metabolic support

    a) Measure oxygen consumption with increased flow until lactic acid level returns to normal.

    b) Provide adequate nutrition. Enteral route is preferred over parenteral using a formula that is high in protein and has medium-chain triglycerides for lipids.

Acute Upper Gastrointestinal Hemorrhage

Acute upper gastrointestinal hemorrhage is the sudden onset of profuse blood loss from lesions in the esophagus, stomach, or duodenum occurring above the Treitz' ligament. The most common causes of upper gastrointestinal bleeding are peptic ulcers, gastritis, esophageal or gastric varices, esophagitis, and Mallory-Weiss tear.

Etiology/Pathophysiology

1. Factors associated with the development of upper gastrointestinal bleeding:
   a. Physiologic stress (i.e., burns, trauma, sepsis, central nervous system [CNS] trauma, shock, serious medical illness)
   b. Use of drugs that may injure the upper gastrointestinal mucosal barrier (i.e., nonsteroidal anti-inflammatory drugs, aspirin, corticosteroids, nicotine, caffeine, alcohol, treatment with cancer chemotherapeutic agents)
   c. Advanced age
   d. Genetic predisposition
   e. Nasogastric suctioning
   f. Bacterial infection (i.e., *Helicobacter pylori* or staphylococcal food poisoning)
   g. Increased gastric acid and pepsin production, decreased production of bicarbonate buffers
   h. Abnormal gastric emptying
   i. Reflux of bile into the stomach
   j. Reduced blood flow to gastric mucosa
   k. Retching; forceful vomiting
   l. Portal hypertension (i.e., cirrhosis or portal venous thrombosis)
   m. Prolonged psychological distress
2. Pathophysiology
   a. Clinical manifestations of gastrointestinal bleeding depend on the rate and amount of blood loss and the coexistence of other diseases.
   b. 10–15% loss of total blood volume (500–700 mL)
      1) Clinical manifestations present in the elderly or patients with anemia.
      2) Sympathetic reflex compensation is initiated.
   c. A 15–30% loss of total blood volume (750–1500 mL) stimulates baroreceptor reflexes and CNS ischemic response causing arterial and venous constriction and stimulating cardiac activity.
   d. A 30–40% loss of total blood volume (1500–2000 mL) initiates angiotensin and vasopressin compensatory mechanisms resulting in the constriction of blood vessels and retention of sodium and water.

e. A >40% loss of total blood (2000 mL or more) will cause a progressive shock state resulting in cardiac and vasomotor failure, intravascular clotting, increased capillary permeability, release of toxins by ischemic tissues, acidosis (blood has an acid excess or base deficit with pH <7.35), cellular demise and ultimately, death.

f. As blood enters the gut, blood protein is digested, resulting in increased blood urea nitrogen (BUN). Blood also irritates the intestines, causing increased peristalsis and diarrhea.

Assessment/Analysis

ASSESSMENT FINDINGS

Subjective

1. Blood in emesis (hematemesis)
2. Shiny, black, tarry stool (melena); bright-red blood or maroon stool per rectum (hematochezia)
3. Syncope and lightheadedness
4. Nausea, vomiting, retching
5. Anorexia, weight loss
6. History of acute abdominal pain which occurs 2 hours after eating and is relieved by eating
7. Diaphoresis
8. Increased thirst

Objective

1. 10–30% blood loss
   a. Anxiety
   b. Abdominal distention
   c. Pink, red, or coffee-ground nasogastric tube aspirate
   d. Guaiac-positive emesis and stool
   e. Near-normal urine output
   f. Mild tachycardia
   g. Tachypnea
   h. Hyperactive bowel sounds
   i. Normal recumbent blood pressure but with orthostatic hypotension >10 mm Hg

    j. Pale palmar creases when fingers are forcibly extended
    k. Capillary refill >3 seconds
2. 30–40% blood loss
    a. State of agitation and confusion
    b. Diminished urine output
    c. Significant tachycardia and tachypnea
    d. Poor skin turgor with dry mucous membranes
3. >40% blood loss
    a. Confusion to lethargy progressing to obtundation
    b. Negligible urine output
    c. Diaphoresis with cool, pale, clammy skin
    d. Extreme tachycardia and tachypnea
    e. Systolic blood pressure <60 mm Hg

SUPPORTING TEST FINDINGS

Laboratory Tests

1. Complete blood count
    Abnormality: Decreased hemoglobin and hematocrit reflecting the true ratio of red blood cells (RBCs) to plasma volume (happens after 24–72 hours, when intravascular volume is restored)
       Increased white blood cell (WBC) count and increased platelet count
2. Prothrombin time (PT)/partial thromboplastin time
    Abnormality: May be elevated in patients with liver disease; detects clotting defects
3. BUN/Creatinine ratio
    Abnormality: Increased ratio of BUN to creatinine (BUN is usually elevated due to the breakdown of blood protein in the gut; creatinine is usually normal)

Diagnostic Tests

1. Gastric content analysis
    Abnormality: Pink, red, or coffee-ground colored aspirant denotes bleeding
2. Esophagogastroduodenoscopy (EGD)
    Abnormality: Performed once patient has been stabilized and stomach has been cleared with lavage; detects bleeding sites in the esophagus, stomach, or duodenum

3. Selective mesenteric arteriography
   Abnormality: Identifies specific bleeding vessels; also may be used to administer intra-arterial vasoconstricting agents or perform embolization of bleeding vessel
4. Barium X-rays
   Abnormality: Identifies duodenal or gastric ulcers

Planning/Intervention

COLLABORATIVE MANAGEMENT

Procedures

1. Patient stabilization
   a. Insert two large-bore, short intravenous (IV) catheters, as ordered.
   b. Administer fluid resuscitation with crystalloid solutions (i.e., normal saline solution or Ringer's solution), as ordered.
   c. Draw blood specimens for baseline laboratory analysis and type and crossmatch, as ordered.
   d. Transfuse to hematocrit of about 30% using packed cells of crossmatched type-specific blood (if patient is exsanguinating, may need to use non-crossmatched type-specific blood), as ordered.
   e. Correct coagulopathy by administering fresh frozen plasma, vitamin K, and platelet packs, as ordered (goal is to correct PT to within 2 seconds of the control and bring platelet count up to 60,000/mm^3).
   f. Assess rate of bleeding and prepare stomach for EGD by inserting a nasogastric tube and lavaging with room temperature saline or tap water, as ordered. (Lavage is also done to reduce the chance of developing hepatic encephalopathy in patients with liver disease.) If aspirant does not clear or clots are aspirated, a large-bore orogastric tube may be inserted (Ewald or Edlich tube) by the physician.
   g. Prevent aspiration by connecting nasogastric tube to low suction, as ordered.
   h. Monitor fluid and electrolyte status by assisting with the insertion of a central venous catheter or a pulmonary artery catheter (need to keep central venous pressure (CVP) <10 mm Hg to prevent variceal bleed-

ing) and inserting an indwelling urinary catheter connected to a urometer, as ordered.

   i. Promote oxygenation by administering supplemental oxygen, as ordered.

   j. Reduce suspected variceal bleeding by administering peripheral IV vasopressin with a nitroglycerin patch, as ordered.

2. Treat underlying cause of bleeding

   a. Measures to control bleeding from peptic ulcer are as follows:

     1) Assist with and prepare patient for laser photocoagulation, bipolar or multipolar electrocoagulation, or heater probe, as ordered.

     2) Assist with and prepare patient for injection of bleeding site with sclerosing agents (i.e., hypertonic saline, epinephrine, or pure ethanol), as ordered.

     3) Prepare patient for intra-arterial infusion of vasoconstricting drug (i.e., vasopressin) via an angiographically placed catheter, as ordered.

     4) Prepare patient for embolization of bleeding artery with gelfoam or autologous clot performed under radiologic control, as ordered.

     5) Prepare patient for surgery to stop bleeding (i.e., oversewing point of bleeding, truncal vagotomy with a pyloroplasty, or antrectomy.

   b. Measures to control bleeding from gastritis are as follows:

     1) Administer acid suppression therapy, as ordered.

     2) Prepare patient for selective infusion of vasopressin or embolization of gelfoam via left gastric artery, as ordered.

     3) Prepare patient for surgery, as ordered.

     4) Administer preventive measures to reduce risk of developing gastritis (antacids and histamine$_2$-receptor antagonist to keep gastric pH between 4–5 or sucralfate 1 g every 4–6 hours), as ordered.

   c. Measures to control bleeding from esophageal varices are as follows:

     1) Administer IV or superior mesenteric artery infusion of vasopressin, as ordered.

     2) Administer concurrent use of sublingual, transder-

mal, or IV nitroglycerin with vasopressin, as ordered.

3) Assist with or prepare patient for endoscopic variceal sclerotherapy or endoscopic band ligation.

4) Assist with insertion of multilumen tamponade tubes.

5) Prepare patient for surgery to stop bleeding.

6) Assist with or prepare patient for percutaneous obliteration of varices or transjugular intrahepatic portacaval shunt.

Drug Therapy

1. Crystalloid solutions

   Examples: Lactated Ringer's solution, normal saline solution

   Action: Expand blood volume; replace fluid and electrolytes lost in hemorrhage

   Caution: Can cause electrolyte imbalance, circulatory overload

2. Blood products

   Example: Packed RBCs

   Action: Replace RBCs lost during hemorrhage to improve the oxygen-carrying capacity of blood

   Caution: Massive blood transfusion (replacement of patient's blood volume within 24 hours) can result in hypothermia, volume overload, decreased serum calcium, metabolic alkalosis, decreased platelet count, coagulopathy, increased serum potassium (especially in patients with renal failure), tighter binding of oxygen to hemoglobin, and transfusion reactions

   Example: Fresh frozen plasma

   Action: Replaces clotting factors V and VIII in patients receiving massive transfusions or in patients with liver disease

   Caution: Can cause volume overload; carries risk of viral transmission

   Example: Platelets

   Action: Replace platelets in patients who are thrombocytopenic or have a coagulopathy during the bleeding episode

   Caution: May sensitize patients to leukocyte and RBC antigens. ABO-incompatible plasma in platelet packs may cause a positive direct antiglobulin test and hemolysis. Also chills, fever, allergic reactions, and transmission of hepatitis and human immunodeficiency virus (HIV)

3. Antidiuretic hormone

   Example: vasopressin (Pitressin)

   Action: Potent vasoconstrictor used to vasoconstrict splanchnic circulation and decrease blood flow to the area to control bleeding; it is also a synthetic antidiuretic hormone

   Caution: If given IV, can cause congestive heart failure, myocardial infarction, hypertension, intracerebral bleed, arrhythmias, nausea, vomiting, abdominal pain, and decreased serum sodium

   If given intra-arterially, causes fewer systemic side effects. Can cause thrombosis or bleeding from the femoral artery, thrombosis of the superior mensenteric artery, mesenteric ischemia

4. Vasodilator

   Example: nitroglycerin (Nitro-Bid IV)

   Action: Reverses the undesirable hemodynamic effects of vasopressin and potentiates vasopressin's ability to decrease portal venous pressure

   Caution: Can cause hypotension, tachycardia, dizziness, and headache

5. Antacids

   Examples: magnesium hydroxide/aluminum hydroxide (Maalox, Mylanta)

   Action: Neutralize gastric acid to promote healing of gastric injury; does not stop bleeding or decrease rate of rebleeding

   Caution: Can cause constipation, diarrhea, increased serum magnesium, and decreased serum phosphate

6. Histamine$_2$-receptor antagonists

   Examples: cimetidine (Tagamet)
   ranitidine (Zantac)
   famotidine (Pepcid)

   Action: Inhibit gastric acid secretion to promote healing of gastric injury; does not stop bleeding or decrease rate of rebleeding. (Note: Research is currently studying the effect of antacids used in combination with histamine$_2$-receptor antagonists on rate of gastric rebleeding.)

Caution: Can cause diarrhea, headache, dizziness, nausea, myalgia, and skin rashes
7. Antiulcer agent
   Example: sucralfate (Carafate) is an aluminum salt of sucrose octasulfate
   Action: Promotes ulcer healing by increasing mucosal blood flow, mucous secretion, and prostaglandin production; also used to prevent stress ulcer formation
   Caution: Can cause constipation, diarrhea, and nausea
8. Vitamin K
   Example: phytonadione (AquaMEPHYTON)
   Action: Replaces vitamin K required by the liver to synthesize prothrombin and factors VII, IX, and X; controls bleeding in patients who have hypoprothrombinemia (patients with liver disease)
   Caution: Can cause rash, pain, or swelling at injection site or allergic reactions

Drugs Currently Being Studied to Prevent or Stop Bleeding

omeprazole (PriLosec)	Inhibits gastric acid production
metoclopramide (Reglan)	Increases lower esophageal sphincter pressure, thereby decreasing variceal blood flow
terlipressin (synthetic analog of vasopressin)	Causes constriction of splanchnic vasculature
glypressin (synthetic analog of vasopressin)	Causes constriction of sphanchnic vasculature
prostaglandins (Cytotec)	Suppresses gastric acid secretion

NURSING MANAGEMENT

Monitoring and Managing Clinical Problems

1. Fluid Volume Deficit or Excess: high risk for
   a. Monitor for hypovolemia due to blood loss.

1) Assess for and report abnormal physical findings, such as:
    a) Tachycardia with a faint thready pulse
    b) Tachypnea
    c) Hypotension in recumbent position or postural hypotension
    d) Cool, pale, or cyanotic clammy skin
    e) Capillary refill > 3 seconds
    f) Poor skin turgor with dry mucous membranes
    g) Hyperactive bowel sounds
    h) Lethargy, confusion, or obtundation
    i) Decreased urine output and guaiac-positive stools and emesis
2) Assess for and report complaints of:
    a) Hematemesis
    b) Melena or hematochezia
    c) Syncope
    d) Weakness
    e) Nausea, vomiting, or retching
    f) Anorexia or weight loss
    g) Abdominal pain
    h) Diaphoresis
    i) Increased thirst
3) Monitor and report serial laboratory values reflecting:
    a) Alterations in serum sodium, potassium, chloride, bicarbonate, and calcium levels
    b) Increased BUN, usually with a normal creatinine
    c) Normal to decreased hemoglobin, hematocrit, and RBC count
    d) Mild increase in WBC count
    e) Increased urine specific gravity
4) Monitor serial hemodynamic parameters for decreased:
    a) CVP
    b) Pulmonary artery pressure (PAP)
    c) Pulmonary capillary wedge pressure (PCWP)
    d) Cardiac output (CO)
b. Promote fluid and electrolyte balance.
    1) Insert two large-bore, short IV catheters peripherally.
    2) Rapidly infuse all crystalloid solutions.

       3) Rapidly infuse packed RBCs or whole blood using pressure-infusing devices (follow hospital policy regarding administration of blood).

       4) Administer fresh frozen plasma, vitamin K, or platelets to correct coagulopathy.

  c. Monitor for hypervolemia due to rapid fluid replacement.

    1) Assess for and report the following abnormal physical findings:

      a) Jugular venous distention

      b) Crackles

      c) Dependent edema

      d) Increased blood pressure

      e) Bounding pulse

      f) Tachycardia, S_3, or S_4

      g) Altered mental status

      h) Tachypnea

      i) Dyspnea

      j) Cough with frothy sputum

      k) Weight gain

      j) Intake greater than output

    2) Monitor serial laboratory values for:

      a) Alterations in serum sodium, chloride, potassium, bicarbonate, and calcium levels; hemoglobin, hematocrit, serum protein, and serum albumin

      b) Decreased urine specific gravity

    3) Monitor serial hemodynamic parameters for increased:

      a) CVP

      b) PAP

      c) PCWP

      d) CO

2. Fluid Volume Deficit

  a. Monitor amount of blood loss.

    1) Assess for and report abnormal physical findings of:

      a) Abdominal distention

      b) Hyperactive bowel sounds

      c) Hematemesis or red or coffee-ground nasogastric tube aspirant

      d) Melena or hematochezia

e) Tachycardia with postural hypotension

2) Record very accurate intake and output, especially noting amount of nasogastric lavage instilled and amount aspirated.

3) Note characteristics of lavage aspirant, particularly color and presence of blood clots. Note if the aspirant becomes clear after lavage. Record amount of lavage used.

4) Guaiac test all nasogastric aspirant and stools.

5) Carefully monitor the number of units of packed RBCs and whole blood the patient has received. For each unit of packed RBCs or whole blood, the patient's hematocrit should increase 3% and the hemoglobin should increase 1 g/dL.

b. Control or stop bleeding.

1) Insert nasogastric tube and irrigate with room temperature normal saline or tap water, as ordered.

2) If irrigant does not clear or many clots are noted, assist physician with insertion of a large-bore orogastric tube (Ewald or Edlich); keep patient in left lateral position to prevent aspiration.

3) Prepare patient for EGD and assist physician with procedure when appropriate; patient may require heat coagulation therapy, sclerotherapy, or banding.

4) Administer vasopressin 20 U per IV bolus then at rate of 0.4–0.6 U/min per continuous IV infusion; monitor patient for cardiovascular side effects and water intoxication.

5) Administer nitroglycerin sublingually, transdermally, or IV to reduce cardiovascular effects of vasopressin.

6) If variceal bleeding is suspected, assist physician with insertion of a multilumen tamponade tube.

7) Prepare patient for ordered radiographic procedures.

8) Prepare patient for vagotomy, antrectomy, or portosystemic shunt, if ordered.

9) Administer antacids, histamine$_2$-receptor antagonists, and sucralfate.

10) Monitor gastric pH and maintain at pH of 4–5, as ordered.

Caring for a Patient with a Tamponade Tube

Inserting the Tube
- Check gastric balloon (300–400 mL air) and esophageal balloon (50–100 mL air) for air leaks before insertion.
- Patient may be intubated endotracheally before insertion.
- Tube may be inserted via the nose or mouth.
- Administer sedative and a local anesthetic for oropharynx/nasopharynx.
- Keep the patient in a semi-Fowler's position.
- Once the tube is inserted to about the 50-cm mark, inflate the gastric balloon with 50 mL of air.
- Check tube placement with a flat plate X-ray of the abdomen.
- After the tube position has been confirmed, inflate the gastric balloon with 150–300 mL of air and double clamp the port.
- Gently pull tube until resistance is met (this means that the tube is at the cardia of the stomach) and secure tube to the face guard of a football helmet.
- Another flat plate X-ray of the abdomen may be done.
- Inflate esophageal balloon to 25-45 mm Hg and double clamp port (pressure is checked using a sphygmomanometer).
- If a Sengstaken-Blakemore tube is used, an nasogastric tube may be inserted alongside or above the esophageal balloon; connect the gastric aspirant and nasogastric tube to low suction.
- If a Minnesota tube is used, connect the gastric aspirant lumen and the esophageal aspirant lumen to low suction.

Care of Patient with a Tamponade Tube
- Suction oropharynx and esophagus frequently.
- Check esophageal balloon pressures every hour with a mercury sphygmomanometer.
- Maintain patency of gastric aspirant lumen; lavage and assess for continued bleeding.

- Never instill anything into the esophageal aspirant portion of the Minnesota tube or nasogastric tube with the Sengstaken-Blakemore tube.
- Assess aspirant for quantity and characteristics.
- Maintain traction on tube at all times.
- Never deflate gastric balloon.
- Deflate/inflate esophageal balloon periodically, as ordered.
- Keep scissors at the bedside to deflate balloons should respiratory distress occur.
- Monitor patient for aspiration, respiratory distress, airway obstruction, and esophageal rupture.

Removing the Tube
- Deflate the esophageal balloon 24–72 hours after it is inflated.

3. Protection: altered
   a. Monitor for coagulopathy.
      1) Coagulopathy can be due to the absence of functioning platelets and factors V and VIII in stored blood, hemodilution, or possibly duration of hypotension.
      2) Monitor platelet count, fibrinogen level, and bleeding time.
      3) Be prepared to administer fresh frozen plasma and platelet packs after patient has received 15–20 U of blood, if ordered.
   b. Monitor for hyperkalemia/hypokalemia.
      1) Each unit of blood may reach 30 mEq/L of potassium after 3 weeks of storage due to leakage of intracellular potassium. Infusion increases serum potassium levels.
      2) Decreased serum potassium levels may result from alkalosis that occurs when citrate is metabolized into bicarbonate.
      3) Identify patients at risk of developing hyperkalemia (patients with compromised renal function, shock and/or acidosis).
      4) Monitor serial potassium levels and report abnormalities.

　　5) Monitor for cardiac arrhythmias that may result from altered potassium levels.

c. Monitor for hypocalcemia (rare).

　　1) Hypocalcemia can occur from the addition of citrate to stored blood, which binds calcium and prevents clotting.

　　2) Assess for patients at risk of developing hypocalcemia (patients with severe liver disease and those receiving 1 U of blood or more every 5 minutes).

　　3) Monitor serial ionized calcium levels and for prolongation of the QT interval.

　　4) Administer supplemental calcium, as ordered (rarely needed and should be administered only in cases of proven hypocalcemia.

d. Monitor for and prevent acid-base alterations.

　　1) Assess for metabolic acidosis in the acute phase. Patients requiring massive blood transfusions are in a low-flow shock state and develop a metabolic acidosis due to an increased lactic acid production.

　　2) Remember that stored blood's pH decreases over time due to an increase in lactic acid and a fall in plasma bicarbonate level; may carry an acid load of 30–40 mEq/L per unit.

　　3) Assess for metabolic alkalosis as patient stabilizes. As tissue perfusion is restored, the citrate in blood and the lactate in resuscitation fluids are metabolized to bicarbonate, causing a metabolic alkalosis; if perfusion and an aerobic metabolism is not restored, acidosis may develop.

　　4) Monitor arterial pH and venous CO_2 for acidosis/alkalosis.

e. Monitor for and prevent administration of alterations in hemoglobin function.

　　1) Monitor for a shift in the oxyhemoglobin dissociation curve to the left. Levels of 2,3-diphosphoglycerate (2,3-DPG) decline to 40% of initial levels after 3 weeks of storage of blood. The low levels result in a tighter binding of oxygen to hemoglobin and impaired tissue oxygenation. RBCs rapidly regenerate 2,3-DPG within 24 hours of transfusion, depending on the patient's metabolic state.

　　2) Assess for alkalosis, hypothermia, and hypoxemia.

Alkalosis and hypothermia combined with low levels of 2,3-DPG enhance the binding of oxygen to hemoglobin, causing hypoxemia.

3) Assess for acidosis, which enhances the release of oxygen from hemoglobin.

4) Use cryopreserved blood or blood that is < 14 days old to ensure an adequate supply of 2,3-DPG, if clinically indicated.

f. Monitor for and prevent hypothermia from the rapid administration of cold, stored blood.

1) Assess for the adverse effects of hypothermia:

   a) Arrhythmias
   b) Decreased CO
   c) Decreased metabolism of citrate and lactate
   d) Tighter binding of oxygen to hemoglobin
   e) Impaired hemostasis
   f) Monitor patient's core temperature.
   g) Administer blood through a heating coil, when possible.

g. Monitor for ammonia intoxication from increased ammonia content in stored blood.

1) Identify patients at risk of developing ammonia intoxication, such as those with severe liver disease.

2) Monitor for signs and symptoms of hepatic encephalopathy/coma.

   a) Changes in the level of consciousness
   b) Behavioral changes
   c) Increased liver function tests

h. Monitor for and prevent administration of microaggregates from the formation of blood clots and cellular debris with increased storage time of blood.

1) Use blood filters to reduce the number of microaggregates that reach the lung.

2) Administer all blood with a standard blood filter of 170- to 260-μg pore size to remove large clots and debris. Change blood filter after every 2 U of blood or packed RBCs.

3) When possible, use a microaggregate blood filter of 20- to 40-μg pore size to remove smaller clots and debris.

4) Always prime blood administration lines with normal saline solution.

5) Use normal saline solution in the blood line.

i. Monitor for and prevent hemolytic transfusion reactions from ABO incompatibility.

1) Check patient and blood identification to prevent administering the incorrect blood. Misidentification of the patient and mismatching of blood results in intravascular hemolysis.

2) Monitor patient for hypotension, chest pain, back pain, chills, fever, pain at the infusion site, shock, nausea, acute renal failure, and bleeding.

3) Prevent this reaction by carefully labeling all blood specimens sent to the laboratory and following hospital policy for blood administration.

j. Monitor for and prevent febrile transfusion reactions from administering platelets or leukocytes to which the patient has antibodies.

1) Monitor patient for fever, chills, and dyspnea.

2) Prevent reaction by administering washed RBCs or leukocyte-poor blood and premedication with antipyretics in patients with history of reaction.

k. Monitor for and prevent allergic transfusions reactions from hypersensitivity to a substance in the donor's plasma.

1) Monitor patient for urticaria and signs and symptoms of an anaphylactic reaction.

2) Prevent reaction by administering antihistamines and washed blood products in patients with history of transfusion reaction.

l. Monitor for and prevent transmission of infections from blood transfusion.

1) Blood transfusion carries the risk of transmitting HIV (acquired immune deficiency syndrome), HIV-II, human T cell lymphomavirus (HTLV-I and HTLV-II), hepatitis B and C bacteria (gram-negative bacteria), cytomegalovirus, Epstein-Barr virus, syphilis, malaria, and parasites.

   a) The current estimate of getting HIV from a blood transfusion is $1:40,000 - 1:200,000$

   b) Incidence of hepatitis ranges from $1-10\%$

2) Prevent infection by aseptic administration of blood, proper blood bank storage, adequate blood bank screening for infection.

4. Pain
   a. Assess patient for pain by observing for the following:
      1) Restlessness
      2) Irritability
      3) Agitation
      4) Diaphoresis
      5) Distressed facial expressions
      6) Rapid, shallow breathing
      7) Tachycardia
      8) Alterations in blood pressure
   b. Assess patient's complaints of pain by noting the following:
      1) Location
      2) Radiation
      3) Severity
      4) Aggravating and mitigating factors
      5) Onset
      6) Associated signs and symptoms
   c. Promote plain relief by:
      1) Administering analgesics, sedatives, antacids, histamine$_2$-receptor antagonists, sucralfate
      2) Assisting patient to find a position of comfort
      3) Securing all drainage tubes
   d. Other comfort measures include:
      1) Providing frequent oral care
      2) Lubricating nares, as needed
      3) Providing extra blankets and keeping environment warm
      4) Reducing environmental stimuli
      5) Providing periods of rest and quiet

Monitoring, Managing, and Preventing Life-Threatening Emergencies

1. Hypovolemic shock
   a. Monitor for hemodynamic instability.
      1) Continuously monitor hemodynamic parameters.
      2) Titrate fluids and inotropic agents to maintain a systolic blood pressure of at least 80 mm Hg.
      3) Position the patient in modified Trendenlenburg position (elevation of the legs at 45 degrees).
   b. Promote adequate oxygenation.

     1) Administer supplemental oxygen, as ordered.

     2) Collect and monitor results of serial arterial blood gases and hemoglobin, and report abnormalities.

     3) Monitor capillary refill and monitor skin color to assess peripheral perfusion.

  c. Monitor for altered organ and tissue perfusion.

     1) Monitor for decreased urine output and elevated renal function tests possibly indicating acute renal failure

     2) Monitor for a falling arterial oxygen concentration possibly indicating adult respiratory distress syndrome

     3) Auscultate for decreased or absent bowel sounds possibly indicating gastroparesis and bright red or coffee ground drainage from the nasogastric tube suggesting stress ulceration

     4) Check temperature every 4 hours to monitor to hypothermia or hyperthermia

     5) Monitor for decreased alertness and attention span, drowsiness, or excessive sleeping indicating downward changes in the level of consciousness.

  d. Monitor for loss of fluid volume from the vasculature

     1) Provide fluid replacement as ordered

     2) Maintain accurate intake and output measurements hourly

     3) Continuously monitor blood pressure

     4) Monitor of skin turgor for signs of dehydration

     5) Observe for fluid volume overload as evidenced by new onset of an S3 heart sound, peripheral edema, and moist crackles in the lungs

     6) Closely monitor pertinent laboratory data (serum electrolytes, urine studies) to assess hydration

PSYCHOSOCIAL ASPECTS

Brain Death and Organ and Tissue Donation in the Intensive Care Unit

Brain death is defined as an irreversible condition occurring when the entire brain and brainstem ceases to function. Criteria for brain death vary from state to state and are used to determine death in organ donors (see the table Criteria for Brain Death).

Once brain death has been diagnosed, it is possible to obtain organs and tissue from the body for transplantation into another living person. Organ donation is the removal of transplantable vital organs, most commonly the heart, liver, lung, kidney, pancreas, and small bowel. The kidneys are the organs in greatest demand.

Tissue donation is the removal of transplantable tissues, particularly corneas, skin, and bone. Persons who do not meet the criteria for organ donation can donate these tissues. (See the table Criteria for Organ and Tissue Donation).

Because of the great need for organs, Congress passed the Organ Donation Request Act of 1987. This act mandates health care professionals to ask families for organ and/or tissue donation following death of a family member.

Organ and tissue donation offers the family of the deceased patient a chance to benefit others. However, families are often not given the option of donating following the death of their loved one, because health care professionals are uncomfortable dealing with death and suggesting donation.

Criteria for Brain Death

1. Absence of spontaneous movement, generalized flaccidity, absence of posturing or shivering, and persistent deep coma for >24 hours
2. Absence of spontaneous respiration
3. Absent brainstem reflexes
   a. Pupils fixed and dilated
   b. No corneal reflex
   c. No gag reflex
   d. No doll's eye phenomenon
   e. No vestibular response to caloric stimulation
4. Absent blood flow to the brain documented using arteriography
5. Absent brain-wave patterns on electroencephalogram (EEG) (isoelectric EEG)
6. Other causes of these responses (hypothermia, drug)

Criteria for Organ and Tissue Donation

For Tissue Donors
a. Age is generally newborn–60.
b. Can be any hospital or emergency department death.
c. The heart may be in asystole, but referrals must be made within 4 hours after the heart stops.

d. The patient must be free from systemic infectious disease.
e. Can have no autoimmune diseases.

For Organ Donors
a. Age generally is newborn – 70.
b. The patient must meet brain death criteria with a heart-beat intact.
c. Vasopressors are acceptable to maintain heartbeat and blood pressure.

Collaborative and Nursing Management

ORGAN AND TISSUE DONATION

1. Have the health care professional who has developed the best rapport with the family approach them for the donation request.
2. Health care professionals must consider the family's cultural and religious beliefs and emotional state when requesting donation.
3. If the physician does not wish the family to be approached about donation, be sure the reasons for this are documented by the physician on the medical record.
4. Be sure the family has the following information before making a decision:
   a. Donation will be carried out promptly with respect for the deceased.
   b. No body deformity results. An open casket funeral can be held following donation.
   c. Procurement of internal organs takes place in an operating room and may take 4–5 hours.
   d. Donated organs are always given to those in greatest need.
   e. As soon as the decision to donate occurs, the expense to the family ends. The family will not receive a bill for organ and tissue procurement.
   f. Confidentiality of the donor and recipients will be maintained.
   g. A follow-up letter may be sent to the donor family by the organ procurement agency, if the family requests one.
   h. Most religious leaders support donation.
   i. Donation often helps the family cope with the loss of a loved one.
5. Support whatever decision the family makes.
6. If the family says "no":
   a. Recognize that families with unresolved guilt or unfinished business with the deceased may not be able to tolerate the request for organ donation.
   b. Reasons why families fail to donate organs:

      1) Belief that the organs might be taken before the patient is dead.

      2) Hope for a miracle that will restore the patient to health.

      3) Belief that organ donation is a violation of the human body and against religious beliefs.

      4) Fear the patient will suffer pain as a result of organ procurement.

7. Brain death certification is equivalent to the pronouncement of death. The time documented for this certification is considered the time of the patient's death.

8. If the family says "yes":

   a. Notify the regional organ procurement agency.

   b. If consent for donation is obtained over the telephone, two witnesses must hear the consent and sign the form.

   c. The next-of-kin makes the ultimate decision about organ and tissue donation. Next-of-kin order of priority:

      1) Spouse

      2) Adult child

      3) Parent

      4) Sibling

      5) Guardian

   d. Three required items must be present in the medical record for donation:

      1) Documentation of death

      2) Next-of-kin's consent for donation

      3) Approval from the medical examiner if required by state law

9. If the deceased is an organ donor:

   a. Maintain vital functions until organ is procured.

      1) Minimum systolic blood pressure of 100 mm Hg

      2) Normal body temperature

      3) Arterial oxygen concentration of 100%

      4) Central venous pressure of 8–12 cm H_2O

      5) Urine output between 100–300 mL/h. Diabetes insipidus is a frequent complication of massive head trauma and should be recognized and treated as quickly as possible.

      6) Hematocrit of at least 30%

      7) Serum electrolytes and blood glucose within normal limits

    b. Protection from nosocomial infection. Prophylactic antibiotics may be started.

    c. Check with the organ procurement agency for a list of appropriate tests to perform on the donor. Obtain required laboratory and diagnostic studies.

10. If the deceased is a tissue donor:

    a. Contact the local organ procurement agency regarding appropriate blood/secretion testing.

    b. Tissue recovery can occur up to 12–16 hours after death.

    c. Expect to obtain:

      1) 4–6 red-topped tubes of blood for serology testing

      2) 1–3 blood cultures

      3) White blood cell count and differential to detect infection

    d. Procure refrigerated morgue space for the body as soon as possible after death, preferably within 4 hours.

11. If the deceased is an eye donor:

    a. Place the body in refrigeration as soon as possible.

    b. Elevate the head 20 degrees.

    c. Tape the eyes shut with paper tape.

    d. Apply cool compresses over the eyes to prevent swelling.

Near-Death Experience in the Intensive Care Unit

In circumstances where interventions by the intensive care staff successfully reverse the process of dying in patients who are near death, such as successful resuscitation from cardiopulmonary arrest, a phenomenon known as near-death experience may occur. If a patient experiences near death, he or she may report:

1. Feeling separated from one's body
2. Moving through a dark tunnel
3. Seeing a bright light
4. Meeting deceased family members or friends
5. Meeting God
6. Having their life pass before them
7. Feeling peaceful, calm, and pain-free
8. Understanding the need to return to his or her body
9. Returning to his or her body
10. Having a sense of all-knowingness

Collaborative and Nursing Management

1. Identify persons at risk.
   a. Any patient who survives close encounters with death, even ones who have attempted suicide
   b. Recognize patient's response to the experience.
      1) May be profoundly affected by the experience.
      2) May consider it the most significant event in his or her life.
      3) May have great difficulty explaining it to anyone.
      4) Usually a positive experience in an overwhelming number of people.
      5) Persons with a negative near-death experience may feel isolation and a sense of being in a void. Some recount scenes of frightening events often associated with society's perception of hell.
      6) May have adjustment difficulties for the first year following the experience.
      7) Patients who feel ignored by others when trying to relate the experience may experience post near-death experience depression.
2. Ensure the patient's best experience by:
   a. Being sensitive to what is said and done during a code situation. The patient may be able to see and hear what is happening.
   b. Providing human contact during and following the close encounter with death.
   c. Recognizing comments indicative of a near-death experience in patients who recover from near death. Comments are often made shortly after the patient regains consciousness.
3. Assist the patient in dealing with the experience.
   a. Nurses are mostly likely to be the first person to be approached by the patient following the experience. Only health care professionals who accept the concept of near-death experience should help the patient deal with it.
      1) Take the story of the experience seriously and do not question the patient's sanity. The patient will

feel very vulnerable following a near-death experience.

2) Be nonjudgmental when listening to a patient describe a near-death experience.

3) Create a trusting, caring environment, so that the patient will feel safe when telling about the experience.

4) Encourage the patient to express emotions and feelings associated with the experience.

5) Let the patient know that others have related similar experiences.

6) Accept the patient's experience without trying to explain it as something else, like hallucination.

7) Provide information for the patient about near-death experience.

8) Consult health care professionals who accept the concept of near-death experience to speak to the patient if referral is warranted.

9) Chart the patient's description of the experience in the medical record.

Death in the Intensive Care Unit

When death occurs in the intensive care units, the family's and staff's responses vary. Patient deaths may be expected or unexpected.

When death is expected, the family and the staff usually have some time to prepare for the loss. But when it is unexpected, deaths may be much more difficult to accept because there is no preparation time.

Collaborative and Nursing Management

1. Caring for a patient when death is expected:
   a. Ask about the presence of a living will and place a copy on the medical record if one exists. Notify the physician of the will.
   b. Allow the patient the opportunity to make his or her own decisions about end-of-life care.
   c. Let the patient and family know that they can change their minds if they desire about end-of-life care. No decision is irrevocable.
   d. Note orders for no resuscitation and for withdrawal of medical treatment that may precede expected death after prolonged unsuccessful treatment. Laws governing "do not resuscitate" orders and withholding of treatment vary from state to state.
   e. Assure the family that the patient will be kept as comfortable as possible until death.
2. Initiating terminal weaning:
   a. Indications for terminal weaning:
      1) The patient wishes the ventilator to be discontinued.
      2) All available treatments have been tried and were unsuccessful.
      3) Prolonging life will only prolong the pain and suffering the patient is experiencing.
   b. Ensure patient comfort by administering pain medication. A morphine drip is the drug of choice and is titrated to relieve signs of distress such as tachypnea, tachycardia, restlessness, or patient's complaints of pain.
   c. Allow family members to be present during terminal weaning.
   d. Provide emotional support to the family during terminal weaning. Remember that family members have two dominant emotions when making the decision to discontinue mechanical ventilation—fear and uncertainty.
3. Dealing with the family in unexpected death:
   a. The news of the unexpected death of a loved one may

be devastating to the family. Allow time for the reality of the situation to be accepted by the family.

b. The more violent the circumstances of death, the more painful the reality is for the family.

c. However, unanticipated grief may not be any greater than anticipated grief.

4. Notifying the family of the death:

a. Use the words "dead" or "died" when notifying the family so there is no misunderstanding.

b. Emphasize to the family that everything possible was done to preserve life and prevent death.

c. Expect any type of emotional response; individuals cope with a crisis in various ways.

d. Provide the family with a quiet, private, comfortable room where they can begin to deal with the death.

e. Encourage the family to spend some time with the decreased as a way of beginning the grieving process.

f. Contact clergy and/or social services personnel to be with the family. Call a priest for Roman Catholic patients before death or as soon as possible after death for Sacrament of the Annointed.

Teaching Needs of the Patient and Family

The teaching/learning interaction between the nurse and the patient/family involves the exchange of information resulting in behavioral changes. In the intensive care unit (ICU) setting, the change in behavior is most often an increased understanding of the ICU environment and a reduction in anxiety.

Teaching and learning are not synonymous. Just because the nurse taught does not mean the patient/family learned. Repetition and reinforcement are often essential, especially when stress levels are high. Assessing the patient's/family's understanding following a teaching session is also essential.

ICU patients and families often have strong barriers to learning, because they are undergoing a crisis. Barriers to learning may include:
1. Poor motivation
2. Low self-esteem
3. Increasing age
4. Inability or limited ability to read and write

5. Individual beliefs about the injury or illness
6. Anxiety, fear, and/or pain
7. Embarrassment about not knowing needed information
8. Unrealistic expectations by the learner or the teacher

Assessment/Analysis

Subjective Findings

1. Verbalizes feeling of fear, anxiety, and loss of control.
2. Increased questioning about hospitalization

Objective Findings

1. Knowledge Deficit
   a. Unfamiliarity with diagnosis and nature of illness
   b. Requests for information
   c. Statements indicating poor understanding, misinterpretation, or misconception
   d. Inappropriate behaviors like hysteria, hostility, agitation, or apathy
2. Noncompliance
   a. Failure to follow prescribed treatment regimen before admission
   b. Failure to keep doctors' appointments before admission
   c. Denial of severity of illness
   d. Hostility or anger
   e. Refusal to participate in self-care
3. Ineffective management of therapeutic regimen
   a. Failure to adhere to regimen restrictions
   b. Failure to take prescribed medicine
   c. Evidence of performance of behaviors detrimental to health
   d. Failure to keep doctor appointments
4. Health-seeking behaviors
   a. Requests information about environmental effects on the disease process.
   b. Expresses a desire to be actively involved in obtaining the most healthy lifestyle possible.
   c. Requests information about the disease process and about changes in lifestyle necessary to manage the disease.
5. Growth and Development: altered
   a. Expressions of concern about physical disability and adjustment to physical disability

b. Evidences regressive behaviors like incontinence and temper tantrums
c. Flat affect, listlessness, decreased verbal and nonverbal responses

Planning/Implementation

NURSING MANAGEMENT

1. Follow the same education principles used in other settings when teaching in critical care.
   a. Assess learning needs before developing a teaching plan.
   b. Provide simple material first and build to complex material.
   c. Give written material during the session to increase retention.
2. Assessing learning needs.
   a. Develop a trusting relationship with the patient/family, to enable them to feel comfortable revealing learning needs.
   b. Determine the patient's/family's level of pre-existing knowledge about the injury/illness to obtain baseline data from which teaching objectives can be developed.
   c. Ascertain the patient's/family's previous experiences with critical illness and ICUs, because the past experiences of the patient/family may increase or decrease the effectiveness of the teaching session.
   d. Identify areas where the patient/family has incorrect knowledge to develop teaching objectives to effectively correct this problem.
3. Develop the teaching plan.
   a. Prioritize teaching needs based on the assessment data as soon as possible.
   b. Include patients/families when setting teaching goals. Plan to address their concerns in initial sessions.
   c. Develop measurable teaching objectives to meet these needs.
   d. Plan teaching/learning sessions to meet the objectives.

4. Content of teaching sessions:
   a. Content presented will vary with each patient/family. Teaching sessions should be guided by patient's/family's needs.
   b. Specific content about the unit should be given to all families and all conscious patients as soon after admission as possible.
      1) Explain environmental noises and machines.
      2) Explain routine procedures that will be performed on the patient, like vital signs, laboratory draws, and monitoring.
      3) Provide necessary information about the injury/illness.
      4) Provide preoperative teaching before all surgical procedures.
      5) Provide preprocedure teaching for all stressful procedures.
      6) Provide information that will be needed when transferring out of the ICU.
5. Teaching the patient or family:
   a. Keep teaching brief and concise.
   b. Focus on what they need to know at the present time to cope with the situation.
   c. Give meaningful, useful information to the patient/family during teaching sessions.
   d. Remember that not all teaching sessions will be successful. For some individuals, learning is a traumatic experience.

Decreasing Fear and Anxiety in the Intensive Care Unit

Becoming ill and being admitted to an intensive care unit can be extremely upsetting and stressful for both the patient and the family. To reduce fear and anxiety, use these interventions.

- Develop a trusting relationship with the patient and the family.
- Allow the patient and family to verbalize their feelings and concerns.
- Explain all procedures.

Continued

**Decreasing Fear and Anxiety in the Intensive
Care Unit — *Continued***

- Involve family members in the patient's care whenever appropriate.
- Provide a calm, quiet environment.
- Assist the patient with activities of daily living.
- Be sure the call bell is within reach and answer calls promptly.
- Provide diversional activities.
- Sedate the patient, as needed, to relieve anxiety.

6. Evaluating the teaching session:
   a. Ask the patient and/or family members for feedback.
   b. Compare actual outcome of the teaching session with the expected outcomes or goals of the session.
   c. Provide additional information if the actual outcome falls short of the expected outcome.
   d. Document each learning session as a way to provide continuity in the patient's/family's education.

Sensory Alterations in the Intensive Care Unit Patient

Sensory alterations are changes in the amount and perception of sensory stimuli received. The two major types of sensory alterations of the intensive care unit (ICU) patient are sensory overload and sensory deprivation.

Sensory overload results when excessive, unfamiliar, uncomfortable, unexpected sensory stimuli are experienced suddenly by the patient. The stimuli are not patterned, are perceived as bothersome or meaningless, and create stress. Patients may respond to the stress by creating a noisy environment, in an attempt to relieve some of the tension caused by the stress.

Sensory deprivation results when the patient experiences a lack of variety and/or intensity of sensory stimuli or a lack of sensory stimuli that are perceived as meaningful. Although it is viewed as the opposite of sensory overload, the two can occur virtually simultaneously.

Etiology/Pathophysiology

1. Types of sensory stimuli that the ICU patient receives include:
   a. Auditory—unfamiliar sounds like alarms, noisy machines, constant talking
   b. Visual—unfamiliar sights that can be altered by drugs
   c. Tactile—invasive procedures, monitoring equipment attached to the patient, uncomfortable tubes
   d. Olfactory—unpleasant odors over which the patient has no control
   e. Gustatory—unpleasant tastes from medications, tubes in the nose and mouth that make swallowing uncomfortable, inability to perform oral hygiene.
2. Sensory alterations can be caused by:
   a. Illness
   b. Drugs that alter consciousness or sensation
   c. Prolonged pain
   d. An unfamiliar environment
   e. Fear
   f. Lack of understanding of the injury or illness
   g. Sleep deprivation
   h. Isolation resulting in lack of contact with significant others

Assessment/Analysis

ASSESSMENT FINDINGS

Subjective

1. May be none if the patient cannot communicate
2. Poor concentration
3. Expresses perceived changes in size, shape, and color of objects
4. Worry
5. Anger

Objective

1. Decreased reasoning and problem-solving skills, resulting in difficulty communicating with others

2. Confusion, disorientation, and possibly hallucinations, delusions, and illusions
3. Behavioral changes, such as combativeness
4. Boredom and daydreaming
5. Restlessness to the point of agitation
6. Fatigue and drowsiness
7. Noncompliance
8. Short-term memory deficit
9. Increased startle response
10. Lethargy or withdrawal
11. Mood swings

Planning/Intervention

COLLABORATIVE MANAGEMENT

Procedures

1. Provide prompt, effective treatment of the injury or illness to minimize the stay in the ICU.
2. Rule out and treat physiologic causes.

Drug Therapy

1. None

Intensive Care Unit Drugs That Alter Sensory Perception

Analgesics
Paralytics
Sedatives
Antianxiety drugs

NURSING MANAGEMENT

Monitoring and Managing Clinical Problems

1. Sensory-Perceptual Alterations
   Monitor for signs of sensory overload when the patient is receiving medications that alter sensory input.
   a. Monitor the patient's environmental noise and decrease noise levels, if possible.

      1) Decrease conversation levels at bedside to as quiet as possible.

      2) Avoid banging equipment.

      3) Turn monitor alarms down to as low as possible.

      4) Provide soft music to cover some of the environmental noise.

  b. Monitor environmental lights.

      1) Dim lights, if possible.

      2) Avoid continuous use of overhead lights.

      3) Cover the patient's eyes to block out some of the light, if possible.

  c. Monitor for environmental odors.

      1) Eliminate unpleasant odors as quickly as possible.

      2) If the odor cannot be eliminated, provide room deodorant to mask it.

      3) Provide frequent mouth care to the patient to eliminate mouth odor.

2. Fear and Anxiety

  a. Provide a calm, supportive atmosphere.

  b. Provide verbal cues before touching the patient.

  c. Be gentle when delivering care.

  d. Explain procedures at the patient's level of understanding. Explain the need for the machinery surrounding the patient, especially the presence of lights and alarms.

  e. Minimize the number and length of invasive procedures, if possible.

  f. Provide measures to promote comfort.

  g. Do not talk about patient within hearing range of patient.

  h. Shield the patient from viewing unpleasant procedures performed on other patients.

  i. Allow the patient to verbalize fears.

  j. Encourage family visitation. This has been identified as the single most important factor for reducing anxiety and fear in ICU patients

3. Sleep Pattern Disturbance: high risk for

  a. Determine patient's normal sleep/rest pattern.

  b. Maintain day/night cycles, if possible, to prevent disruption of circadian rhythms.

  c. Provide care by grouping interventions to allow for uninterrupted sleep/rest periods, if possible.

    d. Dim lights and decrease noise at night.
    e. Be sure wire and tubes connected to the patient are not causing discomfort.
    f. Provide comfort measures at night to promote relaxation/sleep.

4. Thought Processes: altered
    a. Provide calendars and clocks in the patient's room.
    b. Call the patient by name and identify yourself before performing care.
    c. Frequently reorient patient to self, place, time, and situation.
    d. Talk to the patient about current events.
    e. Use touch as a form of communication.
    f. Encourage frequent family visits.
    g. Allow patients to make some decisions about their care, if possible.
    h. Encourage patients to discuss feelings to assist them to find meaning in their experiences.

5. Sensory-Perceptual Alterations
    a. Play tapes of the patient's favorite music or tapes of family voices.
    b. Provide diversional activities, such as television or reading.
    c. Provide a means of communication for intubated patients, such as an alphabet board or pencil and paper
    d. Have family bring familiar items from home for the patient's room.
    e. Talk to the patient frequently.
    f. Teach relaxation techniques to the patient.
    g. Provide patient with his/her eyeglasses and hearing aids to improve sensory input.

Substance Abuse (Drug Overdose)

Substance abuse is the continued, recurrent, frequent use of a psychoactive substance in amounts that cause overt intoxication, in spite of resulting social, occupational, psychological, or physical problems. It is often a symptom of family or social unit dysfunction.

Three Broad Classes of Abused Substances

Depressants ▪ Stimulants ▪ Psychogenics

Substance abuse eventually leads to dependence upon the substance. The elapsed time between substance abuse and substance dependence varies with the type of drug and the psychophysiologic responses in the abuser.

1. Substance dependence occurs when the patient:
   a. Develops tolerance to the substance, resulting in a need for increased amounts of the substance to achieve the desired effect
   b. Wants to or tries to cut down or control substance use
   c. Spends a large amount of time in drug-related activities
   d. Is unable to meet role obligations
   e. Is dysfunctional
   f. Undergoes physical and/or psychological withdrawal when use is stopped, and takes the substance to prevent or relieve the symptoms of withdrawal
2. There are three types of substance abuse:
   a. Accidental overdose of prescribed medication
      1) Inadvertently taking additional pills (a problem encountered in older adults)
      2) Ingestion of prescription drugs belonging to older family members (a problem encountered in young children)
      3) Accumulation of prescribed drugs in the body (may cause overdose if the dosage is too high or blood levels are not monitored)
   b. Recreational drug overdose
      1) More than half the illegal drugs consumed in the world are consumed in the United States.
      2) Drug overdose is often unintentional, because the exact strength of the recreational drug is unknown.
      3) Overdose may result from an attempt to hide drugs from law enforcement officers.
      4) Alcohol is the most commonly abused drug.
      5) Opiate narcotics are used most often by adolescents and young adults.

   c. Suicide attempt

     1) Drug overdose is frequently used to commit suicide.

     2) Often multiple drugs are used. Sedatives are the drugs most often taken.

     3) Alcohol may be used with other drugs in suicide attempts.

     4) The suicide attempt may be:

       a) A means of withdrawal from a situation

       b) A way to win in a perceived no-win situation

       c) A form of punishment

       d) An attempt to secure love

       e) An attempt to cause guilt

Etiology/Pathophysiology

1. There are three categories of etiologic factors associated with substance abuse:

   a. Physiologic factors

     1) A genetic predisposition, as in alcoholism, has been identified.

     2) Further research is needed to identify other drugs that have physiologic etiologic factors

   b. Psychological factors

     1) Insecurity

     2) Anxiety

     3) Chronic malaise

     4) Feelings of inadequacy

     5) Desire to experience altered states of consciousness

     6) Avoidance of stress

     7) Escape from loneliness

     8) A desire for new, exciting experiences

   c. Social factors

     1) Positive familial and/or peer attitudes toward substance abuse

     2) Familial behaviors (drug use or acceptance of drug use) that foster substance abuse

     3) A dependent lifestyle is seen in abusers.

Assessment/Analysis

ASSESSMENT FINDINGS

Subjective

1. Obtaining a history may be difficult due to the patient's:
   a. Having an altered level of consciousness
   b. Giving false information
   c. Giving inaccurate information
   d. Being hostile
   e. Refusing to talk
2. Check for the presence of a precipitating personal crisis.
3. Seek further corroborative data from family and friends, because data from the patient may be unreliable.
4. Certain presenting medical diagnoses are suspicious for substance abuse.
   a. An altered level of consciousness
   b. Cardiac arrhythmias in the young patient
   c. Chest pain in the young patient
   d. Pulmonary edema in the young patient
   e. Acute myocardial infarction in the young patient
   f. Unexplained metabolic acidosis
   g. Gastrointestinal upsets
      1) Nausea
      2) Vomiting
      3) Diarrhea
      4) Abdominal pain
5. Patients with a high index of suspicion of substance abuse:
   a. Trauma victims
   b. Drowning victims
   c. House-fire victims
   d. Alcoholics
   e. Psychiatric patients
   f. Criminals

Objective

1. Patients using depressants
   a. Alcohol

Early Stage	Late Stage
Marked mental and sensory impairment	Coma
	Respiratory failure
Uncoordination	Death
Ataxia	
Slurred speech	
Nystagmus	

   b. Sedatives
      1) Sedation—difficult to arouse
      2) Respiratory depression—decreased rate and depth of respiration
      3) Respiratory arrest
      4) Shock—cold, clammy skin, tachycardia, pallor, decreased urine output
   c. Narcotics
      1) Coma—not arousable to stimuli
      2) Respiratory depression—decreased rate and depth of respiration
      3) Constricted pupils—pinpoint pupils that do not respond to light
      4) Pulmonary edema—dyspnea, moist breath sounds, moist cough, tachycardia, diaphoresis
      5) Seizures—generalized activity
   d. Tricyclic antidepressants
      1) Confusion—unable to correctly answer questions or to reason
      2) Coma—not arousable to stimuli
      3) Cardiac rhythm changes from cardiotoxicity
      4) Generalized seizures that may progress to status epilepticus
      5) Hypotension
      6) Moist lung sounds indicating pulmonary edema
2. Stimulants
   a. Cocaine

Early Stage	Middle Stage	Late Stage
"Fight or flight" reaction	Apprehension	Coma
Excitement	Anxiety	Paralysis
Euphoria	Delirium	Tachycardia
	Hallucinations	Pallor
	Seizures	Hypertension
		Dilated pupils
		Hyperreflexia
		Arrhythmias

- b. Marijuana
    1) Reddened conjunctiva
    2) Impaired coordination
    3) Dry mouth and throat irritation
    4) Cough, dyspnea, and decreased arterial oxygen concentration
    5) Euphoria to acute panic
    6) Changes in sensorium
        a) Heightened perception
        b) Time and space disorientation
        c) Sedation
        d) Lapses in attention and short-term memory loss
        e) Tachycardia
- c. Phencyclidine (PCP)
    1) Disorientation
    2) Inability to concentrate
    3) Altered judgment
    4) Acute psychosis
    5) Violent behavior
    6) Extreme agitation
    7) Hallucinations
    8) Delusions
    9) Catatonia
    10) Coma
    11) Seizures
    12) Severe hypertension leading to hypertensive crisis
    13) Spontaneous vertical and horizontal nystagmus

SUPPORTING TEST FINDINGS

Laboratory Tests

1. Arterial blood gases
   Abnormality: Marijuana:
       Decreased pH
       Decreased Pao_2
       Increased HCO_3
2. Ethanol level
   Abnormality: Presence of ethanol in the blood in patients who have ingested ethanol
3. Methanol level
   Abnormality: Presence of methanol in the blood in patients who have ingested methanol
4. Toxicology level
   Abnormality: Presence of drugs in the gastric aspirate, blood, or urine

Diagnostic Tests

1. Chest X-ray
   Abnormality: Evidence of chronic obstructive pulmonary disease with long-term marijuana use
2. Electrocardiogram (ECG)
   Abnormality: Evidence of rate and rhythm disturbances with stimulants, psychogenics, and depressants

Planning/Intervention

COLLABORATIVE MANAGEMENT

Procedures

1. Neutralize the substance.
   a. Administer large amounts of intravenous fluids, as ordered.
   b. Instill activated charcoal into the stomach through a nasogastric tube or by having the patient drink it, if substance was ingested.
   c. Administer antidotes specific to the substance taken, as ordered.
2. Remove the substance.

    a. Stimulate gastric emptying in patients who have ingested the substance.

       1) Administer ordered emetics, like syrup of ipecac, to patients who are awake and alert to induce vomiting.

       2) Perform gastric lavage and irrigation with a large bore orogastric (36°F Ewald or Edlich tube), as ordered.

    b. Stimulate catharsis in patients who have ingested the substance. Administer ordered laxative to speed the emptying of the substance from the gastrointestinal tract.

    c. Stimulate diuresis.

       1) Administer a diuretic to speed the exit of substances that are excreted in the urine.

       2) Perform forced osmotic diuresis, as ordered, with ethanol, methanol, ethylene glycol, and isoniazid overdoses.

       3) Perform forced alkaline diuresis, as ordered, with salicylate overdose.

       4) Perform forced acid diuresis, as ordered, with overdoses of amphetamines and phencyclidine.

    d. Prepare patient for dialysis and/or hemoperfusion.

       1) Rarely used, but may be beneficial when metabolic acidosis from the substance occurs.

       2) Prepare to use very early in massive, potentially lethal overdose before the drug becomes stored in body deposits.

       3) Prepare to use when the normal route of excretion is impaired.

3. Provide supportive care. Treat any problems caused by the overdose.

    a. Recognize withdrawal signs and symptoms from alcohol or drugs.

    b. Treat withdrawal. Expect to administer the following treatment for drug withdrawal.

Identifying and Treating Drug Overdose

Drug	Signs and Symptoms of Withdrawal	Treatment
Alcohol	Anxiety, agitation, seizures, visual and tactile hallucinations, incontinence, delirium tremens (hypertension, tachycardia, diaphoresis, hallucinosis, tremors, paranoia, extreme restlessness), dehydration, fever, electrolyte imbalances, hypoglycemia, and acidosis	Sedatives (chlordiazepoxide, diazepam), antiseizure drugs (phenytoin, diazepam), ethanol intravenously occasionally to prevent withdrawal
Opioid narcotics	Anxiety, drug craving, rhinorrhea, lacrimation, diaphoresis, yawning,	Fluid replacement, methadone for pain control

	chills, restlessness, irritability, nausea, anorexia, dilated pupils, goose flesh, twitching from central nervous system hyperactivity, muscle spasms with kicking movements, pain, tachycardia, hypertension followed by hypotension, and fetal positioning	
Sedative-Hypnotics	Insomnia, anxiety, twitching, tremors, weakness, orthostatic hypotension, agitation, disorientation, tonic-clonic seizures or status epilepticus, death	Sedative-hypnotic agent, usually a barbiturate, to prevent or minimize withdrawal; slowly taper off once symptoms have subsided
Stimulants	Hyperinsomnia, depression, fatigue, apathy, exhaustion	Sedatives that do not produce dependence for symptomatic treatment
Marijuana	Irritability, sleeping disturbances, nausea	No treatment generally indicated

Drug Therapy

1. Narcotic antagonist
   Example: naloxone (Narcan)
   Action: Completely blocks the effects of narcotics, including central nervous system and respiratory depression, without producing and narcotic-like effects
      Duration of action is 45 minutes
   Caution: Can cause ventricular tachycardia, ventricular fibrillation, and narcotic withdrawal
      May need to repeat dose if drug effect is longer than that of antidote

2. Antidote—absorbent
   Example: Activated charcoal (Acta-Char)
   Action: Binds drugs and chemicals within the gastrointestinal tract, thereby blocking absorption and preventing toxicity
   Caution: Can cause vomiting, so do not use with overdoses of corrosive materials

3. Hypertonic glucose
   Example: 50% dextrose in water
   Action: Increases blood glucose level to treat hypoglycemia caused by insulin, cocaine, or ethanol overdose
   Caution: Can cause hyperglycemia

4. Benzodiazepine antagonist
   Example: flumazenil (Flumazicon)
   Action: Reverses the effects of benzodiazepines
   Caution: Peak effect is in 6–10 minutes with a terminal half-life of about 1 hour; may need to repeat dose

5. Emetics
   Example: syrup of Ipecac
   Action: Stimulates the chemoreceptor trigger zone in the central nervous system and irritates the gastric mucosa, causing vomiting
   Caution: Do not use if corrosive substance has been ingested; use only on alert patients

6. Cholinergic agents
   Example: physostigmine (Antilerium)
   Action: Reverses the central nervous system effect of drugs capable of causing the anticholinergic syndrome like belladonna, phenothiazides, and tricyclic antidepressants

Caution: Can cause seizures, bradycardia, and bronchospasm

NURSING MANAGEMENT

Monitoring and Managing Clinical Problems

1. Breathing Pattern: ineffective
   a. Assess for partial or total airway obstruction.
   b. Assess for an effective breathing pattern.
   c. Monitor for tachypnea.
   d. Assess the mucous membranes of the mouth for burned or discolored areas from oral ingestion.
   e. Smell breath for odor of ingested substance, if the substance has an identifiable odor.
   f. Auscultate the lungs for crackles and/or wheezes.
2. Tissue Perfusion, altered: peripheral
   a. Assess vital signs for abnormalities.
   b. Check peripheral pulses for quality and amplitude.
   c. Monitor ECG, for rhythm disturbances.
3. Tissue Perfusion, altered: cerebral
   a. Assess for a change in the level of consciousness.
   b. Check reflexes for hyperreflexia.
   c. Assess pupil size and reaction.
      1) Pinpoint pupils are seen in overdoses of narcotics, phenothiazides, chloral hydrate, and organophosphates.
      2) Dilated pupils are seen in overdoses of alcohol, amphetamines, cocaine, belladonna derivatives, and tricyclic antidepressants.
      3) Involuntary eye movements are seen in overdoses of alcohol, sedatives, phenytoin, and phencyclidine.
   d. Notify physician of significant alterations and intervene appropriately.
4. Tissue Integrity: impaired
   a. Assess for the presence of needle tracks.
   b. Assess for the presence of pitted scars as a result of "skin popping" (injecting drugs into the subcutaneous tissue).
   c. Assess for the presence of large cutaneous blisters associated with overdoses of barbiturates, sedatives, and carbon monoxide.

    d. Institute appropriate interventions to prevent infection and promote healing.

5. Violence: high risk for, directed at self/others
    a. Assess for guilt and low self-esteem as the patient recovers from the suicide attempt.
    b. Remember that suicidal patient may:
       1) Be ambivalent
       2) Feel helpless
       3) Be self-centered
       4) Have immature thought processes
    c. Promote an environment of acceptance and support, regardless of your personal feelings toward suicide.
    d. Refer patient to alcohol or drug counseling if the patient is a substance abuser.
    e. Protect the patient from subsequent self-inflicted harm. The patient truly wishing death will try again. Psychiatric intervention should begin in the intensive care unit.

6. Injury: high risk for—Remember there may be a repeated suicide attempt.
    a. Ask patients:
       1) If they have contemplated suicide in the past
       2) If they have a concrete plan
    b. Be certain all patients admitted with intentional overdoses have a psychiatric evaluation before leaving the intensive care unit.

Monitoring, Managing, and Preventing of Life-Threatening Emergencies

1. Cardiopulmonary arrest
    a. Call for help
    b. Begin cardiopulmonary resuscitation
    c. Follow with advanced cardiac life support

Family Needs

When an individual undergoes a physiologic crisis and is admitted to an intensive care unit (ICU), the other family members undergo a psychological crisis. Shock and disbelief may be the first emotions experienced by the family. The degree of that crisis experienced by the family is related to the importance of the role held by the patient within the family.

Etiology

1. The major needs of families are:
   a. Relief of anxiety
   b. Assurance that care is competent
   c. Access to the patient
   d. Information about the patient
   e. Emotional support
2. Barriers to meeting family needs include:
   a. An emphasis on technical expertise and efficiency that negates the importance of family relationships
   b. Lack of rewards for the ICU staff for communication with families
   c. Perceived skill deficits in family care by ICU nurses. These are often present in younger, less experienced ICU nurses.
   d. The ICU nurses' attitude toward family needs. A negative attitude by the nurse results in poor communication with the family.
   e. Workload of the nurse caring for the patient. When the choice must be made between family interaction and delivery of essential care, the care will always come first. The busier the ICU nurse is delivering care, the less time available for family interaction.

Assessment/Analysis

1. Fear evidenced by:
   a. Diaphoresis
   b. Feelings of loss of control
   c. Increased blood pressure, pulse, and respiratory rate
   d. Increased questioning about hospitalization
   e. Voice tremors or pitch change
2. Anxiety evidenced by:
   a. Apprehension
   b. Distress
   c. Diaphoresis
   d. Tense posture and facial tension
   e. Restlessness
   f. Trembling, shakiness, or extraneous movements
   g. Uncertainty about outcome

    h. Increased heart rate, blood pressure, respiration, and pupil dilation

    i. Focus on self

Objective Findings

1. Caregiver Role Strain — as evidenced by:
    a. Expressed feelings of inability to perform new role
    b. Expressions of decreased ability to perform usual roles
    c. Denial of the severity of illness/injury
    d. Signs of increased stress — crying, anger, excessive grief, hostility
2. Family Coping: ineffective, compromised — as evidenced by:
    a. Need for excessive information and explanation
    b. Excessive protectiveness
    c. Need to be with the patient at all times
    d. Anger and hostility toward family members and others
    e. Desire for complete control of the situation
3. Family Processes: altered — as evidenced by:
    a. Inability of the family system to meet the emotional needs of the members
    b. Conflict between family members
    c. Failure to designate one person to act as the spokesperson
4. Social Isolation — as evidenced by:
    a. Absence of a family support system
    b. Family failure to visit patient
    c. Lack of knowledge of resources available for help

Planning/Interventions

NURSING MANAGEMENT

1. Provide open visiting or relax visiting hours during the patient's critical phase. The higher the patient acuity, the more frequently the family should be permitted to visit.
2. Provide an information booklet about the ICU that can

be read later, plus an early orientation to the unit and rules regarding families.

3. Provide a comfortable, convenient visitors' lounge with a rest area and easy access to food and drink.

4. Have a hospital volunteer assigned to the lounge to assist families.

5. Promote open communication about the patient between the family and the ICU nurse.

6. Schedule daily interdisciplinary conferences with family members' participation.

7. Have the family select a spokesperson who will phone for information and relay that information to other family members.

8. If possible, assign the same nurse to the patient to reassure the family that consistent, competent care is being given to the patient.

9. Provide written information about the patient's condition to the family, so they have something concrete to refer to, reducing their anxiety.

10. Increase nurse's confidence and competence in family interaction by providing inservice programs teaching the ICU nurse ways to meet family needs.

12. Identify family strengths that will help the ICU nurse to assist the family with coping.

13. Remember that family coping is often more difficult, and negative emotions may be expressed by both the patient and the family members, if the patient has an ambivalent relationship with the family.

14. To decrease fear and anxiety, accompany family to the bedside during the first visit, explain the equipment surrounding the patient, and encourage them to interact with the patient.

Appendices

Appendix P: Cardiac Arrhythmias

Appendix Q: NANDA Nursing Diagnoses

Appendix R: Abbreviations Used in This Book

Appendix A: Calculating Drug Dosages

Drug Dose Calculation

1. $\dfrac{\text{Have}}{\text{Have}} \times \dfrac{\text{Need}}{\text{Need}}$
   a. Cross multiply
   b. Solve for unknown
2. Have : Have : : Need : Need

   a. Multiply insides
   b. Multiply outsides
   c. Solve for unknown

Intravenous (IV) Rate Calculation

$$\dfrac{\text{Amount of solution} \times \text{Drip factor of IV tubing}}{\text{Time of administration in minutes}}$$

Drip Dose Calculation

$$\dfrac{\begin{array}{c}\text{Desired dose in kilogram per minute} \times \\ \text{patient weight in kilograms} \times \text{drip factor of IV tubing}\end{array}}{\text{Concentration of drug per milliliter}}$$

Appendix B: Measurement Conversion Table

From Deglin, J. H. and Vallerand, A. H. 1995. <u>Davis's Drug Guide for Nurses</u>. (4th ed.). Philadelphia: FA Davis, with permission.

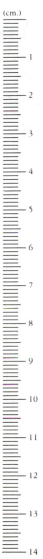

(cm.)

Metric System Equivalents

1 gram (g) = 1000 milligrams (mg)
1000 grams = 1 kilogram (kg)
.001 milligram = 1 microgram (mcg)
1 liter (L) = 1000 milliliters (ml)
1 milliliter = 1 cubic centimeter (cc)
1 meter = 100 centimeters (cm)
1 meter = 1000 millimeters (mm)

Conversion Equivalents

Volume

1 milliliter = 15 minims (M) = 15 drops (gtt)
5 milliliters = 1 fluidram (ℨ) = 1 teaspoon (tsp)
15 milliliters = 4 fluidrams = 1 tablespoon (T)
30 milliliters = 1 ounce (oz) = 2 tablespoons
500 milliliters = 1 pint (pt)
1000 milliliters = 1 quart (qt)

Weight

1 kilogram = 2.2 pound (lb)
1 gram (g) = 1000 milligrams = 15 grains (gr)
0.6 gram = 600 milligrams = 10 grains
0.5 gram = 500 milligrams = 7.5 grains
0.3 gram = 300 milligrams = 5 grains
0.06 gram = 60 milligrams = 1 grain

Length

2.5 centimeters = 1 inch

Centigrade/Fahrenheit Conversions

$C = (F - 32) \times \frac{5}{9}$
$F = (C \times \frac{9}{5}) + 32$

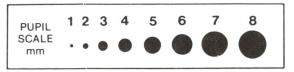

PUPIL
SCALE
mm
1 2 3 4 5 6 7 8

Appendix C: Estimating Body Surface Area in Adults

Reproduced from Lenter, C. (Ed.). Geigy Scientific Tables (8th ed.). Courtesy CIBA-GEIGY, Basle, Switzerland.

Use a straightedge to connect the patient's height in the left-hand column to weight in the right-hand column. The intersection of this line with the center scale estimates the body surface area.

HEIGHT	BODY SURFACE AREA	WEIGHT

HEIGHT

cm 200 — 79 inch
195 — 78
— 77
— 76
190 — 75
— 74
185 — 73
— 72
180 — 71
— 70
175 — 69
— 68
170 — 67
— 66
165 — 65
— 64
160 — 63
— 62
155 — 61
— 60
150 — 59
— 58
145 — 57
— 56
140 — 55
— 54
135 — 53
— 52
130 — 51
— 50
125 — 49
— 48
120 — 47
— 46
115 — 45
— 44
110 — 43
— 42
105 — 41
— 40
cm 100 — 39 in

BODY SURFACE AREA

2.80 m²
2.70
2.60
2.50
2.40
2.30
2.20
2.10
2.00
1.95
1.90
1.85
1.80
1.75
1.70
1.65
1.60
1.55
1.50
1.45
1.40
1.35
1.30
1.25
1.20
1.15
1.10
1.05
1.00
0.95
0.90
0.86 m²

WEIGHT

kg 150 — 330 lb
145 — 320
140 — 310
135 — 300
130 — 290
125 — 280
120 — 270
115 — 260
110 — 250
105 — 240
100 — 230
95 — 220
90 — 210
85 — 200
80 — 190
75 — 180
70 — 170
65 — 160
60 — 150
55 — 140
50 — 130
45 — 120
40 — 110
35 — 105
— 100
— 95
— 90
— 85
— 80
— 75
— 70
kg 30 — 66 lb

Appendix D: Electrolyte Equivalents and Caloric Values of Commonly Used Large-Volume Parenterals

	mEq/Liter								Calories/Liter
Solution	Na	K	Ca	Mg	Cl	Acetate	Lactate		
D5W	—	—	—	—	—	—	—		170
D10W	—	—	—	—	—	—	—		340
0.9% NaCl	154	—	—	—	154	—	—		—
D5/0.9% NaCl	154	—	—	—	154	—	—		170
D5/0.45% NaCl	77	—	—	—	77	—	—		170
D5/0.2% NaCl	38.5	—	—	—	38.5	—	—		170
D5/LR	130	4	3	—	109	—	28		170–180
D5/Ringer's	147.5	4	4	—	156	—	—		170
LR	130	4	3	—	109	—	28		9
Ringer's Injection	147	4	4.5	—	156	—	—		—

D5W = 5% dextrose in water.

D10W = 10% dextrose in water.

0.9% NaCl = 0.9% sodium chloride = normal saline.

D5/0.9% NaCl = 5% dextrose in water with 0.9% sodium chloride = D5 with normal saline.

D5/0.45% NaCl = 5% dextrose in water with 0.45% sodium chloride = D5 with half normal saline.

D5/0.2% NaCl = 5% dextrose in water with 0.2% sodium chloride = D5 with quarter normal saline.

D5/LR = 5% dextrose in water with lactated Ringer's solution.

D5/Ringer's = 5% dextrose in water with Ringer's solution.

LR = Lactated Ringer's solution.

From Deglin, J. H. and Vallerand, A. A. (1995). Davis's Drug Guide for Nurses (4th ed.). Philadelphia: FA Davis, p. 1291, with permission.

Appendix E: Syringe Compatibility Chart

From Deglin, J. H. and Vallerand, A. A. (1995). <u>Davis's Drug Guide for Nurses</u> (4th ed.). Philadelphia: FA Davis, with permission.

Drug Compatibility Charts — **Syringe Compatibility**

Copyright © 1993 F.A. DAVIS CO.

KEY
C = Compatible
L = Compatible for a limited period of time
I = Incompatible
* = Conflicting data
− = Data unavailable
■ = Identical drug

	1. atropine	2. buprenorphine	3. butorphanol	4. chlorpromazine	5. codeine	6. diazepam
1. atropine	■	−	C	L	−	−
2. buprenorphine	−	■	−	−	−	−
3. butorphanol	C	−	■	C	−	−
4. chlorpromazine	L	−	C	■	−	I
5. codeine	−	−	−	−	■	−
6. diazepam	−	−	−	I	−	■
7. diphenhydramine	L	−	C	L	−	−
8. droperidol/fentanyl	−	−	−	L	−	−
9. hydromorphone	C	−	−	C	−	−
10. hydroxyzine	L	−	C	L	C	−
11. meperidine	L	−	C	L	−	−
12. midazolam	L	−	L	L	−	−
13. morphine	L	−	C	L	−	−
14. nalbuphine	C	−	−	−	−	I
15. pentazocine	L	−	C	L	−	−
16. pentobarbital	L	−	I	I	−	−
17. phenobarbital	−	−	−	I	−	−
18. prochlorperazine	L	−	C	L	−	−
19. promethazine	L	−	C	L	−	−
20. scopolamine	L	−	C	L	−	−
21. secobarbital	−	−	−	−	−	−

	7. diphenhydramine	8. droperidol/fentanyl	9. hydromorphone	10. hydroxyzine	11. meperidine	12. midazolam	13. morphine	14. nalbuphine	15. pentazocine	16. pentobarbital	17. phenobarbital	18. prochlorperazine	19. promethazine	20. scopolamine	21. secobarbital
1	L	–	C	L	L	L	L	C	L	L	–	L	L	L	–
2	–	–	–	–	–	–	–	–	–	–	–	–	–	–	–
3	C	–	–	C	C	L	C	–	C	I	–	C	C	C	–
4	L	L	C	L	L	L	L	–	L	I	I	L	L	L	–
5	–	–	–	C	–	–	–	–	–	–	–	–	–	–	–
6	–	–	–	–	–	–	–	I	–	–	–	–	–	–	–
7	■	L	C	L	L	L	L	–	L	I	–	L	L	L	–
8	L	■	–	–	–	–	–	–	–	–	–	–	–	–	–
9	C	–	■	C	–	L	–	–	C	C	–	*	C	C	–
10	L	–	C	■	L	L	L	C	L	I	I	L	L	L	–
11	L	–	–	L	■	L	I	–	L	I	–	L	L	L	–
12	L	–	L	L	L	■	L	L	–	I	L	I	L	L	–
13	L	–	–	L	I	L	■	–	L	*	–	*	*	L	–
14	–	–	–	C	–	L	–	■	–	I	–	C	C	C	–
15	L	–	C	L	L	–	L	–	■	I	–	L	L	L	–
16	I	–	C	I	I	I	*	I	I	■	–	I	I	L	–
17	–	–	–	L	–	–	–	–	–	–	■	I	–	–	–
18	L	–	*	L	L	I	*	C	L	I	I	■	L	L	–
19	L	–	C	L	L	L	*	C	L	I	–	L	■	L	–
20	L	–	C	L	L	L	L	C	L	L	–	L	L	■	–
21	–	–	–	–	–	–	–	–	–	–	–	–	–	–	■

Appendix F:
IV Admixture
Compatibility Chart

From Deglin, J. H. and Vallerand, A. A. (1993). Davis's Drug Guide for Nurses (3rd ed.). Philadelphia: FA Davis, p. 1258–1259, with permission.

Copyright © 1993 F.A. DAVIS CO.

Drug Compatibility Charts

IV Admixture Compatibility

KEY

C = Compatible
L = Compatible for a limited period of time
I = Incompatible
* = Conflicting data
– = Data unavailable
■ = Identical drug

Column headings (1–15):
1. amikacin
2. aminophylline
3. amphotericin B
4. ampicillin
5. calcium chloride
6. calcium gluconate
7. cefamandole
8. cefazolin
9. cefoxitin
10. chloramphenicol
11. cimetidine
12. clindamycin
13. dexamethasone
14. diphenhydramine
15. gentamicin

Drug	1	2	3	4	5	6	7	8	9	10	11	12	13	14	15
1. amikacin	■	*	I	I	C	C	–	I	C	C	C	C	*	C	–
2. aminophylline	*	■	–	–	–	C	–	–	–	C	I	I	C	C	–
3. amphotericin B	I	–	■	I	I	I	–	–	–	–	I	–	–	I	I
4. ampicillin	I	–	I	■	–	I	–	–	–	–	*	*	–	–	I
5. calcium chloride	C	–	I	–	■	–	–	–	–	C	–	–	–	–	–
6. calcium gluconate	C	C	I	I	–	■	I	I	–	C	–	I	C	C	I
7. cefamandole	–	–	–	–	–	I	■	–	–	–	*	C	–	–	I
8. cefazolin	I	–	–	–	–	I	–	■	–	L	I	C	C	–	I
9. cefoxitin	C	–	–	–	–	–	–	–	■	–	C	C	–	–	I
10. chloramphenicol	C	C	–	–	C	C	–	L	–	■	–	–	C	C	I
11. cimetidine	C	I	I	*	–	–	*	*	C	–	■	C	C	–	C
12. clindamycin	C	I	–	*	–	I	C	C	C	–	C	■	–	–	C
13. dexamethasone	*	C	–	–	–	C	–	C	–	C	C	–	■	I	I
14. diphenhydramine	C	C	I	–	–	C	–	–	–	C	–	C	–	■	I
15. gentamicin	–	–	I	I	–	I	I	I	I	I	C	C	I	I	■
16. heparin	I	C	C	*	–	C	–	–	L	C	–	C	L	–	I
17. hydrocortisone	C	C	C	*	C	C	–	–	–	C	–	C	L	L	I
18. insulin, regular	–	I	–	–	–	–	–	–	C	–	C	–	–	–	I
19. lidocaine	–	C	–	*	C	C	C	–	–	C	C	–	C	C	C
20. methicillin	I	C	–	I	C	C	–	–	–	I	–	–	C	C	I
21. methylprednisolone	–	*	–	–	–	I	–	–	–	C	–	C	–	–	–
22. metoclopramide	–	–	–	–	–	I	–	–	–	C	C	C	–	–	–
23. metronidazole	C	C	–	*	–	–	*	C	*	C	–	C	–	–	C
24. mezlocillin	–	–	–	–	–	–	–	–	–	–	–	–	–	–	I
25. multivitamin infusion	–	–	–	–	–	–	–	–	C	–	–	–	–	–	–
26. nafcillin	–	*	–	–	–	–	–	–	–	C	–	–	C	C	–
27. oxacillin	*	–	–	–	–	–	–	–	–	C	–	–	–	–	–
28. oxytocin	–	–	–	–	–	–	–	–	–	C	–	–	–	–	–
29. penicillin G	*	I	I	–	C	C	–	–	–	C	C	C	–	C	*
30. piperacillin	–	–	–	–	–	–	–	–	–	–	C	–	–	–	–
31. potassium chloride	*	C	I	–	–	C	–	–	–	C	C	C	–	–	–
32. procainamide	–	–	–	–	–	–	–	–	–	–	–	–	–	–	–
33. ranitidine	C	–	I	*	–	–	–	*	–	C	–	I	C	–	C
34. ticarcillin	–	–	I	–	–	–	–	–	–	–	–	–	–	–	–
35. tobramycin	–	–	–	–	C	I	–	C	–	–	*	–	–	–	–
36. vancomycin	C	*	–	–	–	C	–	–	–	I	C	–	I	–	–
37. verapamil	C	C	I	*	C	C	C	C	C	C	C	C	C	–	C

	16. heparin	17. hydrocortisone	18. insulin, regular	19. lidocaine	20. methicillin	21. methylprednisolone	22. metoclopramide	23. metronidazole	24. mezlocillin	25. multivitamin infusion	26. nafcillin	27. oxacillin	28. oxytocin	29. penicillin G	30. piperacillin	31. potassium chloride	32. procainamide	33. ranitidine	34. ticarcillin	35. tobramycin	36. vancomycin	37. verapamil
1.	I	C	–	–	I	–	–	–	C	–	–	–	*	–	*	–	–	C	–	–	C	C
2.	C	C	I	C	C	*	–	C	–	–	*	–	–	I	–	C	–	–	–	–	*	C
3.	C	C	–	–	–	–	–	–	–	–	–	–	–	I	–	I	–	I	–	–	–	I
4.	*	*	–	*	I	–	–	*	–	–	–	–	–	–	–	–	–	*	–	–	–	*
5.	–	C	–	C	I	–	–	–	–	–	–	–	–	C	–	–	–	–	–	–	–	C
6.	C	L	–	C	C	I	I	–	–	–	–	–	C	–	C	–	–	–	–	C	C	C
7.	–	–	–	C	–	–	–	*	–	–	–	–	–	–	–	–	–	–	–	I	–	C
8.	–	–	–	–	–	–	–	C	–	–	–	–	–	–	–	–	–	*	–	–	–	C
9.	L	C	–	–	–	–	–	*	–	C	–	–	–	–	–	–	–	–	–	C	–	C
10.	C	C	–	C	I	C	–	C	–	–	C	C	C	C	–	C	–	C	–	–	I	C
11.	–	–	C	C	–	C	C	–	–	–	–	–	C	–	C	–	–	–	–	–	C	C
12.	C	C	–	–	C	C	C	–	–	–	–	–	C	C	C	–	I	–	*	–	–	C
13.	L	L	–	C	C	–	C	–	–	–	C	–	–	–	–	–	–	C	–	–	I	C
14.	–	I	–	C	C	–	–	–	–	–	C	–	C	–	–	–	–	–	–	–	–	–
15.	I	I	I	C	I	–	–	C	I	–	–	–	–	*	–	–	–	C	–	–	–	C
16.	■	*	I	C	*	C	–	C	–	–	C	–	–	*	–	C	–	–	–	–	I	C
17.	*	■	L	C	*	–	–	*	–	–	I	–	–	C	C	C	–	–	–	–	C	C
18.	I	L	■	C	–	I	–	–	–	–	–	–	–	–	–	–	–	–	–	–	–	C
19.	C	C	C	■	–	–	–	–	–	–	–	–	C	–	C	C	–	–	–	–	–	C
20.	*	*	–	–	■	–	–	–	–	–	–	C	–	C	–	C	–	–	–	–	I	C
21.	C	–	I	–	–	■	C	–	–	–	I	–	–	*	–	–	–	–	–	–	–	C
22.	–	–	–	–	C	–	■	–	–	C	–	–	–	–	C	–	–	–	–	–	–	–
23.	C	*	–	–	–	–	–	■	–	C	–	–	–	C	–	–	–	–	–	C	–	–
24.	–	–	–	–	–	–	–	–	■	–	–	–	–	–	–	–	–	–	–	–	–	*
25.	–	–	–	–	C	C	–	–	–	■	–	–	L	–	–	–	–	–	–	–	–	C
26.	C	I	–	–	–	I	–	–	–	–	■	–	–	–	–	C	–	–	–	–	–	*
27.	–	–	–	–	–	–	–	–	–	–	–	■	–	–	–	C	–	–	–	–	–	*
28.	–	–	–	–	–	–	–	–	–	–	–	–	■	–	–	–	–	–	–	–	–	C
29.	*	C	–	C	C	*	–	*	–	L	–	–	–	■	–	*	–	C	–	–	–	C
30.	–	C	–	–	–	–	–	–	–	–	–	–	–	–	■	C	–	–	–	–	–	C
31.	C	C	–	C	C	–	C	–	–	C	C	–	*	C	–	■	–	–	–	–	C	C
32.	–	–	–	C	–	–	–	–	–	–	–	–	–	–	–	–	■	–	–	–	–	C
33.	–	–	–	–	–	–	–	–	–	–	–	–	–	C	–	–	–	■	C	C	C	–
34.	–	–	–	–	–	–	–	–	C	–	–	–	–	–	–	–	–	C	■	–	–	C
35.	–	–	–	–	–	–	C	–	–	–	–	–	–	–	–	C	–	C	–	■	–	C
36.	I	C	–	–	I	–	–	–	–	–	–	–	C	–	C	–	–	C	–	–	■	C
37.	C	C	C	C	C	C	–	*	C	*	*	C	C	C	C	C	–	C	C	C	C	■

Appendix G: Infusion Rate Tables

From Deglin, J. H. and Vallerand, A. A. (1995). Davis's Drug Guide for Nurses (4th ed.). Philadelphia: FA Davis, p. 1264, with permission.

ALTEPLASE (Activase)

Dilution: 20-mg vial with 20 ml diluent or 50-mg vial with 50 ml diluent = 1 mg/ml.

Alteplase 1 mg/ml pt >65 kg	dose (vol) first hr* 60 mg (60 ml)	dose (vol) second hr 20 mg (20 ml)	dose (vol) third hr 20 mg (20 ml)
Alteplase 1 mg/ml pt <65 kg	dose (mg/kg) first hr† 0.75 mg/kg	dose (mg/kg) second hr 0.25 mg/kg	dose (mg/kg) third hr 0.25 mg/kg

* Give 6–10 mg (6–10 ml) as a bolus over first 1–2 min.

† 0.075–0.125 mg/kg of this given as a bolus over the first 1–2 min.

AMINOPHYLLINE

Dilution: 250 mg in 250 ml or 500 mg in 500 ml or 1000 mg in 1000 ml = 1 mg/ml.
Loading dose in patients who have not received aminophylline in preceding 24 hr = 5.6 mg/kg (5.6 ml/kg) of above dilution administered over 20 min.

Aminophylline Infusion Rates (ml/hr)
Concentration = 1 mg/ml

	Patient Weight					
Dose	50 kg	60 kg	70 kg	80 kg	90 kg	100 kg
loading dose (mg)*	280 mg	336 mg	392 mg	448 mg	504 mg	560 mg
0.9 mg/kg/hr	45 ml/hr	54 ml/hr	63 ml/hr	72 ml/hr	81 ml/hr	90 ml/hr
0.8 mg/kg/hr	40 ml/hr	48 ml/hr	56 ml/hr	64 ml/hr	72 ml/hr	80 ml/hr
0.7 mg/kg/hr	35 ml/hr	42 ml/hr	49 ml/hr	56 ml/hr	63 ml/hr	70 ml/hr
0.6 mg/kg/hr	30 ml/hr	36 ml/hr	42 ml/hr	48 ml/hr	54 ml/hr	60 ml/hr
0.5 mg/kg/hr	25 ml/hr	30 ml/hr	35 ml/hr	40 ml/hr	45 ml/hr	50 ml/hr
0.4 mg/kg/hr	20 ml/hr	24 ml/hr	28 ml/hr	32 ml/hr	36 ml/hr	40 ml/hr
0.3 mg/kg/hr	15 ml/hr	18 ml/hr	21 ml/hr	24 ml/hr	27 ml/hr	30 ml/hr
0.2 mg/kg/hr	10 ml/hr	12 ml/hr	14 ml/hr	16 ml/hr	18 ml/hr	20 ml/hr
0.1 mg/kg/hr	5 ml/hr	6 ml/hr	7 ml/hr	8 ml/hr	9 ml/hr	10 ml/hr

*Loading dose administered over 20 min.

AMRINONE (Inocor)

Dilution: 100 mg/100 ml = 1 mg/ml.
Dilute with 0.45% or 0.9% sodium chloride.
Loading dose: 0.75 mg/kg (0.75 ml/kg) over 2–3 min.
To calculate infusion rate (ml/min), multiply patient's weight (kg) by dose in ml/kg/min.
To calculate infusion rate (ml/hr), multiply patient's weight (kg) by dose in mg/kg/min × 60.

Amrinone Infusion Rates
(ml/hr)
Concentration = 1 mg/ml

	Patient Weight					
Dose	50 kg	60 kg	70 kg	80 kg	90 kg	100 kg
loading dose (mg)*	37.5 mg	45 mg	52.5 mg	60 mg	67.5 mg	75 mg
5 mcg/kg/min	15 ml/hr	18 ml/hr	21 ml/hr	24 ml/hr	27 ml/hr	30 ml/hr

Amrinone Infusion Rates
(ml/hr)
Concentration = 1 mg/ml

Dose	Patient Weight					
	50 kg	60 kg	70 kg	80 kg	90 kg	100 kg
6 mcg/kg/min	18 ml/hr	21.6 ml/hr	25.5 ml/hr	28.8 ml/hr	32.4 ml/hr	36 ml/hr
7 mcg/kg/min	21 ml/hr	25.2 ml/hr	29.4 ml/hr	33.6 ml/hr	37.8 ml/hr	42 ml/hr
8 mcg/kg/min	24 ml/hr	28.8 ml/hr	33.6 ml/hr	38.4 ml/hr	43.2 ml/hr	48 ml/hr
9 mcg/kg/min	27 ml/hr	32.4 ml/hr	37.8 ml/hr	43.2 ml/hr	48.6 ml/hr	54 ml/hr
10 mcg/kg/min	30 ml/hr	36 ml/hr	42 ml/hr	48 ml/hr	54 ml/hr	60 ml/hr

* Given over 2–3 min.

BRETYLIUM (Bretylol)

A. For life-threatening ventricular arrhythmias: (V Fib. or hemodynamically unstable V Tach). Administer 5 mg/kg (0.1 ml/kg) of *undiluted* drug by rapid IV injection. *Undiluted* drug concentration = 50 mg/1 ml.

Rapid IV Injection of Undiluted Bretylium
Doses given in volume of undiluted bretylium injection
50 mg/1 ml

Dose	Patient Weight					
	50 kg	60 kg	70 kg	80 kg	90 kg	100 kg
5 mg/kg	5 ml	6 ml	7 ml	8 ml	9 ml	10 ml

B. For other ventricular arrhythmias: Dilution; 2 g/500 ml = 4 mg/ml. Administer as 5–10 mg/kg (1.25–2.5 ml/kg) IV over 10–30 min, may be repeated q 6 hr or administered as a continuous infusion at 1–2 mg/min.

Bretylium Intermittent Infusion Rates
Volume of diluted bretylium
to infuse over 10–30 min
Concentration = 4 mg/ml

Dose	Patient Weight					
	50 kg	60 kg	70 kg	80 kg	90 kg	100 kg
5 mg/kg	62.5 ml	75 ml	87.5 ml	100 ml	112.5 ml	125 ml
6 mg/kg	75 ml	90 ml	105 ml	120 ml	135 ml	150 ml
7 mg/kg	87.5 ml	105 ml	122.5 ml	140 ml	157.5 ml	175 ml
8 mg/kg	100 ml	120 ml	140 ml	160 ml	180 ml	200 ml
9 mg/kg	112.5 ml	135 ml	157.5 ml	180 ml	202.5 ml	225 ml
10 mg/kg	125 ml	150 ml	175 ml	200 ml	225 ml	250 ml

Bretylium Continuous Infusion Rates
Concentration = 4 mg/ml

Dose mg/min	Dose ml/hr
1.0 mg/min	15 ml/hr
1.5 mg/min	23 ml/hr
2.0 mg/min	30 ml/hr

DOBUTAMINE (Dobutrex)

Dilution: May be prepared as 250 mg/1000 ml = 250 mcg/ml.
500 mg/1000 ml = 500 mcg/ml.
1000 mg/1000 ml = 1000 mcg/ml.
To calculate infusion rate (ml/min), multiply patient's weight (kg) by dose in ml/kg/min.
To calculate infusion rate (ml/hr), multiply patient's weight (kg) by dose in ml/kg/min × 60.

Dobutamine Infusion Rates (ml/hr)
Concentration = 250 mcg/ml

	Patient Weight					
Dose	50 kg	60 kg	70 kg	80 kg	90 kg	100 kg
2.5 mcg/kg/min	30 ml/hr	36 ml/hr	42 ml/hr	48 ml/hr	54 ml/hr	60 ml/hr
5 mcg/kg/min	60 ml/hr	72 ml/hr	84 ml/hr	96 ml/hr	108 ml/hr	120 ml/hr
7.5 mcg/kg/min	90 ml/hr	108 ml/hr	126 ml/hr	144 ml/hr	162 ml/hr	180 ml/hr
10 mcg/kg/min	120 ml/hr	144 ml/hr	168 ml/hr	192 ml/hr	216 ml/hr	240 ml/hr

Dobutamine Infusion Rates (ml/hr)
Concentration = 500 mcg/ml

	Patient Weight					
Dose	50 kg	60 kg	70 kg	80 kg	90 kg	100 kg
2.5 mcg/kg/min	15 ml/hr	18 ml/hr	21 ml/hr	24 ml/hr	22.5 ml/hr	30 ml/hr
5 mcg/kg/min	30 ml/hr	36 ml/hr	42 ml/hr	48 ml/hr	54 ml/hr	60 ml/hr
7.5 mcg/kg/min	45 ml/hr	54 ml/hr	63 ml/hr	72 ml/hr	81 ml/hr	90 ml/hr
10 mcg/kg/min	60 ml/hr	72 ml/hr	84 ml/hr	96 ml/hr	108 ml/hr	120 ml/hr

Dobutamine Infusion Rates (ml/hr)
Concentration = 1000 mcg/ml

	Patient Weight					
Dose	50 kg	60 kg	70 kg	80 kg	90 kg	100 kg
2.5 mcg/kg/min	7.5 ml/hr	9 ml/hr	10.5 ml/hr	12 ml/hr	11.3 ml/hr	15 ml/hr
5 mcg/kg/min	15 ml/hr	18 ml/hr	21 ml/hr	24 ml/hr	27 ml/hr	30 ml/hr
7.5 mcg/kg/min	22.3 ml/hr	27 ml/hr	31.5 ml/hr	36 ml/hr	40.5 ml/hr	45 ml/hr
10 mcg/kg/min	30 ml/hr	36 ml/hr	41 ml/hr	48 ml/hr	54 ml/hr	60 ml/hr

DOPAMINE (Intropin)

Dilution: May be prepared as 200 mg/500 ml = 400 mcg/ml.
400 mg/500 ml = 800 mcg/ml.
800 mg/500 ml = 1600 mcg/ml†.
To calculate infusion rate (ml/min), multiply patient's weight (kg) by dose in ml/kg/min.
To calculate infusion rate (ml/hr), multiply patient's weight (kg) by dose in ml/kg/min × 60.

Dopamine Infusion Rates (ml/hr)
400 mcg/ml Concentration

	Patient Weight					
Dose	50 kg	60 kg	70 kg	80 kg	90 kg	100 kg
2 mcg/kg/min	15 ml/hr	18 ml/hr	21 ml/hr	24 ml/hr	27 ml/hr	30 ml/hr
5 mcg/kg/min	37.5 ml/hr	45 ml/hr	52.5 ml/hr	60 ml/hr	67.5 ml/hr	75 ml/hr

Dopamine Infusion Rates (ml/hr)
400 mcg/ml Concentration

Dose	Patient Weight					
	50 kg	60 kg	70 kg	80 kg	90 kg	100 kg
10 mcg/kg/min	75 ml/hr	90 ml/hr	105 ml/hr	120 ml/hr	135 ml/hr	150 ml/hr
20 mcg/kg/min	150 ml/hr	180 ml/hr	210 ml/hr	240 ml/hr	270 ml/hr	300 ml/hr
30 mcg/kg/min	225 ml/hr	270 ml/hr	315 ml/hr	360 ml/hr	405 ml/hr	450 ml/hr
40 mcg/kg/min	300 ml/hr	360 ml/hr	420 ml/hr	480 ml/hr	540 ml/hr	600 ml/hr
50 mcg/kg/min	375 ml/hr	450 ml/hr	525 ml/hr	600 ml/hr	675 ml/hr	750 ml/hr

Dopamine Infusion Rates (ml/hr)
800 mcg/ml Concentration

Dose	Patient Weight					
	50 kg	60 kg	70 kg	80 kg	90 kg	100 kg
2 mcg/kg/min	7.5 ml/hr	9 ml/hr	10.5 ml/hr	12 ml/hr	13.5 ml/hr	15 ml/hr
5 mcg/kg/min	18.8 ml/hr	22.5 ml/hr	26.3 ml/hr	30 ml/hr	33.8 ml/hr	37.5 ml/hr
10 mcg/kg/min	37.5 ml/hr	45 ml/hr	52.5 ml/hr	60 ml/hr	67.5 ml/hr	75 ml/hr
20 mcg/kg/min	75 ml/hr	90 ml/hr	105 ml/hr	120 ml/hr	135 ml/hr	150 ml/hr
30 mcg/kg/min	112.5 ml/hr	135 ml/hr	157.5 ml/hr	180 ml/hr	202.5 ml/hr	225 ml/hr
40 mcg/kg/min	150 ml/hr	180 ml/hr	210 ml/hr	240 ml/hr	270 ml/hr	300 ml/hr
50 mcg/kg/min	187.5 ml/hr	225 ml/hr	262.5 ml/hr	300 ml/hr	337.5 ml/hr	375 ml/hr

Dopamine Infusion Rates (ml/hr)
1600 mcg/ml Concentration*

Dose	Patient Weight					
	50 kg	60 kg	70 kg	80 kg	90 kg	100 kg
2 mcg/kg/min	3.8 ml/hr	4.5 ml/hr	5.3 ml/hr	6 ml/hr	6.8 ml/hr	7.5 ml/hr
5 mcg/kg/min	9.4 ml/hr	11.2 ml/hr	13.1 ml/hr	15.0 ml/hr	16.9 ml/hr	18.7 ml/hr
10 mcg/kg/min	18.8 ml/hr	22.5 ml/hr	26.3 ml/hr	30 ml/hr	33.8 ml/hr	37.5 ml/hr
20 mcg/kg/min	37.5 ml/hr	45 ml/hr	52.5 ml/hr	60 ml/hr	67.5 ml/hr	75 ml/hr
30 mcg/kg/min	56.3 ml/hr	67.5 ml/hr	78.8 ml/hr	90 ml/hr	101.3 ml/hr	112.5 ml/hr
40 mcg/kg/min	75 ml/hr	90 ml/hr	105 ml/hr	120 ml/hr	135 ml/hr	150 ml/hr
50 mcg/kg/min	93.8 ml/hr	112.5 ml/hr	131.3 ml/hr	150 ml/hr	168.8 ml/hr	187.5 ml/hr

* Appropriate concentration for patients with fluid restriction.

EPINEPHRINE

Dilution: 1 mg/250 ml = 4 mcg/ml.

Epinephrine Infusion Rates (ml/hr)
Concentration = 4 mcg/ml

Dose (mcg/ml)	Dose (ml/hr)
1 mcg/min	15 ml/hr
2 mcg/min	30 ml/hr
3 mcg/min	45 ml/hr
4 mcg/min	60 ml/hr

ESMOLOL (Brevibloc)

Dilution: 5 g/500 ml = 10 mg/ml.
Loading regimen = 500 mcg/kg (0.05 ml/kg) loading dose over 1 min, followed by 50 mcg/kg/min

(0.005 ml/kg/min) infusion over 4 min. If no response, repeat loading dose over 1 min and increase infusion rate to 100 mcg/kg/min for 4–10 min. If no response, loading dose may be repeated before increasing infusion rates in 50 mcg/kg/min increments.

Esmolol Infusion Rates
Concentration = 10 mg/ml

Dose	Patient Weight					
	50 kg	60 kg	70 kg	80 kg	90 kg	100 kg
loading dose (ml)*	2.5 ml	3 ml	3.5 ml	4 ml	4.5 ml	5 ml
50 mcg/kg/min	15 ml/hr	18 ml/hr	21 ml/hr	24 ml/hr	27 ml/hr	30 ml/hr
75 mcg/kg/min	22.5 ml/hr	27 ml/hr	31.5 ml/hr	36 ml/hr	40.5 ml/hr	45 ml/hr
100 mcg/kg/min	30 ml/hr	36 ml/hr	42 ml/hr	48 ml/hr	54 ml/hr	60 ml/hr
125 mcg/kg/min	37.5 ml/hr	45 ml/hr	52.5 ml/hr	60 ml/hr	67.5 ml/hr	75 ml/hr
150 mcg/kg/min	38 ml/hr	54 ml/hr	63 ml/hr	72 ml/hr	81 ml/hr	90 ml/hr
175 mcg/kg/min	52.5 ml/hr	63 ml/hr	73.5 ml/hr	84 ml/hr	94.5 ml/hr	105 ml/hr
200 mcg/kg/min	60 ml/hr	72 ml/hr	84 ml/hr	96 ml/hr	108 ml/hr	120 ml/hr

* Loading dose given over 1 min.

HEPARIN

Dilution: 20,000 units/1000 ml = 20 units/ml.
Loading dose: 1000–2000 units as a bolus.

Heparin Infusion Rates (ml/hr)
Concentration = 20 units/ml

Dose (units/hr)	Dose (ml/hr)
500 units/hr	25 ml/hr
750 units/hr	37.5 ml/hr
1000 units/hr	50 ml/hr
1250 units/hr	62.5 ml/hr
1500 units/hr	75 ml/hr
1750 units/hr	87.5 ml/hr
2000 units/hr	100 ml/hr

ISOPROTERENOL (Isuprel)

Dilution: 2 mg/500 ml.

Isoproterenol Infusion Rates (ml/hr)
Concentration = 4 mcg/ml

Dose (mcg/min)	Dose (ml/hr)
2 mcg/min	30 ml/hr
5 mcg/min	75 ml/hr
10 mcg/min	150 ml/hr
15 mcg/min	225 ml/hr
20 mcg/min	300 ml/hr

LIDOCAINE (Xylocaine)

Dilution: May be prepared as 1 g/1000 ml = 1 mg/ml.
2 g/1000 ml = 2 mg/ml.
4 g/1000 ml = 4 mg/ml.
8 g/1000 ml = 8 mg/ml.
Loading dose: 50–100 mg at 25–50 mg/min.

Lidocaine Infusion Rates (ml/hr)

Dose (mg/min)	1 mg/ml concentration	2 mg/ml concentration	4 mg/ml concentration	8 mg/ml concentration
1 mg/min	60 ml/hr	30 ml/hr	15 ml/hr	7.5 ml/hr
2 mg/min	120 ml/hr	60 ml/hr	30 ml/hr	15 ml/hr
3 mg/min	180 ml/hr	90 ml/hr	45 ml/hr	22.5 ml/hr
4 mg/min	240 ml/hr	120 ml/hr	60 ml/hr	30 ml/hr

MILRINONE

Loading dose: 50 mcg/kg given over 10 min.

Milrinone Infusion Rates (ml/hr)

	Patient Weight					
Dose	50 kg	60 kg	70 kg	80 kg	90 kg	100 kg
loading dose (mg)	2.5 mg	3.0 mg	3.5 mg	4.0 mg	4.5 mg	5.0 mg

Milrinone Infusion Rates (ml/hr)
Concentration = 100 mcg/ml

	Patient Weight					
Dose	50 kg	60 kg	70 kg	80 kg	90 kg	100 kg
0.375 mcg/kg/min	11 ml/hr	13.2 ml/hr	15.4 ml/hr	17.6 ml/hr	19.8 ml/hr	22.0 ml/hr
0.400 mcg/kg/min	12 ml/hr	14.4 ml/hr	16.8 ml/hr	19.2 ml/hr	21.6 ml/hr	24.0 ml/hr
0.500 mcg/kg/min	15.0 ml/hr	18.0 ml/hr	21.0 ml/hr	24.0 ml/hr	27.0 ml/hr	30.0 ml/hr
0.600 mcg/kg/min	18.0 ml/hr	21.6 ml/hr	25.2 ml/hr	28.8 ml/hr	32.4 ml/hr	36.0 ml/hr
0.700 mcg/kg/min	21.0 ml/hr	25.2 ml/hr	29.4 ml/hr	33.6 ml/hr	37.8 ml/hr	42.0 ml/hr
0.750 mcg/kg/min	22.5 ml/hr	27.0 ml/hr	31.5 ml/hr	36.0 ml/hr	40.5 ml/hr	45.0 ml/hr

Concentration = 150 mcg/ml

	Patient Weight					
Dose	50 kg	60 kg	70 kg	80 kg	90 kg	100 kg
0.375 mcg/kg/min	7.5 ml/hr	9.0 ml/hr	10.5 ml/hr	12.0 ml/hr	13.4 ml/hr	15.0 ml/hr
0.400 mcg/kg/min	8.0 ml/hr	9.6 ml/hr	11.2 ml/hr	12.8 ml/hr	14.4 ml/hr	16.0 ml/hr
0.500 mcg/kg/min	10.0 ml/hr	12.0 ml/hr	14.0 ml/hr	16.0 ml/hr	18.0 ml/hr	20.0 ml/hr
0.600 mcg/kg/min	12.0 ml/hr	14.4 ml/hr	16.8 ml/hr	19.2 ml/hr	21.6 ml/hr	24.0 ml/hr
0.700 mcg/kg/min	14.0 ml/hr	16.8 ml/hr	19.6 ml/hr	22.4 ml/hr	25.2 ml/hr	28.0 ml/hr
0.750 mcg/kg/min	15.0 ml/hr	18.0 ml/hr	21.0 ml/hr	24.0 ml/hr	27.0 ml/hr	30.0 ml/hr

Concentration = 200 mcg/ml

	Patient Weight					
Dose	50 kg	60 kg	70 kg	80 kg	90 kg	100 kg
0.375 mcg/kg/min	5.5 ml/hr	6.6 ml/hr	7.7 ml/hr	8.8 ml/hr	9.9 ml/hr	11.1 ml/hr
0.400 mcg/kg/min	6.0 ml/hr	7.2 ml/hr	8.4 ml/hr	9.6 ml/hr	10.8 ml/hr	12.0 ml/hr
0.500 mcg/kg/min	7.5 ml/hr	9.0 ml/hr	10.5 ml/hr	12.0 ml/hr	13.5 ml/hr	15.0 ml/hr
0.600 mcg/kg/min	9.0 ml/hr	10.8 ml/hr	12.6 ml/hr	14.4 ml/hr	16.2 ml/hr	18.0 ml/hr
0.700 mcg/kg/min	10.5 ml/hr	12.6 ml/hr	14.7 ml/hr	16.8 ml/hr	18.9 ml/hr	21.0 ml/hr
0.750 mcg/kg/min	11.0 ml/hr	13.5 ml/hr	15.4 ml/hr	17.6 ml/hr	19.8 ml/hr	22.0 ml/hr

NITROGLYCERIN (Nitro-bid, Nitrol, Nitrostat, Tridil)

Dilution: May be prepared as 5 mg/100 ml (25 mg/500 ml, 50 mg/1000 ml) = 50 mcg/ml.
25 mg/250 ml (50 mg/500 ml, 100 mg/1000 ml) = 100 mcg/ml.
50 mg/250 ml (100 mg/500 ml, 200 mg/1000 ml = 200 mcg/ml.

Note that different products are available in different concentrated solutions and should be used with appropriate infusion tubing. Changes in tubing may result in altered response to a given dose.

Dose (mcg/min)	Nitroglycerin Infusion Rates (ml/hr)		
	50 mcg/ml concentration	100 mcg/ml concentration	200 mcg/ml concentration
2.5 mcg/min	3 ml/hr	1.5 ml/hr	0.75 ml/hr
5 mcg/min	6 ml/hr	3 ml/hr	1.5 ml/hr
10 mcg/min	12 ml/hr	6 ml/hr	3 ml/hr
15 mcg/min	18 ml/hr	9 ml/hr	4.5 ml/hr
20 mcg/min	24 ml/hr	12 ml/hr	6 ml/hr
30 mcg/min	36 ml/hr	18 ml/hr	9 ml/hr
40 mcg/min	48 ml/hr	24 ml/hr	12 ml/hr
50 mcg/min	60 ml/hr	30 ml/hr	15 ml/hr
60 mcg/min	72 ml/hr	36 ml/hr	18 ml/hr

NITROPRUSSIDE (Nipride, Nitropress)

Dilution: May be prepared as 50 mg/1000 ml = 50 mcg/ml.
100 mg/1000 ml = 100 mcg/ml.
200 mg/1000 ml = 200 mcg/ml.

To calculate infusion rate (ml/min), multiply patient's weight (kg) by dose in ml/kg/min.
To calculate infusion rate (ml/hr), multiply patient's weight (kg) by dose in ml/kg/min $\times$ 60.
Dosing range: 0.3 mcg/kg/min–10 mcg/kg/min.

Dose (mcg/kg/min)	Nitroprusside Infusion Rates (ml/kg/min)		
	50 mcg/ml concentration	100 mcg/ml concentration	200 mcg/ml concentration
0.3 mcg/kg/min	0.006 ml/kg/min	—	—
0.5 mcg/kg/min	0.01 ml/kg/min	—	—
1 mcg/kg/min	0.02 ml/kg/min	0.01 ml/kg/min	—
2 mcg/kg/min	0.04 ml/kg/min	0.02 ml/kg/min	0.01 ml/kg/min
3 mcg/kg/min	0.06 ml/kg/min	0.03 ml/kg/min	0.015 ml/kg/min
4 mcg/kg/min	0.08 ml/kg/min	0.04 ml/kg/min	0.02 ml/kg/min
5 mcg/kg/min	0.1 ml/kg/min	0.05 ml/kg/min	0.025 ml/kg/min
6 mcg/kg/min	0.12 ml/kg/min	0.06 ml/kg/min	0.03 ml/kg/min
7 mcg/kg/min	0.14 ml/kg/min	0.07 ml/kg/min	0.035 ml/kg/min
8 mcg/kg/min	0.16 ml/kg/min	0.08 ml/kg/min	0.04 ml/kg/min
9 mcg/kg/min	0.18 ml/kg/min	0.09 ml/kg/min	0.045 ml/kg/min
10 mcg/kg/min	0.2 ml/kg/min	0.1 ml/kg/min	0.05 ml/kg/min

Nitroprusside Infusion Rates (ml/hr)
50 mcg/ml Concentration

Patient Weight

Dose	50 kg	60 kg	70 kg	80 kg	90 kg	100 kg
0.3 mcg/kg/min	18 ml/hr	22 ml/hr	25 ml/hr	29 ml/hr	32 ml/hr	36 ml/hr
0.5 mcg/kg/min	30 ml/hr	36 ml/hr	42 ml/hr	48 ml/hr	54 ml/hr	60 ml/hr
1 mcg/kg/min	60 ml/hr	72 ml/hr	84 ml/hr	96 ml/hr	108 ml/hr	120 ml/hr
2 mcg/kg/min	120 ml/hr	144 ml/hr	168 ml/hr	192 ml/hr	216 ml/hr	240 ml/hr
3 mcg/kg/min	180 ml/hr	216 ml/hr	252 ml/hr	288 ml/hr	324 ml/hr	360 ml/hr
4 mcg/kg/min	240 ml/hr	288 ml/hr	336 ml/hr	384 ml/hr	432 ml/hr	480 ml/hr
5 mcg/kg/min	300 ml/hr	360 ml/hr	420 ml/hr	480 ml/hr	540 ml/hr	600 ml/hr
6 mcg/kg/min	360 ml/hr	432 ml/hr	504 ml/hr	576 ml/hr	648 ml/hr	720 ml/hr
7 mcg/kg/min	420 ml/hr	504 ml/hr	588 ml/hr	672 ml/hr	756 ml/hr	840 ml/hr
8 mcg/kg/min	480 ml/hr	576 ml/hr	672 ml/hr	768 ml/hr	864 ml/hr	960 ml/hr
9 mcg/kg/min	540 ml/hr	648 ml/hr	672 ml/hr	864 ml/hr	972 ml/hr	1080 ml/hr
10 mcg/kg/min	600 ml/hr	720 ml/hr	840 ml/hr	960 ml/hr	1080 ml/hr	1200 ml/hr

Nitroprusside Infusion Rates (ml/hr)
100 mcg/ml Concentration

Patient Weight

Dose	50 kg	60 kg	70 kg	80 kg	90 kg	100 kg
0.3 mcg/kg/min	9 ml/hr	11 ml/hr	13 ml/hr	14 ml/hr	16 ml/hr	18 ml/hr
0.5 mcg/kg/min	15 ml/hr	18 ml/hr	21 ml/hr	24 ml/hr	27 ml/hr	30 ml/hr
1 mcg/kg/min	30 ml/hr	36 ml/hr	42 ml/hr	48 ml/hr	54 ml/hr	60 ml/hr
2 mcg/kg/min	60 ml/hr	72 ml/hr	84 ml/hr	96 ml/hr	108 ml/hr	120 ml/hr
3 mcg/kg/min	90 ml/hr	108 ml/hr	126 ml/hr	144 ml/hr	162 ml/hr	180 ml/hr
4 mcg/kg/min	120 ml/hr	144 ml/hr	168 ml/hr	192 ml/hr	216 ml/hr	240 ml/hr
5 mcg/kg/min	150 ml/hr	180 ml/hr	210 ml/hr	240 ml/hr	270 ml/hr	300 ml/hr
6 mcg/kg/min	180 ml/hr	216 ml/hr	252 ml/hr	288 ml/hr	324 ml/hr	360 ml/hr
7 mcg/kg/min	210 ml/hr	252 ml/hr	294 ml/hr	336 ml/hr	378 ml/hr	420 ml/hr
8 mcg/kg/min	240 ml/hr	288 ml/hr	336 ml/hr	384 ml/hr	432 ml/hr	480 ml/hr
9 mcg/kg/min	270 ml/hr	324 ml/hr	336 ml/hr	432 ml/hr	486 ml/hr	540 ml/hr
10 mcg/kg/min	300 ml/hr	360 ml/hr	420 ml/hr	480 ml/hr	540 ml/hr	600 ml/hr

Nitroprusside Infusion Rates (ml/hr)
200 mcg/ml Concentration

Patient Weight

Dose	50 kg	60 kg	70 kg	80 kg	90 kg	100 kg
0.3 mcg/kg/min	5 ml/hr	5 ml/hr	6 ml/hr	7 ml/hr	8 ml/hr	9 ml/hr
0.5 mcg/kg/min	7.5 ml/hr	9 ml/hr	10.5 ml/hr	12 ml/hr	13.5 ml/hr	15 ml/hr
1 mcg/kg/min	15 ml/hr	18 ml/hr	21 ml/hr	24 ml/hr	27 ml/hr	30 ml/hr
2 mcg/kg/min	30 ml/hr	36 ml/hr	42 ml/hr	48 ml/hr	54 ml/hr	60 ml/hr
3 mcg/kg/min	45 ml/hr	54 ml/hr	63 ml/hr	72 ml/hr	81 ml/hr	90 ml/hr
4 mcg/kg/min	60 ml/hr	72 ml/hr	84 ml/hr	96 ml/hr	108 ml/hr	120 ml/hr
5 mcg/kg/min	75 ml/hr	90 ml/hr	105 ml/hr	120 ml/hr	135 ml/hr	150 ml/hr
6 mcg/kg/min	90 ml/hr	108 ml/hr	126 ml/hr	144 ml/hr	162 ml/hr	180 ml/hr
7 mcg/kg/min	105 ml/hr	126 ml/hr	147 ml/hr	168 ml/hr	189 ml/hr	210 ml/hr
8 mcg/kg/min	120 ml/hr	144 ml/hr	168 ml/hr	192 ml/hr	216 ml/hr	240 ml/hr
9 mcg/kg/min	135 ml/hr	162 ml/hr	168 ml/hr	216 ml/hr	243 ml/hr	270 ml/⫶
10 mcg/kg/min	150 ml/hr	180 ml/hr	210 ml/hr	240 ml/hr	270 ml/hr	300 m′

NOREPINEPHRINE (Levophed)

Dilution: May be prepared as 1 mg/250 ml = 4 mcg/ml.
To calculate infusion rate (ml/hr), multiply infusion rate in ml/min × 60.

Norepinephrine Infusion Rates (ml/hr)
Concentration = 4 mcg/ml

Dose (mcg/min)	Dose (ml/hr)
8 mcg/min	120 ml/hr
9 mcg/min	135 ml/hr
10 mcg/min	150 ml/hr
11 mcg/min	165 ml/hr
12 mcg/min	180 ml/hr

PHENYLEPHRINE (Neo-Synephrine)

Dilution: 10 mg/500 ml = 20 mcg/ml.

Phenylephrine Infusion Rates (ml/hr)
Concentration = 20 mcg/ml

Dose (mg/min)	Dose (ml/hr)
0.04 mg/min	120 ml/hr
0.06 mg/min	180 ml/hr
0.08 mg/min	240 ml/hr
0.10 mg/min	300 ml/hr
0.12 mg/min	360 ml/hr
0.14 mg/min	420 ml/hr
0.16 mg/min	480 ml/hr
0.18 mg/min	540 ml/hr

PROCAINAMIDE (Pronestyl)

Dilution: May be prepared as 1000 mg/500 ml = 2 mg/ml.
Loading dose: 50–100 mg q 5 min until arrhythmia is controlled; adverse reaction occurs, or 500 mg has been given, or 500–600 mg as a loading infusion over 25–30 min.

Procainamide Infusion Rates (ml/hr)
Concentration = 2 mg/ml

Dose (mg/min)	Dose (ml/hr)
1 mg/min	30 ml/hr
2 mg/min	60 ml/hr
3 mg/min	90 ml/hr
4 mg/min	120 ml/hr
5 mg/min	150 ml/hr
6 mg/min	180 ml/hr

Appendix H: Equianalgesic Tables

From Deglin, J. H. and Vallerand, A. A. (1995). <u>Davis's Drug Guide for Nurses</u> (4th ed.). Philadelphia: FA Davis, p. 1258, with permission.

OPIOID ANALGESICS COMMONLY USED FOR SEVERE PAIN

Equianalgesic doses are equivalent to 10 mg of IM morphine (i.e., morphine 10 mg IM = meperidine 75 mg IM = oxycodone 30 mg PO).

| NAME | EQUIANALGESIC DOSE (mg) | | STARTING ORAL DOSE | | COMMENTS | PRECAUTIONS AND CONTRAINDICATIONS |
	ORAL	PARENTERAL*	ADULTS (mg)	CHILDREN (mg/kg)		
Morphine	30†	10	15–30	0.3	Standard of comparison for opioid analgesics; sustained-release preparations (MS Contin, Oramorph-SR) release drug over 8–12 hr.	For all opioids, caution in patients with impaired ventilation, bronchial asthma, increased intracranial pressure, liver failure.
Hydromorphone (Dilaudid)	7.5	1.5	4–8	0.06	Slightly shorter duration than morphine.	
Oxycodone	30	—	15–30	0.3		
Methadone (Dolophine)	20	10	5–10	0.2	Good oral potency; long plasma half-life (24–36 hr).	Accumulates with repetitive dosing, causing excessive sedation (on days 2–5).
Levorphanol (Levo-Dromoman)	4	2	2–4	0.04	Long plasma half-life (12–16 hr).	Accumulates on days 2–3.
Fentanyl	—	0.1	—	—	Transdermal fentanyl (Duragesic) 25–50 mcg/hr roughly equivalent to 30 mg sustained-release morphine q 8 hr.	Because of skin reservoir of drug, 12-hr delay in onset and offset of transdermal patch; fever increases rate of absorption.

Drug						
Oxymorphone (Numorphan)	—	1	—	—	5 mg rectal suppository = 5 mg morphine IM.	Like IM morphine.
Meperidine (Demerol)	300	75	Not recommended		Slightly shorter acting than morphine.	Normeperidine (toxic metabolite) accumulates with repetitive dosing, causing CNS excitation; avoid in patients with impaired renal function or who are receiving monoamine oxidase inhibitors, irritating to tissues with repeated IM injection.
Opioid Agonist-Antagonists						
Nalbuphine (Nubain)	—	10	—	—	Not available orally; not scheduled under Controlled Substances Act.	Incidence of psychotomimetic effects lower than with pentazocine; may precipitate withdrawal in opioid-dependent patients.
Butorphanol (Stadol)	—	2	—	—	Like nalbuphine.	Like nalbuphine.
Dezocine (Dalgan)	—	10	—	—	Like nalbuphine.	May precipitate withdrawal in opioid-dependent patients; SC injection irritating.
Buprenorphine (Buprenex)	—	0.4	—	—	Not available orally; sublingual preparation not yet in US; less abuse liability than morphine; does not produce psychotomimetic effects.	May precipitate withdrawal in opioid-dependent patients; not readily reversed by naloxone; avoid in labor.

*These are standard IM doses for acute pain in adults and also may be used to convert doses for IV infusions and repeated small IV boluses. For single IV boluses, use half the IM dose. IV doses for children >6 mo = parenteral equianalgesic dose × weight (kg)/100.

†Some experts argue that 60 mg of oral morphine is the more accurate equivalent dose and suggest caution in converting patients from high doses of oral morphine to other drugs if the 30-mg equivalent is used.

Appendix I: Normal Values of Common Laboratory Tests

SERUM TESTS

Hematologic	Male ♂/♀	Female
Hemoglobin	13.5–18 g/dL	12–16 g/dL
Hematocrit	40–54%	38–47%
Red Blood Cells (RBC)	4.6–6.2 million/mm^3	4.2–5.4 million/mm^3
Leukocytes (WBC)	5,000–10,000/mm^3	
Neutrophils	54–75% (3,000–7,500/mm^3)	
Bands	3–8% (150–700/mm^3)	
Eosinophils	1–4% (50–400/mm^3)	
Basophils	0–1% (25–100/mm^3)	
Monocytes	2–8% (100–500/mm^3)	
Lymphocytes	25–40% (1,500–4,500/mm^3)	
T-lymphocytes	60–80% of lymphocytes	
B-lymphocytes	10–20% of lymphocytes	
Platelets	150,000–450,000/mm^3	
Prothrombin Time (PT)	9.6–11.8 sec	9.5–11.3 sec
Partial Thromboplastin Time (PTT)	30–45 sec	
Bleeding Time (Duke)	1–3 min	
(Ivy)	3–6 min	
(Template)	3–6 min	
Clotting Time (Lee-White)	4–8 min	

658

Chemistry	Male ♂/♀	Female
Sodium	135–145 mEq/L	
Potassium	3.5–5.0 mEq/L	
Chloride	95–105 mEq/L	
Bicarbonate (HCO_3)	19–25 mEq/L	
Total Calcium	9–11 mg/dL or 4.5–5.5 mEq/L	
Ionized Calcium	4.2–5.4 mg/dL or 2.1–2.6 mEq/L	
Phosphorous/Phosphate	2.4–4.7 mg/dL	
Magnesium	1.8–3.0 mg/dL or 1.5–2.5 mEq/L	
Glucose	70–110 mg/dL	
Osmolality	285–310 mOsm/kg	

Cardiac	Male ♂/♀	Female
Total Creatinine Phosphokinase (CPK)	12–70 U/mL	10–55 U/mL
CPK-MM	100%	
CPK-MB	0%	
CPK-BB	0%	
SGOT (AST)	8–20 U/L	
Lactic Dehydrogensase (LDH)	45–90 U/L	
LDH-1	17–27%	
LDH-2	27–37%	

Continued

659

SERUM TESTS — Continued

Cardiac	Male ♂/♀	Female
LDH-3		18–25%
LDH-4		3–8%
LDH-5		0–5%

Hepatic	Male ♂/♀	Female
SGOT (AST)	8–46 U/L	7–34 U/L
SGPT (ALT)		
Total Bilirubin		10–30 IU/mL
Conjugated Bilirubin		0.3–1.2 mg/dL
Unconjugated (Indirect) Bilirubin		0.0–0.2 mg/dL
Alkaline Phosphatase		0.2–0.8 mg/dL
		20–90 U/L

Renal	Male ♂/♀	Female
BUN		6–20 mg/dL
Creatinine	0.6–1.3 mg/dL	0.5–1.0 mg/dL
Uric Acid	4.0–8.5 mg/dL	2.7–7.3 mg/dL

Arterial Blood Gases	Male ♂/♀	Female
pH	7.35 – 7.45	
pO$_2$	80 – 100 mmHg	
pCO$_2$	35 – 45 mmHg	
O$_2$ Saturation	95 – 97%	
Base Excess	+2 – (−2)	
Bicarbonate (HCO$_3$)	22 – 26 mEq/L	

URINE TESTS

Urine	Male ♂/♀	Female
pH	4.5 – 8.0	
Specific Gravity	1.010 – 1.025	

Modified from Deglin, J. H. and Vallerand, A. A. (1995). Davis's Drug Guide for Nurses (4th ed.). Philadelphia: FA Davis, pp. 1284 – 1285, with permission.

Appendix J:
Blood Gases in
Acid-Base Imbalance

Disorder	pH	PaCO₂	HCO₃⁻
Respiratory acidosis	Decreased	Increased	Normal
With compensation	Slightly decreased or normal	Increased	Increased
Respiratory alkalosis	Increased	Decreased	Normal
With compensation	Slightly increased or normal	Decreased	Decreased
Metabolic acidosis	Decreased	Normal	Decreased
With compensation	Slightly decreased or normal	Decreased	Decreased
Metabolic alkalosis	Increased	Normal	Increased
With compensation	Slightly increased or normal	Increased	Increased
Mixed respiratory and metabolic acidosis	Decreased	Increased	Decreased

Appendix K: Causes of Altered Oxygen Saturation

Oxygen Saturation Value	Physiologic Alteration	Causes
■ High (80–90%)	■ Decreased oxygen consumption	■ Hypothermia ■ Anesthesia ■ Iatrogenic muscle paralysis ■ Sepsis
	■ Increased oxygen delivery	■ Hyperoxygen-ation
	■ Mechanical interference	■ Wedged pulmonary artery catheter ■ Left-to-right shunt
■ Normal (60–80%)	■ Oxygen supply equals oxygen demand	■ Adequate perfusion
■ Low (<60%)	■ Increased consumption	■ Shivering ■ Pain ■ Seizures ■ Activity ■ Hyperthermia ■ Anxiety
	■ Decreased oxygen delivery	■ Hypoperfusion ■ Anemia ■ Hypoxemia

Appendix L: Oxygen-Hemoglobin Dissociation Curve

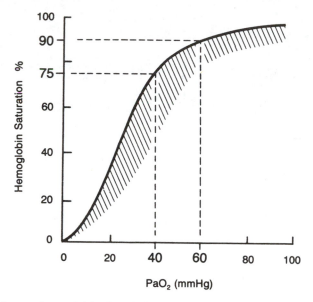

Oxygen-hemoglobin dissociation curve, relating the percent hemoglobin saturation and the partial pressure of oxygen (PO_2). The unique structure of the hemoglobin molecule accounts for the unusual affinity this molecule has for oxygen. When the PO_2 is high as in the lungs (plateau portion), oxygen readily binds with hemoglobin; when the PO_2 is low as in the tissue (steep portion), oxygen is readily released. Note that at a PaO_2 of 60, approximately 90% of the hemoglobin is saturated. Thus, clinically, oxygen therapy is often instituted to maintain a PaO_2 of 60 minimally, in the patient with compromised pulmonary function. Oxygen unloading at the cellular level is enhanced when the oxyhemoglobin dissociation curve is shifted to the right (*striped area*). The presence of acidemia (i.e., an increase in hydrogen-ion concentration), increase in body temperature, and increased levels of 2,3-DPG, all function to shift the curve to the right. Alkalemia, hypothermia, and reduced levels of 2,3-DPG function to shift the curve in the opposite direction, thereby reducing the release of oxygen at the cellular level. (Adapted from Dolan, J. T. (1991). Critical Care Nursing: Clinical Management Through the Nursing Process (2nd ed.). Philadelphia: FA Davis, p. 570, with permission.)

Appendix M:
Calculated
Hemodynamic
Parameters

Parameter	Formula	Normal Values
Arteriovenous oxygen difference (a-vDO$_2$)	Arterial O$_2$ content—venous O$_2$ content	3.5–5.5 vol%
Cardiac output (CO)	Heart rate × stroke volume	4–8 liters/minute
Cardiac index (CI)	$\dfrac{\text{Cardiac output}}{\text{BSA}}$	2.5–4 liters/minute
Coronary artery perfusion pressure (CAPP)	MAP—LVedp (or PAWm)	60–80 mmHg
Left ventricular stroke work index (LVSWI)	SI × (MAP – PAWm) × 0.0136	30–50 g/beat/m^2
Mean arterial pressure (MAP)	$\dfrac{\text{Systolic blood pressure} + (\text{diastolic pressure} \times 2)}{3}$	70–90 mmHg

Oxygen content of blood	% Saturation × hemoglobin × 1.34	17.5–20.5 vol% (arterial) 12.5–16.5 vol% (venous)
Oxygen consumption (VO_2)	CO × hemoglobin × 1.34 × (arterial O_2 saturation —venous O_2 saturation) × 10	200–250 mL/minute
Oxygen delivery (DO_2)	CO × arterial O_2 content	900–1100 mL/minute
Right ventricular stroke work index (RVSWI)	SI × (PAm–RAm) × 0.0136	5–10 g/beat/m^2
Stroke index (SI)	$\dfrac{\text{Stroke volume}}{\text{BSA}}$	40–50 mL/beat/m^2
Stroke volume (SV)	$\dfrac{\text{CO}}{\text{Heart rate}}$	70–130 mL/beat

From Dolan, J. T. (1991). Critical Care Nursing: Clinical Management Through the Nursing Process (2nd ed.). Philadelphia: FA Davis, p. 841, with permission.

Appendix N: Glasgow Coma Scale

A quick way to assess a patient's level of consciousness and ensure consistency in assessment by all persons caring for the patient is to use the Glasgow Coma Scale. The assessment tool grades the level of consciousness by evaluating eye opening, best verbal response, and best motor response. Using this scale, trends in neurologic status can be monitored.

Select the score for each response by matching the patient's response with the best description listed. Maximum score is 15 and minimum is 3.

Response	Patient Response	Score
Eyes open	Spontaneously	4
	To speech	3
	To pain	2
	None	1
Best verbal response	Oriented	5
	Confused	4
	Inappropriate words	3
	Incomprehensible sounds	2
	None	1
Best motor response	Obeys commands	6
	Localizes	5
	Flexion withdrawal	4
	Abnormal flexion	3
	Abnormal extension	2
	None	1

Appendix O: ACLS Algorithms

THE ALGORITHM APPROACH TO EMERGENCY CARDIAC CARE

These guidelines use algorithms as an educational tool. They are an illustrative method to summarize information. Providers of emergency care should view algorithms as a summary and a memory aid. They provide a way to treat a broad range of patients. Algorithms, by nature, oversimplify. The effective teacher and care provider will use them wisely, not blindly. Some patients may require care not specified in the algorithms. When clinically appropriate, flexibility is accepted and encouraged. Many interventions and actions are listed as "considerations" to help providers think. These lists should not be considered endorsements or requirements or "standard of care" in a legal sense. Algorithms do not replace clinical understanding. Although the algorithms provide a good "cookbook," the patient always requires a "thinking cook."

The following clinical recommendations apply to all treatment algorithms:

- First, treat the patient, not the monitor.
- Algorithms for cardiac arrest presume that the condition under discussion continually persists, that the patient remains in cardiac arrest, and that CPR is always performed.
- Apply different interventions whenever appropriate indications exist.
- The flow diagrams present mostly Class I (acceptable, definitely effective) recommendations. The footnotes present Class IIa (acceptable, probably effective), Class IIb (acceptable, possibly effective), and Class III (not indicated, may be harmful) recommendations.
- Adequate airway, ventilation, oxygenation, chest compressions, and defibrillation are more important than administration of medications and take precedence over initiating an intravenous line or injecting pharmacologic agents.
- Several medications (epinephrine, lidocaine, and atropine) can be administered via the endotracheal tube, but clinicians must use an endotracheal dose 2 to 2.5 times the intravenous dose.
- With a few exceptions, intravenous medications should always be administered rapidly, in bolus method.
- After each intravenous medication, give a 20- to 30-mL bolus of intravenous fluid and immediately elevate the extremity. This will enhance delivery of drugs to the central circulation, which may take 1 to 2 minutes.
- Last, treat the patient, not the monitor.

(Reproduced with permission, CPR Issue of *JAMA*, October 28, 1992. Copyright American Heart Association.)

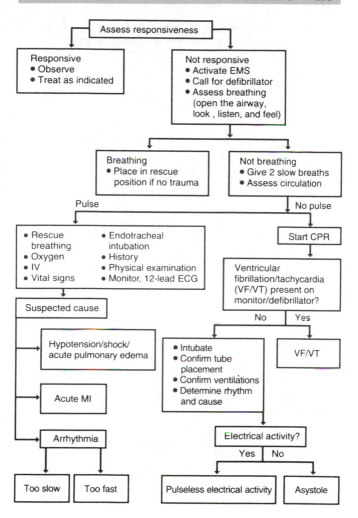

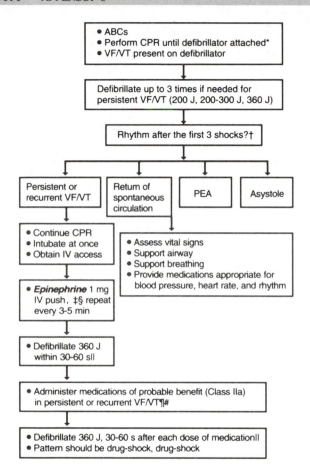

- ABCs
- Perform CPR until defibrillator attached*
- VF/VT present on defibrillator

Defibrillate up to 3 times if needed for persistent VF/VT (200 J, 200-300 J, 360 J)

Rhythm after the first 3 shocks?†

| Persistent or recurrent VF/VT | Return of spontaneous circulation | PEA | Asystole |

- Continue CPR
- Intubate at once
- Obtain IV access

- Assess vital signs
- Support airway
- Support breathing
- Provide medications appropriate for blood pressure, heart rate, and rhythm

- *Epinephrine* 1 mg IV push, ‡§ repeat every 3-5 min

- Defibrillate 360 J within 30-60 s‖

- Administer medications of probable benefit (Class IIa) in persistent or recurrent VF/VT¶#

- Defibrillate 360 J, 30-60 s after each dose of medication‖
- Pattern should be drug-shock, drug-shock

Class I: definitely helpful
Class IIa: acceptable, probably helpful
Class IIb: acceptable, possibly helpful
Class III: not indicated, may be harmful

*Precordial thump is a Class IIb action in witnessed arrest, no pulse, and no defibrillator immediately available.

†Hypothermic cardiac arrest is treated differently after this point. See section on hypothermia.

‡The recommended dose of *epinephrine* is 1 mg IV push every 3-5 min. If this approach fails, several Class IIb dosing regimens can be considered:
- Intermediate: *epinephrine* 2-5 mg IV push, every 3-5 min
- Escalating: *epinephrine* 1 mg-3 mg-5 mg IV push (3 min apart)
- High: *epinephrine* 0.1 mg/kg IV push, every 3-5 min

§ *Sodium bicarbonate* (1 mEq/kg) is Class I if patient has known preexisting hyperkalemia

‖Multiple sequenced shocks (200J, 200-300J, 360 J) are acceptable here (Class I), especially when medications are delayed

¶
- *Lidocaine* 1.5 mg/kg IV push. Repeat in 3-5 min to total loading dose of 3 mg/kg; then use
- *Bretylium* 5 mg/kg IV push. Repeat in 5 min at 10 mg/kg
- *Magnesium sulfate* 1-2 g IV in torsades de pointes or suspected hypomagnesemic state or severe refractory VF
- *Procainamide* 30 mg/min in refractory VF (maximum total 17 mg/kg)
- *Sodium bicarbonate* (1 mEq/kg IV):

\# Class IIa
- if known preexisting bicarbonate-responsive acidosis
- if overdose with tricyclic antidepressants
- to alkalinize the urine in drug overdoses

Class IIb
- if intubated and continued long arrest interval
- upon return of spontaneous circulation after long arrest interval

Class III
- hypoxic lactic acidosis

PEA includes
- Electromechanical dissociation (EMD)
- Pseudo-EMD
- Idioventricular rhythms
- Ventricular escape rhythms
- Bradyasystolic rhythms
- Postdefibrillation idioventricular rhythms

- Continue CPR
- Intubate at once
- Obtain IV access
- Assess blood flow using Doppler ultrasound

↓

Consider possible causes
(Parentheses=possible therapies and treatments)
- Hypovolemia (volume infusion)
- Hypoxia (ventilation)
- Cardiac tamponade (pericardiocentesis)
- Tension pneumothorax (needle decompression)
- Hypothermia (see hypothermia algorithm, Section IV)
- Massive pulmonary embolism (surgery, *thrombolytics*)
- Drug overdoses such as tricyclics, digitalis, β-blockers, calcium channel blockers
- Hyperkalemia*
- Acidosis†
- Massive acute myocardial infarction (go to Fig 9)

- *Epinephrine* 1 mg IV push, *‡ repeat every 3-5 min

- If absolute bradycardia (<60 beats/min) or relative bradycardia, give *atropine* 1 mg IV
- Repeat every 3-5 min up to a total of 0.04 mg/kg§

Class I: definitely helpful
Class IIa: acceptable, probably helpful
Class IIb: acceptable, possibly helpful
Class III: not indicated, may be harmful
*__Sodium bicarbonate__ 1 mEq/kg is Class I if patient has known preexisting
  hyperkalemia.
†__Sodium bicarbonate__ 1 mEq/kg:
  Class IIa
  • if known preexisting bicarbonate-responsive acidosis
  • if overdose with tricyclic antidepressants
  • to alkalinize the urine in drug overdoses
  Class IIb
  • if intubated and long arrest interval
  • upon return of spontaneous circulation after long arrest interval
  Class III
  • hypoxic lactic acidosis
‡The recommended dose of __epinephrine__ is 1 mg IV push every 3-5 min.
  If this approach fails, several Class IIb dosing regimens can be considered.
  • Intermediate: __epinephrine__ 2-5 mg IV push, every 3-5 min
  • Escalating: __epinephrine__ 1 mg-3 mg-5 mg IV push (3 min apart)
  • High: __epinephrine__ 0.1 mg/kg IV push, every 3-5 min
§ Shorter __atropine__ dosing intervals are possibly helpful
  in cardiac arrest (Class IIb).

- Continue CPR
- Intubate at once
- Obtain IV access
- Confirm asystole in more than one lead

↓

Consider possible causes
- Hypoxia
- Hyperkalemia
- Hypokalemia
- Preexisting acidosis
- Drug overdose
- Hypothermia

↓

Consider immediate transcutaneous pacing (TCP)*

↓

- *Epinephrine* 1 mg IV push, †‡ repeat every 3-5 min

↓

- *Atropine* 1 mg IV, repeat every 3-5 min up to a total of 0.04 mg/kg§ǁ

↓

Consider
- Termination of efforts¶

Class I: definitely helpful
Class IIa: acceptable, probably helpful
Class IIb: acceptable, possibly helpful
Class III: not indicated, may be harmful

*TCP is a Class IIb intervention. Lack of success may be due to delays in pacing. To be effective TCP must be performed early, simultaneously with drugs. Evidence does not support routine use of TCP for asystole.

†The recommended dose of *epinephrine* is 1 mg IV push every 3-5 min. If this approach fails, several Class IIb dosing regimens can be considered:

- Intermediate: *epinephrine* 2-5 mg IV push, every 3-5 min
- Escalating: *epinephrine* 1 mg-3 mg-5 mg IV push (3 min apart)
- High: *epinephrine* 0.1 mg/kg IV push, every 3-5 min

‡*Sodium bicarbonate* 1 mEq/kg is Class I if patient has known preexisting hyperkalemia.

§Shorter *atropine* dosing intervals are Class IIb in asystolic arrest.

‖*Sodium bicarbonate* 1 mEq/kg:

Class IIa
- if known preexisting bicarbonate-responsive acidosis
- if overdose with tricyclic antidepressants
- to alkalinize the urine in drug overdoses

Class IIb
- if intubated and continued long arrest interval
- upon return of spontaneous circulation after long arrest interval

Class III
- hypoxic lactic acidosis

¶If patient remains in asystole or other agonal rhythms after successful intubation and initial medications and no reversible causes are identified, consider termination of resuscitative efforts by a physician. Consider interval since arrest.

679

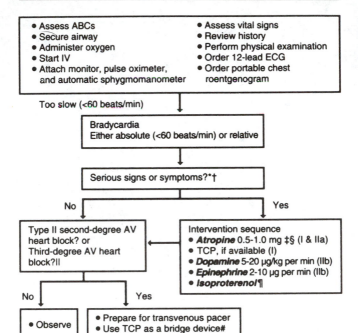

- Assess ABCs
- Secure airway
- Administer oxygen
- Start IV
- Attach monitor, pulse oximeter, and automatic sphygmomanometer

- Assess vital signs
- Review history
- Perform physical examination
- Order 12-lead ECG
- Order portable chest roentgenogram

Too slow (<60 beats/min)

Bradycardia
Either absolute (<60 beats/min) or relative

Serious signs or symptoms?*†

No — Yes

Type II second-degree AV heart block? or
Third-degree AV heart block?‖

Intervention sequence
- *Atropine* 0.5-1.0 mg ‡§ (I & IIa)
- TCP, if available (I)
- *Dopamine* 5-20 µg/kg per min (IIb)
- *Epinephrine* 2-10 µg per min (IIb)
- *Isoproterenol*¶

No — Yes

- Observe

- Prepare for transvenous pacer
- Use TCP as a bridge device#

*Serious signs or symptoms must be related to the slow rate.
Clinical manifestations include:
symptoms (chest pain, shortness of breath, decreased level of
consciousness) and
signs (low BP, shock, pulmonary congestion, CHF, acute MI).
†Do not delay TCP while awaiting IV access or for *atropine* to take
effect if patient is symptomatic.
‡Denervated transplanted hearts will not respond to *atropine*. Go at once
to pacing, *catecholamine* infusion, or both.
§*Atropine* should be given in repeat doses in 3-5 min up to total of 0.04
mg/kg. Consider shorter dosing intervals in severe clinical conditions.
It has been suggested that atropine should be used with caution in
atrioventricular (AV) block at the His-Purkinje level (type II AV block
and new third-degree block with wide QRS complexes) (Class IIb).
∥Never treat third-degree heart block plus ventricular escape
beats with *lidocaine*.
¶*Isoproterenol* should be used, if at all, with externe caution. At low doses
it is Class IIb (possibly helpful); at higher doses it is Class III (harmful).
#Verify patient tolerance and mechanical capture. Use analgesia and
sedation as needed.

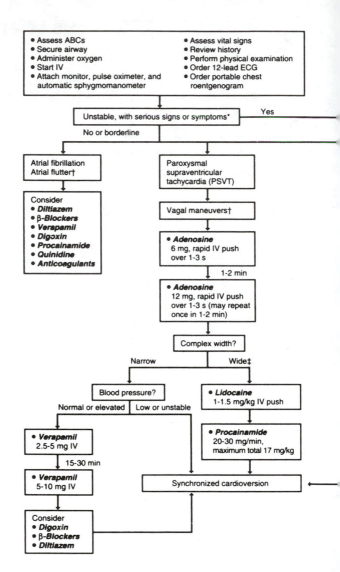

- Assess ABCs
- Secure airway
- Administer oxygen
- Start IV
- Attach monitor, pulse oximeter, and automatic sphygmomanometer

- Assess vital signs
- Review history
- Perform physical examination
- Order 12-lead ECG
- Order portable chest roentgenogram

Unstable, with serious signs or symptoms*   Yes

No or borderline

Atrial fibrillation Atrial flutter†

Consider
- *Diltiazem*
- β-*Blockers*
- *Verapamil*
- *Digoxin*
- *Procainamide*
- *Quinidine*
- *Anticoagulants*

Paroxysmal supraventricular tachycardia (PSVT)

Vagal maneuvers†

- *Adenosine* 6 mg, rapid IV push over 1-3 s

1-2 min

- *Adenosine* 12 mg, rapid IV push over 1-3 s (may repeat once in 1-2 min)

Complex width?

Narrow   Wide‡

Blood pressure?

Normal or elevated | Low or unstable

- *Verapamil* 2.5-5 mg IV

15-30 min

- *Verapamil* 5-10 mg IV

Consider
- *Digoxin*
- β-*Blockers*
- *Diltiazem*

- *Lidocaine* 1-1.5 mg/kg IV push

- *Procainamide* 20-30 mg/min, maximum total 17 mg/kg

Synchronized cardioversion

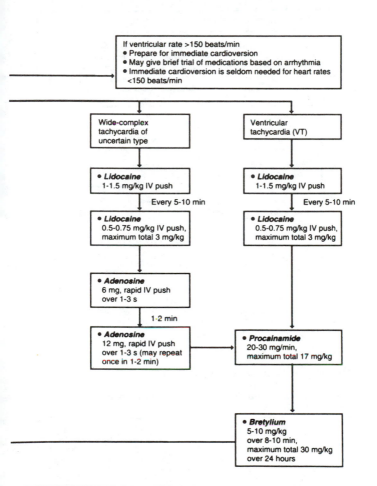

If ventricular rate >150 beats/min
- Prepare for immediate cardioversion
- May give brief trial of medications based on arrhythmia
- Immediate cardioversion is seldom needed for heart rates <150 beats/min

Wide-complex tachycardia of uncertain type

- *Lidocaine*
  1-1.5 mg/kg IV push

Every 5-10 min

- *Lidocaine*
  0.5-0.75 mg/kg IV push, maximum total 3 mg/kg

- *Adenosine*
  6 mg, rapid IV push over 1-3 s

1-2 min

- *Adenosine*
  12 mg, rapid IV push over 1-3 s (may repeat once in 1-2 min)

Ventricular tachycardia (VT)

- *Lidocaine*
  1-1.5 mg/kg IV push

Every 5-10 min

- *Lidocaine*
  0.5-0.75 mg/kg IV push, maximum total 3 mg/kg

- *Procainamide*
  20-30 mg/min, maximum total 17 mg/kg

- *Bretylium*
  5-10 mg/kg over 8-10 min, maximum total 30 mg/kg over 24 hours

*Unstable condition must be related to the tachycardia. Signs and symptoms may include chest pain, shortness of breath, decreased level of consciousness, low blood pressure (BP), shock, pulmonary congestion, congestive heart failure, acute myocardial infarction.
†Carotid sinus pressure is contraindicated in patients with carotid bruits; avoid ice water immersion in patients with ischemic heart disease.
‡If the wide-complex tachycardia is known with certainty to be PSVT and BP is normal/elevated, sequence can include *verapamil*.

683

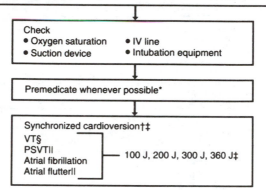

Tachycardia with serious signs and symptoms related to the tachycardia

If ventricular rate is >150 beats/min, prepare for immediate cardioversion.
May give brief trial of medications based on specific arrhythmias.
Immediate cardioversion is generally not needed for rates <150 beats/min.

Check
- Oxygen saturation   • IV line
- Suction device   • Intubation equipment

Premedicate whenever possible*

Synchronized cardioversion†‡
VT§
PSVT‖ ⎤
Atrial fibrillation ⎬ — 100 J, 200 J, 300 J, 360 J‡
Atrial flutter‖ ⎦

---

*Effective regimens have included a sedative (eg, *diazepam,
midazolam, barbiturates, etomidate, ketamine, methohexital*) with
or without an analgesic agent (eg, *fentanyl, morphine, meperidine*).
Many experts recommend anesthesia if service is readily available.
†Note possible need to resynchronize after each cardioversion.
‡If delays in synchronization occur and clinical conditions are critical,
go to immediate unsynchronized shocks.
§Treat polymorphic VT (irregular form and rate) like VF:
200 J, 200-300 J, 360 J.
‖PSVT and atrial flutter often respond to lower energy levels
(start with 50 J).

Community
- Community emphasis on "call first/call fast, call 911"
- National Heart Attack Alert Program

EMS System
EMS system approach that should address
- Oxygen-IV-cardiac monitor-vital signs
- *Nitroglycerin*
- Pain relief with narcotics
- Notification of emergency department
- Rapid transport to emergency department
- Prehospital screening for *thrombolytic* therapy*
- 12-lead ECG, computer analysis, transmission to emergency department*
- Initiation of *thrombolytic* therapy*

Emergency Department
"Door-to-drug" team protocol approach
- Rapid triage of patients with chest pain
- Clinical decision maker established (emergency physician, cardiologist, or other)

Time interval in emergency department

Assessment
Immediate:
- Vital signs with automatic BP
- Oxygen saturation
- Start IV
- 12-lead ECG (MD review)
- Brief, targeted history and physical
- Decide on eligibility for *thrombolytic* therapy
Soon:
- Chest roentgenogram
- Blood studies (electrolytes, enzymes, coagulation studies)
- Consult as needed

Treatments to consider if there is evidence of coronary thrombosis plus no reasons for exclusion (some but not all may be appropriate)
- Oxygen at 4 L/min
- *Nitroglycerin* SL, paste or spray (if systolic blood pressure >90 mm Hg)
- *Morphine* IV
- *Aspirin* PO
- *Thrombolytic* agents
- *Nitroglycerin* IV (limit systolic BP drop to 10% if normotensive; 30% drop if hypertensive; never drop below 90 mm Hg systolic)
- β-*Blockers* IV
- *Heparin* IV
- Percutaneous transluminal coronary angioplasty
- Routine *lidocaine* administration is not recommended for all patients with AMI

30-60 min to *thrombolytic* therapy

*Optional guidelines

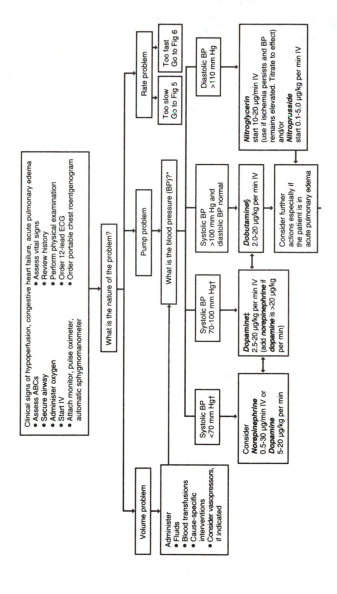

Clinical signs of hypoperfusion, congestive heart failure, acute pulmonary edema

- Assess ABCs
- Secure airway
- Administer oxygen
- Start IV
- Attach monitor, pulse oximeter, automatic sphygmomanometer
- Assess vital signs
- Review history
- Perform physical examination
- Order 12-lead ECG
- Order portable chest roentgenogram

What is the nature of the problem?

| Volume problem | Pump problem | Rate problem |

Volume problem

Administer
- Fluids
- Blood transfusions
- Cause-specific interventions
- Consider vasopressors, if indicated

Pump problem

What is the blood pressure (BP)?*

| Systolic BP <70 mm Hg† | Systolic BP 70-100 mm Hg† | Systolic BP >100 mm Hg and diastolic BP normal |

Consider
Norepinephrine
0.5-30 µg/min IV or
Dopamine
5-20 µg/kg per min

Dopamine†
2.5-20 µg/kg per min IV
(add ***norepinephrine*** if ***dopamine*** is >20 µg/kg per min)

Dobutamine§
2.0-20 µg/kg per min IV

Consider further actions especially if the patient is in acute pulmonary edema

Rate problem

| Too slow Go to Fig 5 | Too fast Go to Fig 6 |

Diastolic BP >110 mm Hg

Nitroglycerin
start 10-20 µg/min IV
(use if ischemia persists and BP remains elevated. Titrate to effect)
and/or
Nitroprusside
start 0.1-5.0 µg/kg per min IV

First-line actions
- **Furosemide** IV 0.5-1.0 mg/kg
- **Morphine** IV 1-3 mg
- **Nitroglycerin** SL
- Oxygen/intubate PRN

Second-line actions
- **Nitroglycerin** IV (if BP >100 mm Hg)
- **Nitroprusside** IV (if BP >100 mm Hg)
- **Dopamine** (if BP <100 mm Hg)
- **Dobutamine** (if BP >100 mm Hg)
- Positive end-expiratory pressure (PEEP)
- Continuous positive airway pressure (CPAP)

Third-line actions
- **Amrinone** 0.75 mg/kg then 5-15 µg/kg per min (if other drugs fail)
- **Aminophylline** 5 mg/kg (if wheezing)
- **Thrombolytic** therapy (if not in shock)
- **Digoxin** (if atrial fibrillation, supraventricular tachycardias)
- Angioplasty (if drugs fail)
- Intra-aortic balloon pump (bridge to surgery)
- Surgical interventions (valves, coronary artery bypass grafts, heart transplant)

*Base management after this point on invasive hemodynamic monitoring if possible.
†Fluid bolus of 250-500 mL normal saline should be tried. If no response, consider sympathomimetics.
‡Move to **dopamine** and stop **norepinephrine** when BP improves.
§Add **dopamine** when BP improves. Avoid **dobutamine** when systolic BP <100 mm Hg.

687

Appendix P: Cardiac Arrhythmias

NORMAL SINUS RHYTHM
Rate
Ventricular 60–100

Atrial 60–100

Rhythm
R-R regular

P-P regular

Duration
PR Interval .12–.20 sec

QRS Complex .06–.10 sec

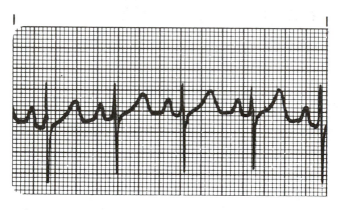

Lead II

SINUS BRADYCARDIA
Rate
Ventricular less than 60

Atrial same as ventricular

Rhythm
R-R regular

P-P regular

Duration
PR Interval .12–.20 sec

QRS Complex .06–.10 sec

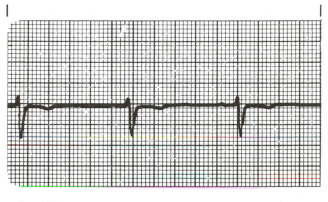

Lead II

SINUS TACHYCARDIA
Rate
Ventricular greater than 100

Atrial same as ventricular

Rhythm
R-R regular

P-P regular

Duration
PR Interval .12-.20 sec

QRS Complex .06-.10 sec

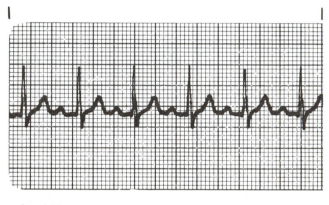

Lead II

SINUS ARRHYTHMIA
Rate
Ventricular increases and decreases with respiration

Atrial same as ventricular

Rhythm
R-R irregular

P-P irregular

Duration
PR Interval .12–.20 sec

QRS Complex .06–.10 sec

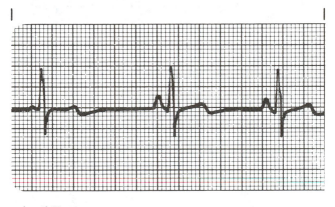

Lead II

ATRIAL FIBRILLATION
Rate
Ventricular 100 controlled
            100 uncontrolled

Atrial greater than 350

Rhythm
R-R irregular

P-P absent

Duration
PR Interval absent due to fibrillation waves

QRS Complex .06 – .10 sec

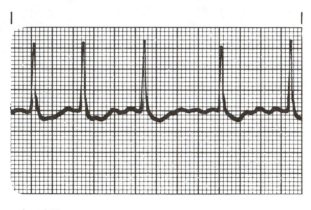

Lead II

ATRIAL FLUTTER
Rate
Ventricular <u>variable depending on degree of block</u>

Atrial <u>less than or equal to 350</u>

Rhythm
R-R <u>regular/irregular</u>

P-P <u>absent</u>

Duration
PR Interval <u>absent due to flutter waves</u>

QRS Complex <u>.06–.10 sec</u>

Note: A variable flutter rate will cause the R-R interval to become *irregular*. Ventricular response can be less than or greater than 100.

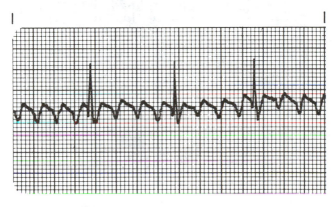

Lead II

PAROXYSMAL ATRIAL TACHYCARDIA
Rate
Ventricular 150–250

Atrial same as ventricular

Rhythm
R-R regular

P-P regular

Duration
PR Interval .12–.20 sec

QRS Complex .06–.10 sec

Note: This rhythm is always of sudden onset.

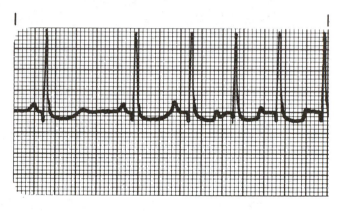

Lead II

JUNCTIONAL RHYTHM
Rate
Ventricular 40–60

Atrial usually less than or equal to ventricular rate

Rhythm
R-R regular

P-P absent; inverted in leads II, III, aV_F; or "buried" in QRS
complex

Duration
PR Interval absent

QRS Complex .06–.10 sec

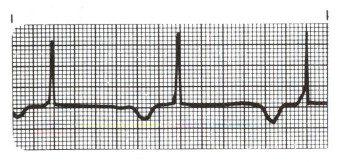

Lead MCL₁

Adapted from Dolan, J. T. (1991). Critical Care Nursing: Clinical Management Through the Nursing Process (2nd ed.). Philadelphia: FA Davis, pp 807–815, with permission.

JUNCTIONAL TACHYCARDIA

Rate

Ventricular 60 – 130

Atrial same as ventricular (if visible)

Rhythm

R-R regular

P-P same as in junctional rhythm

Duration

PR Interval absent

QRS Complex .06 – .10 sec; may show widening

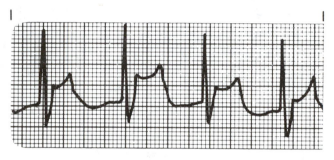

Lead II

PAROXYSMAL JUNCTIONAL TACHYCARDIA
Rate
Ventricular greater than 130

Atrial same as ventricular (if visible)

Rhythm
R-R regular

P-P same as in junctional rhythm

Duration
PR Interval absent

QRS Complex .06 – .10 sec

Note: This rhythm is always of sudden onset.

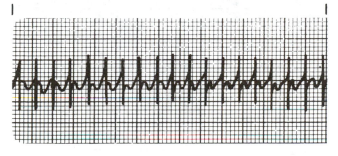

Lead II

PREMATURE VENTRICULAR CONTRACTION
Rate
Ventricular 60–100

Atrial 60–100

Rhythm
R-R irregular due to PVCs

P-P irregular due to PVCs

Duration
PR Interval absent in ectopic beats; remaining beats conducted normally

QRS Complex PVCs widened greater than .12 sec

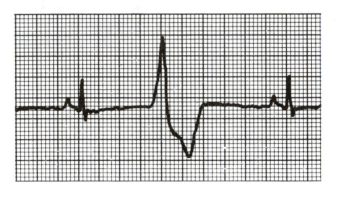

Lead II

VENTRICULAR TACHYCARDIA
Rate
Ventricular greater than 150

Atrial absent

Rhythm
R-R regular

P-P absent

Duration
PR Interval absent

QRS Complex widened and bizarre

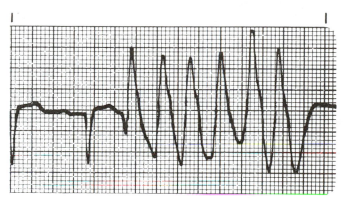

Lead MCL$_1$

VENTRICULAR FIBRILLATION
Rate
Ventricular indeterminable

Atrial absent

Rhythm
R-R chaotic rhythm

P-P absent

Duration
PR Interval absent

QRS Complex bizarre in configuration; no uniformity

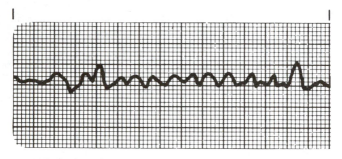

Lead MCL$_1$

FIRST-DEGREE AV BLOCK
Rate
Ventricular usually normal

Atrial same as ventricular

Rhythm
R-R regular

P-P regular

Duration
PR Interval greater than .20 sec

QRS Complex .06–.10 sec

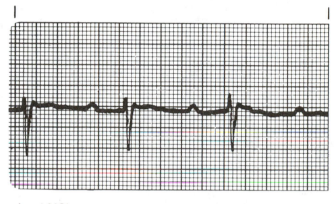

Lead MCL$_1$

SECOND-DEGREE AV BLOCK (WENCKEBACH, MOBITZ TYPE I)

Rate

Ventricular normal or slow

Atrial greater than ventricular

Rhythm

R-R irregular

P-P regular

Duration

PR Interval progressive lengthening until one P wave is blocked, and the cycle repeats

QRS Complex .06–.10 sec

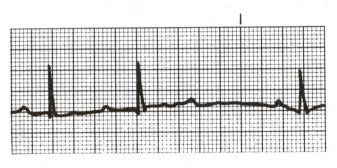

Lead II

SECOND-DEGREE AV BLOCK (MOBITZ TYPE II)

Rate
Ventricular usually slow

Atrial greater than ventricular

Rhythm
R-R irregular

P-P regular

Duration
PR Interval normal or prolonged

QRS Complex normal

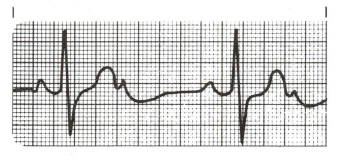

Lead II

THIRD-DEGREE AV BLOCK (COMPLETE HEART BLOCK)
Rate
Ventricular usually 20–40

Atrial usually 60–100

Rhythm
R-R regular

P-P regular

Duration
PR Interval constantly changing

QRS Complex normal or widened

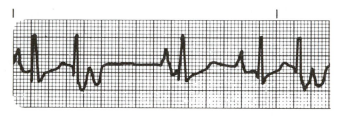

Lead II

Appendix Q: NANDA Nursing Diagnoses

Activity Intolerance
Activity Intolerance: high
  risk for
Adjustment: impaired
Airway Clearance:
  ineffective
Anxiety
Aspiration: high risk for
Body Image Disturbance
Body Temperature:
  altered, high risk for
Bowel Incontinence
Breastfeeding: effective
Breastfeeding: ineffective
Breastfeeding: interrupted
Breathing Pattern:
  ineffective
Cardiac Output: decreased
Caregiver Role Strain
Caregiver Role Strain:
  high risk for
Communication: impaired
  verbal
Constipation
Constipation: colonic
Constipation: perceived
Coping: defensive
Coping, Individual:
  ineffective
Decisional Conflict
  (specify)

Denial: ineffective
Diarrhea
Disuse Syndrome: high
  risk for
Diversional Activity
  Deficit
Dysreflexia
Family Coping:
  ineffective,
  compromised
Family Coping:
  ineffective, disabling
Family Coping: potential
  for growth
Family Processes: altered
Fatigue
Fear
Fluid Volume Deficit
Fluid Volume Deficit: high
  risk for
Fluid Volume Excess
Gas Exchange:
  impaired
Grieving: anticipatory
Grieving: dysfunctional
Growth and Development:
  altered
Health Maintenance:
  altered
Health-Seeking Behaviors
  (specify)

Home Maintenance Management: impaired
Hopelessness
Hyperthermia
Hypothermia
Incontinence: functional
Incontinence: reflex
Incontinence: stress
Incontinence: total
Incontinence: urge
Infant Feeding Pattern: ineffective
Infection: high risk for
Injury: high risk for
Knowledge Deficit (specify)
Noncompliance (specify)
Nutrition: altered, less than body requirements
Nutrition: altered, more than body requirements
Nutrition: altered, high risk for more than body requirements
Oral Mucous Membrane: altered
Pain
Pain: chronic
Parental Role Conflict
Parenting: altered
Parenting: altered, high risk for
Peripheral Neurovascular Dysfunction: high risk for
Personal Identity Disturbance
Physical Mobility: impaired
Poisoning: high risk for
Post-Trauma Response
Powerlessness
Protection: altered

Rape Trauma Syndrome
Rape Trauma Syndrome: compound reaction
Rape Trauma Syndrome: silent reaction
Relocation Stress Syndrome
Role Performance: altered
Self-Care Deficit: feeding, bathing/hygiene, dressing/grooming, toileting
Self-Esteem: chronic low
Self-Esteem Disturbance
Self-Esteem: situational low
Self-Mutilation: high risk for
Sensory-Perceptual Alterations (specify): visual, auditory, kinesthetic, gustatory, tactile, olfactory
Sexual Dysfunction
Sexuality Patterns: altered
Skin Integrity: impaired
Skin Integrity: impaired, high risk for
Sleep Pattern Disturbance
Social Interaction: Impaired
Social Isolation
Spiritual Distress (distress of the human spirit)
Spontaneous Ventilation: inability to sustain
Suffocation: high risk for
Swallowing Impaired
Therapeutic Regimen, Individuals: ineffective management of

Thermoregulation: ineffective

Thought Processes: altered

Tissue Integrity: impaired

Tissue Perfusion, altered (specify): cerebral, cardiopulmonary, renal, gastrointestinal, peripheral

Trauma: high risk for

Unilateral Neglect

Urinary Elimination: altered

Urinary Retention

Ventilatory Weaning Response: dysfunctional (DVWR)

Violence: high risk for, directed at self/others

Appendix R: Abbreviations Used in This Book

ABGs	arterial blood gases
ABO	abbreviation for blood type
ACE	angiotensin-converting enzyme inhibitors
ACTH	adrenocorticotropic hormone
ADH	antidiuretic hormone
AICD	automatic implantable cardiac defibrillator
A-JVO$_2$	arterial and jugular venous oxygen gradient
ALT	alanine aminotransferase
AMI	acute myocardial infarction
ARDS	acute respiratory distress syndrome, adult respiratory distress syndrome
ARF	acute renal failure
AST	aspartate aminotransferase
ATG	antithymocyte globulin
A-V	atrioventricular
AVM	arteriovenous malformation
BUN	blood urea nitrogen
C5, C6	vertebrae (cervical)
CABG	coronary artery bypass graft surgery
CBC	complete blood count
CBF	cerebral blood flow
CBV	cerebral blood volume
CHF	congestive heart failure
CK	creatine kinase

$CMRO_2$	cerebral oxygen consumption
CMV	cytomegalovirus
CN I, II, III, etc.	cranial nerve I, II, III, etc.
CNS	central nervous system
CO	cardiac output
COPD	chronic obstructive pulmonary disease
CPAP	controlled positive airway pressure
CPP	cerebral perfusion pressure
CRF	chronic renal failure
CRRT	continuous renal replacement therapy
CSF	cerebrospinal fluid
CT	computed tomography
CVA	cerebrovascular accident
CVP	central venous pressure
DIC	disseminated intravascular coagulopathy
DKA	diabetic ketoacidosis
DNA	deoxyribonucleic acid
2, 3-DPG	2, 3-diphosphoglycerate
DPTA	diethylenetriamine penta-acetic acid
DVT	deep vein thrombosis
ECG	electrocardiogram
ECHO	extracorporeal membrane oxygenation
EEG	electroencephalography
EGD	esophagogastroduodenoscopy
ESRD	end-stage renal disease
EV	expiratory volume
GRF	glomerular filtration rate
H & H	hematocrit and hemoglobin
HIV	human immunodeficiency virus
HTLV	human T cell lymphoma virus
ICP	intracranial pressure
ICU	intensive care unit

IgE	immunoglobulin E
IHSS	idiopathic hypertrophic subaortic stenosis
IICP	increased intracranial pressure
IM	intramuscular
IMV/SIMV	intermittent mandatory ventilation with or without synchronization
IV	intravenous
IVP	intravenous pyelogram
JVO_2	jugular venous oxygen content
KUB	kidneys, ureters, bladder
L1	vertebra (lumbar)
LDH	lactic dehydrogenase
LDH_1, LDH_2	LDH isoenzymes
LOC	level of consciousness
MAP	mean arterial pressure
MAST	medical antishock trousers
MI	myocardial infarction
MMI	methimazole
MODS	multiple organ dysfunction syndrome
MSOF	multiple system organ failure
NaCl	sodium chloride solution
NSAIDs	nonsteroidal anti-inflammatory drugs
PAP	pulmonary artery pressure
PCWP	pulmonary capillary wedge pressure
PE	pulmonary embolism
PEEP	positive end-expiratory pressure
PEG-SOD	polyethylene glycol conjugated superoxide dismutase
PETT	positron emission transaxial tomography scan
PFTs	pulmonary function tests
PMI	point of maximal impulse

PT	prothrombin time
PTCA	percutaneous transluminal coronary angioplasty
PTT	partial thromboplastin time
PTU	propylthiouracil
RAP	right atrial pressure
RBC	red blood cell
RNA	ribonucleic acid
RRT	renal replacement therapy
rT_3	serum reverse triiodothyronine
RV	residual volume
SGOT	serum glutamic oxaloacetic transaminase
SGPT	serum glutamic pyruvic transaminase
SIADH	syndrome of inappropriate secretion of antidiuretic hormone
SIRS	systemic inflammatory response syndrome
SLE	systemic lupus erythematosus
SMA	superior mesenteric artery
SOD	superoxide dismutase
STSH	sensitive thyroid – stimulating hormone
T_3	serum triiodothyronine
T_3-RIA	triiodothyroxine by radioimmune assay
T_4	serum thyroxine
T11, T12	vertebrae (thoracic)
TENS	transcutaneous electrical nerve stimulation
THAM	tromethamine
TIG	tetanus immune globulin
TIPS	transjugular intrahepatic portacaval shunt
TLC	total lung capacity
TSH	thyroid-stimulating hormone
UF	ultrafiltrate

VC	vital capacity
WBC	white blood cell

References

Ahrens, T. (1993). The cutting edge in pulmonary critical care. Critical Care Nurse (Suppl.), 4–5.

Ali, J. (1992). Torso trauma. In J. B. Hall, G. A. Schmidt, & L. D. H. Wood (Eds.), Principles of critical care (pp. 736–755). New York: McGraw-Hill.

Alspach, J. G. (1991). American association of critical-care nurses core curriculum for critical care nursing. Philadelphia: WB Saunders.

Austin, J. J., & Shragge, B. W. (1992) Aortic dissection. In J. B. Hall, G. A. Schmidt, & L. D. H. Wood, (Eds.), Principles of critical care (pp. 1572–1583). New York: McGraw-Hill.

Baron, B. W., & Baron, J. M. (1992). Blood products and plasmaphoresis. In J. B. Hall, G. A. Schmidt, & L. D. H. Wood (Eds.), Principles of critical care (pp. 453–463). New York: McGraw-Hill.

Barron, J. T., & Parrillo, J. E. (1992). Myocardial ischemia. In critical illness. In J. B. Hall, G. A. Schmidt, & L. D. H. Wood (Eds.), Principles of critical care (pp. 1437–1453). New York: McGraw-Hill.

Bayley, E. W., & Turcke, S. A. (1992). A comprehensive curriculum for trauma nursing. Boston: Jones & Bartlett Publishers.

Bernhard, J. D. (1992). Pruritus: Pathophysiology and clinical aspects. In S. L. Moschella, & H. J. Hurley (Eds.), Dermatology (pp. 2042–2046). Philadelphia: WB Saunders.

Brandt, L. J., & Boley, S. J. (1993). Ischemic and vascular lesions of the bowel. In M. H. Sleisenger, & J. S. Fordtran (Eds.), Gastrointestinal disease pathophysiology/diagnosis/ management (pp. 1927–1948). Philadelphia: WB Saunders.

Broscious, S. K. (1991). Toxic shock syndrome and its potential complications. Critical Care Nurse, 11(2), 28–35.

Brown, A. (1991). Acute pancreatitis: Pathophysiology, nursing diagnoses, and collaborative problems. Focus on Critical Care, 18(2), 121–130.

Brown, K. A., & Sheagren, J. N. (1990). Recognition and emergent treatment of septic shock/multiple systems organ failure syndrome. Internal Medicine, 11(2), 3–11.

Brown, B. M. (1992). Heart failure. In L. Burrell (Ed.), Adult nursing in hospital and community settings. Norwalk, CT: Appleton & Lange.

Braunwald, E., & Grossman, W. (1992). Clinical aspects of heart failure. In E. Braunwald (Ed.). Heart disease: A text of cardiovascular medicine (4th ed.) (pp. 444–463). Philadelphia: WB Saunders.

Burns, D. (1993). Review of thrombolytic use in acute myocardial infarction, pulmonary embolism, and cerebral thrombosis. Critical Care Nursing Quarterly, 15(4), 1–12.

Burrell, L. O. (1992). Nursing management of adults with disorders of the biliary tract and exocrine pancreas. In L. O. Burrell (Ed.), Adult nursing in hospital and community settings (pp. 1527–1533). Norwalk, CT: Appleton & Lange.

Campbell, M. L., & Carlson, R. W. (1992). Terminal weaning from mechanical ventilation: Ethical and practical considerations for patient management. American Journal of Critical Care, 1(3), 52–56.

Cardona, V. D., Hurn, P. D., Mason, P. J. B., Scanlon-Schilpp, A. M., & Veise-Berry, S. W. (1988). Trauma nursing from resuscitation through rehabilitation. Philadelphia: WB Saunders.

Case, S. C., & Sabo, C. E. (1992). Adult respiratory distress syndrome: A deadly complication of trauma. Focus on Critical Care, 19(2), 116–121.

Cayten, C. G. (1992). Abdominal trauma. In G. R. Schwartz, C. G. Cayten, M. A. Mangelsen, T. A. Mayer, & B. K. Hanke (Eds.). Principles and practice of emergency medicine (pp. 1064–1077). Philadelphia: Lea & Febiger.

Cella, J. H., & Watson, J. (1989). Nurse's manual of laboratory tests. Philadelphia: FA Davis.

Cerney, M. S. (1993). Solving the organ donor shortage by meeting the bereaved family's needs. Critical Care Nurse, (13) 1, 32–36.

Cerra, F. B. (1992). Multiple system organ failure. Disease-a-Month, 38(12), 847–889.

Clark, E. T., & Gewertz, B. L. (1992). Mesenteric ischemia. In J. B. Hall, G. A. Schmidt, & L. D. H. Wood (Eds.), Principles of critical care (pp. 2043–2049). New York: McGraw-Hill.

Clevenger, F. W. (1993). Nutritional support in the patient with systemic inflammatory response syndrome. The American Journal of Surgery, 165(2A), 68S–73S.

Coburn, K. (1992). Traumatic brain injury: The silent epidemic. American Association of Critical Care Nurses Clinical Issues, 3(1), 9–17.

Coen, S. D. (1992). Spinal cord injury: Preventing secondary injury. AACN Clinical Issues, 3, (1) 44–54.

Corcoran, D. K. (1988). Helping patients who've had near-death experiences. Nursing 88, (15)4, 34–39.

Cotran, R. S., Kumar, V., & Robbins, S. L. (1989). Robbins pathologic basis of disease (4th ed.). Philadelphia: WB Saunders.

Cronin, L. A. (1993). Beat the clock: Saving the heart with thrombolytic drugs. Nursing 93, August, 34–42.

Dandan, I. S. (1992). Trauma in the elderly patient. Topics in Emergency Medicine, 14(3), 39–45.

Daly, B. J., Newlon, B., Montenegro, H. D., & Langdon, T. (1993). Withdrawal of mechanical ventilation: Ethical principles and guidelines for terminal weaning. American Journal of Critical Care, 2(3), 217–223.

Davenport, A., Will, E. J., & Davison, A. M. (1990). Effect of position on intracranial pressure in patients with fulminant hepatic and renal failure after acetaminophen self-poisoning. Critical Care Medicine, 18(3), 286–289.

Deglin, J. H., & Vallerand, A. H. (1993). Davis's drug guide for nurses (3rd ed.). Philadelphia: FA Davis.

Dickerman, M. (1988). Anaphylaxis and anaphylactic shock. Critical Care Quarterly, 11(1), 68–74.

Dolan, J. T. (1991). Critical care nursing: Clinical management through the nursing process. Philadelphia: FA Davis.

Dossey, B. M., Guzetta, C. E., & Kenner, C. V. (1992). Critical care nursing body-mind-spirit. Philadelphia: JB Lippincott.

Doyle, E. (1991). GI emergencies: GI bleeding and abdominal trauma. In K. E. Goldberg (Ed.), Nurse review a clinical update system (pp. 133–141). Springhouse, PA: Springhouse Corp.

Dracup, K. (1993). Helping patients and families cope. Critical Care Nurse, (Suppl. 8), 4–13.

Dracup, K., Bryan-Brown, C. W. (1992). An open door policy in ICU. American Journal of Critical Care, 1(2), 16–18.

Dupuis, R. E., & Miranda-Massari, J. (1991). Anticonvulsants; Pharmacotherapeutic issues in the critically ill patient. AACN Clinical Issues, 2(4), 639–655.

Eckhauser, F. E., Raper, S. E., & Knol, J. A. (1992). Upper gastrointestinal bleeding. In G. R. Schwartz, C. G. Cayten, M. A. Mangelsen, T. A. Mayer, & B. K. Hanke (Eds.), Principles and practice of emergency medicine (pp. 1735–1745). Philadelphia: Lea & Febiger.

Elliott, W. J. (1992). Malignant hypertension. In J. B. Hall, G. A. Schmidt, & L. D. H. Wood, (Eds.), Principles of critical care (pp. 1563–1571). New York: McGraw-Hill.

Feinsilver, S. H. (1989). Respiratory failure in asthma and COPD. Emergency Medicine, April 15, 90–96.

Fink, M. E. (1992). Coma, persistent vegetative state, and brain death. In J. B. Hall, G. A. Schmidt, & L. D. H. Wood (Eds.), Principles of critical care (pp. 1793–1804.) New York: McGraw-Hill.

Finocchiaro, D. N., & Herzfeld, S. T. (1990). Understanding autonomic dysreflexia. American Journal of Nursing, 90, (9), 56–59.

Fischbach, F. (1992). A manual of laboratory and diagnostic tests. (4th ed.). Philadelphia: JB Lippincott.

Follman, D., & and Sobotka, P. (1992). Valvular heart disease. In J. B. Hall, G. A. Schmidt, & L. D. H. Wood (Eds.), Principles of critical care (pp. 1542–1560). New York: McGraw-Hill.

Fontaine, D. K. (1993). The cutting edge in trauma. Critical Care Nurse, (Suppl. 6), 14–15.

Hassar, D. (1993). New drugs. Nursing '93, May, 57–64.

Gilman, A. G., Rall, T. W., Nies, A. S., & Taylor P. (Eds.). (1990). Goodman and Gilman's the pharmacological basis of therapeutics. New York: Pergamon Press.

Goldberg, K. (1989). Nurse review. Springhouse, PA: Springhouse Corp.

Greenberger, N. J., Toskes, P. P., & Isselbacher, K. J. (1991). Acute and chronic pancreatitis. In J. D. Wilson, E. Braunwald, K. J. Issebacher, R. G. Petersdorf, J. B. Martin, A. S. Fauci, & R. K. Root (Eds.), Harrison's principles of internal medicine (pp. 1372–1378). New York: McGraw-Hill.

Gueldner, S. H. (1992). Nursing management of adults with common problems of the hematologic system. In L. O. Burrell (Ed.), Adult nursing in hospital and community settings (pp. 548–573). Norwalk, CT: Appleton & Lange.

Guyton, A. C. (1991). Textbook of medical physiology (8th ed.). Philadelphia: WB Saunders.

Hadley, S. A., & Fitzsimmons, L. (1990). Acute pancreatitis: A potential life-threatening emergency. Topics in Emergency Medicine, 12(2), 39–47.

Hanan, I. M. (1992). Gastrointestinal hemorrhage. In J. B. Hall, G. A. Schmidt, & L. D. H. Wood (Eds.), Principles of critical care (pp. 2001–2013). New York: McGraw-Hill.

Halfman-Franey, M. (1988). Current trends in hemodynamic monitoring of patients in shock. Critical Care Quarterly, 11(1), 9–18.

Hancock, B. G., & Eberhard, N. K. (1988). The pharmacologic management of shock. Critical Care Quarterly, 11(1), 19–29.

Hanisch, P. J. (1991). Identification and treatment of acute myocardial infarction by electrocardiographic site classification. Focus on Critical Care 18(6), 480–488.

Harford, W. (1991). Intestinal ischemia. Unpublished manuscript, Medical Grand Rounds, U.T. Southwestern Medical School, Dallas.

Hazinski, M. F., Iberti, T. J., MacIntyre, N. R., Parker, M. M., Tribett, D., Prion, S., & Chmel, H. (1993). Epidemiology, pathophysiology, and clinical presentation of gram-negative sepsis. American Journal of Critical Care, 2(3), 224–234.

Henneman, E. A. (1991). The art and science of weaning from mechanical ventilation. Focus on Critical Care, 18(6), 490–501.

Henneman, E. A., McKenzie, J. B., & Dewa, C. S. (1992). An evaluation of interventions for meeting the information needs of families of critically ill patients. American Journal of Critical Care, 1(3), 85–93.

Hickey, J V. (1992). Neurological and neurosurgical nursing (3rd ed.). Philadelphia: JB Lippincott.

Hilton, G. (1991). Review of neurobehavioral assessment tools. Heart and Lung, 20(5), 436–442.

Hilton, G. & Frei, J. (1991). High-dose methylprednisolone in the treatment of spinal cord injuries. Heart and Lung, 20(6), 675–679.

Holloway, N. M., (1993). Nursing the critically ill adult (4th ed.). Redwood City, CA: Addison-Wesley.

Hudak, C. M., Gallo, B. M., & Benz, J. J. (1990). Critical care nursing: A holist approach (5th ed.). Philadelphia: JB Lippincott.

Huggins, B. (1990). Trauma physiology. Nursing Clinics of North America, 25(1), 1–9.

Ignativicius, D. D., & Bayne, M. V. (1991). Medical-surgical nursing: A nursing process approach. Philadelphia: WB Saunders.

Jeffres, C. (1989). Complications of acute pancreatitis. Critical Care Nurse, 9(4), 38–49.

Jeffries, P. R., & Whelan, S. K. (1988). Cardiogenic shock: Current management. Critical Care Quarterly, 11(1), 48–56.

Johanson, B. C., Wells, S. J., Dungca, C. U., & Hoffmeister, D. (1988). Standards for critical care (3rd ed.). St. Louis: Mosby Year Book.

Johnson, G. E. (1992). Spine injuries. In J. B. Hall, G. A. Schmidt, & L. D. H. Wood (Eds.), Principles of critical care (pp. 715–743.) New York: McGraw-Hill.

Jordan, K. (1990). Chest trauma how to detect—and react to—serious trouble. Nursing 90, 17(9), 34–41.

Kaleya, R. N., Sammartano, R. J., & Boley, S. J. (1992). Aggressive approach to acute mesenteric ischemia. Surgical Clinics of North America, 72(1), 157–181.

Keamy M. F. III, & Hall, J. (1992). Hypothermia. In J. B. Hall, G. A. Schmidt, & L. D. H. Wood (Eds.), Principles of critical care (pp. 848–857). New York: McGraw-Hill.

Kennedy, G. T. (1992). Acute congestive heart failure: Pharmacologic intervention. Critical Care Nursing Clinics of North America, 4(2), 365–375.

Klein, H. G. (1992). When is transfusion the best option? Emergency Medicine, 24(4), 59–66.

Kinney, M. R., Pacha, D. R. & Dunbar, S. B. (1993). AACN's clinical reference for critical care nursing (3rd ed.). St. Louis: CV Mosby.

Kitt, S., & Kaiser, J. (1990). Emergency nursing: A physiologic and clinical perspective. Philadelphia: WB Saunders.

Kollef, M. H. (1992). Lung hyperinflation caused by inappropriate ventilation resulting in electromechanical dissociation: A case report. Heart and Lung, 21(1), 74-77.

Kramer, D. J., Aggarwal, S., Martin, M., Darbey, J., Obrist, W., Rosenbloom, A., Murray, G., & Linden, P. (1991). Management options in fulminant hepatic failure. Transplantation Proceedings, 23(3), 1895-1898.

Lee, B. C. P., M.D. (1987). Computerized tomography of intracranial lesions. Hospital Medicine. May.

Lee, W. M. (1992). Acute liver failure: "Be published or perish." Unpublished manuscript, University of Texas Southwestern Medical School Grand Rounds, Dallas.

Leor, J., Goldbourt, U., Reicher-Reiss, H., Kaplinsky, E., & Behar, S. (1993). Cardiogenic shock complicating acute myocardial infarction in patients without heart failure on admission: Incidence, risk factors, and outcome. American Journal of Medicine, 94(3), 265-272.

Leppik, I. E. (1992). Status epilepticus and serial seizures. In J. B. Hall, G. A. Schmidt, & L. D. H. Wood (eds.), Principles of critical care (pp. 1777-1782). New York: McGraw-Hill.

Leske, J. S. (1991). Family member intervention: Research challenges. Heart and Lung, 20(4), 391-393.

Lewis, T. H. & Schmidt, G. A. (1992). Acute and chronic hepatic disease. In J. B. Hall, G. A. Schmidt, & L. D. H. Wood (Eds.), Principles of critical care (pp. 2014-2027). New York: McGraw-Hill.

Littleton, M. T. (1988). Pathophysiology and assessment of sepsis and septic shock. Critical Care Quarterly, 11(1), 30-47.

Littleton, M. T. (1993). Trends in agents used for the management of sepsis. Critical Care Nurse Quarterly, 15(4), 33-46.

Lower, J. (1992). Rapid neuro assessment. American Journal of Nursing, June, 38-48.

Luce, J. M. (1992). Neuromuscular diseases leading to respiratory failure. In J. B. Hall, G. A. Schmidt, & L. D. H. Wood (Eds.), Principles of critical care (pp. 1783-1791). New York: McGraw-Hill.

Luquire, R., & Houston, S. (1993). Cardiomyopathy: How to buy time. RN, May, 29-33.

Lutchefeld, W. B. (1990). Pulmonary contusion. Focus on Critical Care, 17(6), 482-488.

Marino, P. L. (1991). The ICU book. Philadelphia: Lea & Febiger.

Marsden, C. (1992). Family centered critical care: An option or obligation? American Journal of Critical Care, 1(3), 115-117.

Mason, P., & Bastnagel, J. (1992). Neurodiagnostic testing in critically injured adults. Critical Care Nurse. August, 64-75.

Matloff, D. S. (1992). Treatment of acute variceal bleeding. Gastroenterology Clinics of North America, 21(3), 103-118.

McAnena, O. J., Moore, E. E., & Marx, J. A. (1990). Initial

evaluation of the patient with blunt abdominal trauma. Surgical Clinics of North America, 70, 495–511.

McArthur, K. E. (1991). Acute pancreatitis diagnosis and treatment. Unpublished manuscript, The University of Texas Southwestern Medical Center at Dallas, Medical Grand Rounds, Dallas. (official date October 24, 1991).

McCance, K. L., & Huether, S. E. (1994). Pathophysiology: The biologic basis for disease in adults and children. St. Louis: CV Mosby.

McGoldrick, J. P., & Wallwork, J. (1992). Postoperative cardiac surgical care. In J. Tinker & W. M. Zapop (Eds.), Care of the critically ill patient (2nd ed.). (pp. 315–326). New York: Springer Verlag.

McQuillan, K. A. (1991). Intracranial pressure monitoring: Technical imperatives. AACN Clinical Issues, 2(4), 623–635.

McSwain, N. E. (1992). Traumatology and trauma systems. In G. R. Schwartz, C. G. Cayten, M. Q. Mangelsen, T. A. Mayer, & B. K. Hanke (Eds.), Principles and practice of emergency medicine (pp. 886–889). Philadelphia: Lea & Febiger.

Meyer, C. (1993). End-of-life care: Patients' choices, nurses' challenges. American Journal of Nursing, 93(2), 40–47.

Meyers, K. A., & Hickey, M. K. (1988). Nursing management of hypovolemic shock. Critical Care Quarterly, 11(1), 57–67.

Mitchell, P. H. (1993). Neurological data acquisition. In M. R. Kinney, D. R. Pacha, & S. B. Dunbar, (eds.). AACN's clinical reference for critical care nursing (3rd ed.) (pp. 781–802). St. Louis: CV Mosby.

Mitchell, P. H. (1994). Closed head injuries. In V. Cardona, P. D. Hurn, P. J. B. Mason, A. M. Scanlon-Schlipp & S. W. Veise-Berry (Eds.) Trauma nursing from resuscitation through rehabilitation (2nd ed.) (Ch. 17). Philadelphia: WB Saunders.

Moulton, R. J. (1992). Closed and open head injury. In J. B. Hall, G. A. Schmidt, & L. D. H. Wood (Eds.), Principles of critical care (pp. 702–713). New York: McGraw-Hill.

Mudge, C., & Carlson, L. (1992). Hepatorenal syndrome. AACN Clinical Issues in Critical Care Nursing, 3(3), 614–632.

Muizelaar, J. P. (1993). Improving the outcome of severe head injury with the oxygen radical scavenger polyethylene glycol-conjugated superoside dismutase: A Phase II trial. Journal of Neurosurgery, 78, 375–382.

O'Malley, P., Favalore, R., Anderson, B., Anderson, M. L., Siewe, S., Benson-Landau, M., Deane, E., Feeney, J., Gmeiner, J., Keefer, N., Mains, J., & Riddle, K. (1991). Critical care nurse perceptions of family needs. Heart and Lung, 20(2), 189–201.

Paul, S., & York, D. (1992). Cocaine abuse: An expanding healthcare problem for the 1990s. American Journal of Critical Care, 1(1), 109–112.

Peterson, W. L., & Laine, L. (1993). Gastrointestinal bleeding. In M. H. Sleisenger, & J. S. Fordtran (Eds.). Gastrointestinal disease, pathophysiology/diagnosis/management (pp. 162–180). Philadelphia: WB Saunders.

Perry, A. G. (1988). Shock complications: Recognition and management. Critical Care Quarterly, 11(1), 1–8.

Podolsky, D. K., & Isselbacher, K. J. (1991). Cirrhosis of the liver. In J. D. Wilson, E. Braunwald, K. J. Isselbacher, R. G. Petersdorf, J. B. Martin, A. S. Fauci, & R. K. Root (Eds.), Harrison's principles of internal medicine (pp. 1340–1350). New York: McGraw-Hill.

Rice, V. (1991). Shock, a clinical syndrome: An update. Part 1: An overview of shock. Critical Care Nurse, 11(4), 20–27.

Ruben, B. H., & Greenberg, J., (1992). Neurologic Injury: Prevention and initial care. In J. M. Civetta, R. W. Taylor, & R. R. Kirby (Eds.), Critical Care (2nd ed.) (pp. 740–743.) Philadelphia: JB Lippincott.

Rudolph, R., & Boyd, C. R. (1990). Massive transfusion: Complications and their management. Southern Medical Journal, 83(9), 1065–1070.

Schell, K. H. (1993). Current trends in antimicrobial therapy for the critically ill patient. Critical Care Nurse Quarterly, 15(4), 23–32.

Schmidt, G. (1992). Anticoagulants and thrombolytic agents in critical illness. In J. B. Hall, G. A. Schmidt, & L. D. H. Wood (Eds.) Principles of critical care (pp. 1493–1501). New York: McGraw-Hill.

Schoenbeck, S. B. (1993). Exploring the mystery of near-death experiences. American Journal of Nursing, 93(5), 43–46.

Schumann, L. L., & Remington, M. A. (1990). The use of naloxone in treating endotoxic shock. Critical Care Nurse, 10(2), 63–71.

Sheehy, S. B. (1992). Emergency nursing principles and practice (3rd ed.). St. Louis: Mosby Year Book.

Sherlock, S., & Dooley, J. (1993). Diseases of the liver and biliary system (9th ed.). London: Blackwell Scientific Publications.

Slater, A. L., Fassnacht-Hanrahan, K., Slater, H., & Goldfarb, I. W. (1991). From hopeful to hopeless. When do we write "do not resuscitate"? Focus on Critical Care Nursing, 18(6), 476–479.

Smith, A. (1991). When the pancreas self-destructs. American Journal of Nursing, September, 38–52.

Smith, T. W., Braunwald, E., & Kelly, R. (1992). The management of heart failure. In E. Braunwald (Ed.). Heart disease: A textbook of cardiovascular medicine (4th ed.) (pp. 464–510). Philadelphia: WB Saunders.

Soergel, K. H. (1993). Acute pancreatitis. In M. H. Sleisenger, & J. S. Fordtran (Eds.), Gastrointestinal disease pathophysiology/

diagnosis/management (pp. 1628–1650). Philadelphia: WB Saunders.

Spady, D. K. (1991). Hepatic encephalopathy: Role of benzodiazepine receptor ligands. Unpublished manuscript. University of Texas Southwestern Medical Center, Dallas.

Staub, C. (1990). Complications of massive transfusion. Physician Assistant, 14(3), 51–63.

Steigmann, G. Z., Goff, J. S., Michaletz-Onody, P. A., Korula, J., Lieberman, D., Saeed, Z., Reveille, M., Sun, J. H., & Lowenstein, S. R. (1992). Endoscopic sclerotherapy as compared with endoscopic ligation for bleeding esophageal varices. New England Journal of Medicine, 326(23), 1527–1532.

Steffes, C., & Fromm, D. (1992). The current diagnosis and management of upper gastrointestinal bleeding. Advances in Surgery, 25, 331–361.

Stewart, C. (1989). Acute pancreatitis. Emergency Care Quarterly, 5(3), 71–83.

Sympson, G. M. (1991). CATR: A new generation of autologous blood transfusion. Critical Care Nurse, 11(4), 60–64.

Szaflarski, N. L., & Cohen, N. H. (1991). Use of capnography in critically ill adults. Heart and Lung 20(4), 363–371.

Tauen, C. A. (1992). Trauma and the elderly: The impact on critical care. AACN Clinical Issues in Critical Care, 3(1), 149–154.

Thelan, L. A., Davie, J. K., & Urden, L. D. (1990). Textbook of critical care nursing diagnosis and management. St. Louis: Mosby Year Book.

Urden, L. D., Davie, J. K., & Thelan, L. A. (1992). Essentials of critical care nursing. St. Louis: Mosby Year Book.

Vos, H. R. (1993). Making headway with intracranial hypertension. AJN, February, 28–35.

Walleck, C. A. (February 1992). Preventing secondary brain injury. American Journal of Nursing Clinical Issues. 3(1), 19–27.

Walleck, C. A. (1990). Controversies in the management of the head injured patient. Critical Care Nursing Clinics of North America, 1(2), 67–74.

Walker, B. A. (1989). Health care professionals and the near-death experience. Death Studies, 13(13), 63–71.

Walley, K. R., & Wood, L. D. H. (1992). Ventricular dysfunction in critical illness. In J. B. Hall, G. H. Schmidt, & L. D. H. Wood (Eds.), Principles of critical care (pp. 1417–1434). New York: McGraw-Hill.

Weil, M. H., & Desai, V. (1992). Measuring the severity of shock. Emergency Medicine, 24(4), 207–209.

White, K. M. (1993). Sepsis and the systemic inflammatory response syndrome. Lecture notes from 1993 National Teaching Institute and Critical Care Exposition, Anaheim, CA.

Wilson, R. F. (1992). Critical care manual: Applied physiology and principles of therapy. Philadelphia: FA Davis.

Wilson, B. A., Shannon, M. T., & Stang, C. (1993). Govoni and Hayes nurse's drug guide. Norwalk, CT: Appleton & Lange.

Wolf, A. L., et al. (1993). Effect of THAM upon outcome in severe head injury: A randomized prospective clinical trial. Journal of Neurosurgery 78, 54–59.

Wright, J. E., & Shelton, B. K. (1993). Desk reference for critical care nursing. Boston: Jones & Bartlett Publishers.

Index

A page number followed by a "t" indicates a table.